ENVIRONMENTAL HEALTH
2nd EDITION

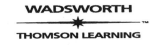

P9-BZT-380

Monroe T. Morgan, B.A., M.S.P.H., Dr. P.H.
East Tennessee State University

CONTRIBUTING AUTHORS:

Darryl B. Barnett, Dr.P.H.
Eastern Kentucky University

Franklin B. Carver, Ph.D.
Ohio University

Lawrence R. Curtis, Ph.D.
East Tennessee State University

Trenton G. Davis, Dr. P.H.
East Carolina University

Larry Gordon, M.S., M.P.H.
University of New Mexico

Albert F. Iglar, M.D.
East Tennessee State University

Rallie McAllister, M.D.
East Tennessee State University

Bailus Walker, Jr., Ph.D.
Howard University

WADSWORTH
THOMSON LEARNING

Australia • Canada • Mexico • Singapore • Spain • United Kingdom • United States

This book is dedicated to
Monroe T. Morgan, Jr., Marcus T. Morgan, Katrien and Natasha, Shirley L. Morgan,
and all of my former students.

This generation's contributions to society will not be determined by the height of our buildings, by how far we have traveled into space, by the depth of ocean explorations, by how many atomic bombs we have or by how advanced our technology, but, rather, by how fast we learn to live together as human beings and how well we manage our fragile environment.

We environmentalists are partially responsible for overpopulation by controlling the vectors of and the causative agents of death. Therefore, it is incumbent upon us to be the advocators of family planning (preventing unwanted pregnancies) lest humanity become a hungry mass of people living in poverty with a pitiable quality of life.

Senior Editor: Ruth Horton
Production Manager/Designer: Joanne Saliger
Copy Editor: Carolyn Acheson
Cover Design: Bob Schram, Bookends

Manufactured in the United States of America

10 9 8 7 6 5 4 3

ISBN: 0-89582-373-X

Preface

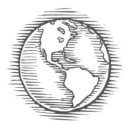

I wrote the first edition of this book in an attempt to place in one convenient volume the more important principles of environmental health. The book does not concentrate on practice because practices change. The principles, however, seldom do. This book "Environmental Health" is aimed at the human population rather than just the environmental sciences. The book attempts to portray the requirements for human life with emphasis on providing things that support human life. Also, this book emphasizes the need to control factors that are harmful to human life. Thus, there is the need to control factors that cause disease (dis-ease, discomfort, deviation from normal). Therefore, chapters outline the requisites of life, water, air, food, space, and shelter. They also address ways of controlling agents that cause disease i.e., communicable disease control, wastewater treatment, swimming pool guidelines, solid waste management, insect and rodent control, radiation control, and environmental issues. In Chapter 16, "Environmental Laws and Health Planning" utilizes planning methods as they apply to environmental management. The goal of environmental management is to improve the quality of life for all people by creating a sustainable society.

Community health educators, public health officers, nurses, engineers, physicians, epidemiologists, veterinarians, physical education majors, environmentalists, and many other health professionals, I hope, will benefit from this knowledge of the role of environmental health in public health and the health care system.

The chapters build upon each other. For example, everything prior to Chapter 12 applies to food management. Thus, in Chapter 11 (Food Quality Control) we do not have to discuss water supplies, sewage disposal, solid waste management, insects and rodents, and radiation because these topics have been addressed in preceding chapters.

Acknowledgments

I hope this book serves as a medium for the transfer of knowledge to the keen minds of our future much needed environmental and public health professionals. In preparing this book, I received much encouragement from professionals throughout the United States. Friends, environmentalists, engineers, health educators, professors of public health and other health professionals made valuable, logical, and well-founded suggestions. Without their help the book would be of far less value. I am grateful to many friends for suggestions and contributions.

The major contributors to the book are Dr. Albert F. Iglar, Professor of Environmental Health, East Tennessee State University; Dr. Trenton G. Davis, Professor at East Carolina University, my son Monroe T. (Monte) Morgan, Jr., and my wife, Dr. Shirley L. Morgan, MPH, M.S.E.H., Professor of Public Health at ETSU. Without their help, this book would not have become a reality. The assistance provided by Alex Broyles, MPH, and Dr. Carolyn Harvey, Assistant Professor of Environmental Health at ETSU, is much appreciated. I am grateful to the graduate assistants who assisted in the preparation of this book, particularly Rhonda Cook and Hollie Williamson. The photographs used were provided by ETSU. The contributing authors are some of the top environmental and public health practitioners and professors in the world.

Contents

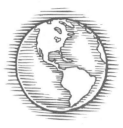

v

7 Solid and Hazardous Waste Management   107

8 Vectors and Their Control   127

9 Principles of Toxicology   141

10 Radiological Health   147

11 Food Quality Control   157

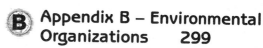

World Population

Key Terms

Biosphere

Doubling time

Growth rate

ZPG

Objectives

- 🌐 Explore the historical aspects of population growth.

- 🌐 Define *doubling time* and explain its meaning.

- 🌐 Discuss why the population explosion occurred.

- 🌐 Explain the effects of urbanization.

- 🌐 Express the need for family planning and describe planning programs.

- 🌐 Describe ideal population levels.

- 🌐 Discuss how to manage human environments.

The world is approximately 4 billion years old. It has taken that many years to form the earth, develop its resources, store energy in various forms, and enable living organisms to adapt to the planet. More human-caused environmental degradation has taken place in the last 2,000 years than in all the previous years combined. Hence, we have a need for courses in planet management, ecosystems management, and human environment management. Humans should become the environment's protecting manager rather than its self-serving destroyer.

For almost 300,000 years, human overpopulation was not a problem. Drought, floods, famine, plagues, pestilence, and war kept early populations in check, as did the lack of heating for homes, the inability to preserve food, and the harsh wilderness. Couples had large families to be certain that some children survived these hazards.

When the Europeans discovered America, approximately 250 million people lived on the earth. By 1650, about 150 years later, the population had increased to about 500 million. In 1850, approximately 1.2 billion people lived on the earth. The population increased 70 years later (1920) to just under 2 billion people. In 1950, another one-half billion inhabitants were added to the earth. By 1980, the earth's population had reached approximately 4.5 billion. That is a more than fivefold increase in 300 years.

As the world population base became larger, the chance of a population increase became much greater. Today, the world population is approximately 5.8 billion and is increasing at a rate of 11.5 new children every second, which equates to 215,000 per day or 78 million people per year. This means future population increases will be even greater than from 1950 to 1980, when the increase amounted to only three times the population of the world in 1650. By 2000, there will be 21 cities in the world with more than 10 million people, 17 of these in developing countries. By 2030, global urban populations will be twice the size of rural populations. Over this period, developing countries will grow by 160%.

DOUBLING TIME

The world population increased more rapidly about 200 years ago with the "Great Awakening," followed quickly by the industrial-medical-scientific revolution. At this time, sanitation, immunization, and other measures of environmental and public health greatly reduced the incidence of childhood and other communicable diseases. As three cases in point:

- In 1796 Edward Jenner demonstrated that immunizations could prevent smallpox.
- Walter Reed discovered that the *Aedes* mosquito spread yellow fever.
- Alexander Fleming later discovered penicillin.

Scientists refined flood control, improved agricultural and food technology, and developed public and environmental health practices. All of this activity served to control plagues and epidemics, which led to fewer children dying and a longer life expectancy. As a result, the world population grew rapidly. At the same time, a culture characterized by large families

continued, with few of the children dying. Instead of two of twelve children surviving, now eight, nine, and ten, or more survived.

The **doubling time** for the world population is decreasing. Table 1.1 highlights this concept. To find the doubling time, we have to know the **growth rate**. The relationship between growth rate and doubling time is shown in Table 1.2.

As the graphs in Figure 1.1 and Figure 1.2 reveal, developing nations tend to have greater potential than developed countries for population increase. This is because the potential for population increase becomes greater as more females enter childbearing ages. The women have babies, and the population base and growth potential increase even further. Many developing countries have a "stairstep" or "Christmas tree" graph. In contrast, when the population of developed nations is plotted, it gives a "stovepipe" effect. More babies are born in countries that are less able to provide food and the other requirements of life.

TABLE 1.1 World Population Doubling Time

Year	Estimated World Population	Years To Double
800 B.C.	5 million	1,500
AD 1650	500 million	200
AD 1850	1 billion	80
AD 1930	2 billion	45
AD 1975	4 billion	36
AD ??	8 billion	??

TABLE 1.2 Relationship Between Growth Rate and Doubling Time

Growth Rate	Years to Double
0.5%	140
0.8%	87
1.0%	70
2.0%	35
3.0%	24
4.0%	18
5.0%	14
7.0%	10
10.0%	7

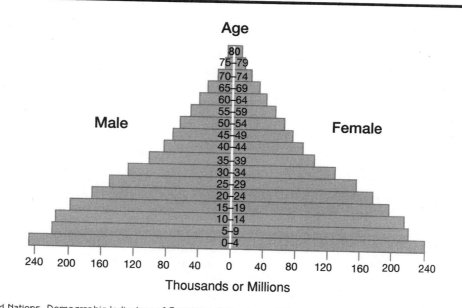

Age

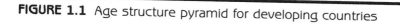

Male   **Female**

Thousands or Millions

Source: United Nations, Demographic Indicators of Countries: Estimates and Projections, as assessed in 1980

FIGURE 1.1 Age structure pyramid for developing countries

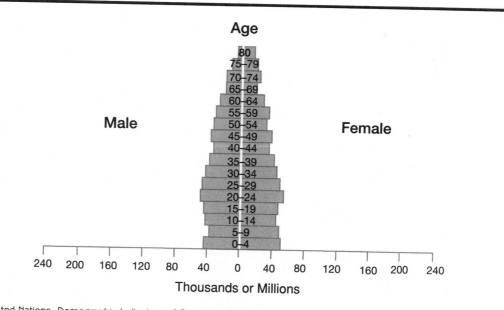

Age

Male   **Female**

Thousands or Millions

Source: United Nations, Demographic Indicators of Countries: Estimates and Projections, as assessed in 1980

FIGURE 1.2 Age structure pyramid for developed countries.

WHY THE POPULATION EXPLOSION?

Most microorganisms multiply by simple division. One organism divides into two. Each of the two divides into four, four into eight, and so on. Let's assume that these organisms are being grown in a test tube that will hold only a certain number of organisms. Also assume that the organisms divide every 24 hours. If the test tube were inoculated with one organism on day one and the test tube, because of available life requirements, would support only 365 days of growth, then one year (365 days) after inoculation the test tube would have reached its maximum carrying capacity. If asked when the test tube would be one-half full, the answer would be on the 364th day.

Now let's assume that on the 200th day one-fourth of the microorganisms were to die. In that case the population on day 365 would not have filled the test tube. A longer incubation period would be required to fill the test tube. If, then, on day 240 another one-fourth of the population were to die, it would take an even longer period of time to fill the test tube. The death rate slows population growth. Expressed simply, more deaths equate to a smaller population base.

The preceding analogy can be related to the history of the earth's human population. Floods, droughts, famine, war, and disease have all decreased the population. A prime example of population reduction is the pandemic of bubonic plague, which occurred in 430 B.C., and again in the A.D. 1340s, destroying approximately one-fourth of the world's population each time. Now think of the epidemics and pandemics of smallpox, cholera, typhoid fever, malaria, yellow fever, typhus, tuberculosis, rabies, and others that have occurred. Imagine how these diseases have kept the world population in check until recent years.

Modern knowledge in medicine, public and environmental health, and agriculture have started to control epidemics. More and more people are living, and living longer. This includes more unwanted, unplanned babies living, and living longer than ever before. Thus, the world is experiencing a human population explosion. Table 1.3 gives population data for selected countries. In 1996, one-third of humanity was under 15 years of age. The most populous nations are shown in Figure 1.3. The four most populous nations provide a study in contrasts. First-rated China has an average of 338 people per square mile, and India has a crowded 811. By comparison, the former Soviet Union and the United States have only 102 and 74 people per square mile, respectively.

TABLE 1.3 Population Data for Selected Countries, 1995

Country/ Region	Population (Millions)	Birth Rate (%)	Death Rate (%)	Growth Rate (%)	Doubling Time (Years)	Population (sq. mi.)
WORLD	5,702	24	9	1.5	45	—
AFRICA	720	41	13	2.8	24	—
Egypt	61.9	30	8	2.3	31	161
Ethiopia	56.0	46	16	3.1	23	149
Ghana	17.5	42	12	3.0	23	197
Kenya	28.3	45	12	3.3	21	128
Nigeria	101.2	43	12	3.1	22	288
South Africa	43.5	31	8	2.3	30	92
Tanzania	28.5	45	15	3.0	23	83
Zaire	44.1	48	16	3.2	22	50

(Continued)

TABLE 1.3 (Continued)

Country/Region	Population (Millions)	Birth Rate (%)	Death Rate (%)	Growth Rate (%)	Doubling Time (Years)	Population (sq. mi.)
ASIA	3,451	24	8	1.7	42	—
Bangladesh	119.2	36	12	2.4	29	2,371
China	1,218.8	18	6	1.1	62	338
India	930.6	29	9	1.9	36	811
Iran	61.3	36	7	2.9	24	97
Japan	125.2	10	7	0.3	277	861
Philippines	68.4	30	9	2.1	33	594
Saudi Arabia	18.5	36	4	3.2	22	22
Thailand	60.2	20	6	1.4	48	305
Turkey	61.4	23	7	1.6	44	207
Vietnam	75.0	30	7	2.3	30	597
LATIN AMERICA	481	26	7	1.9	36	—
Argentina	34.6	21	8	1.3	55	33
Brazil	157.8	25	8	1.7	41	48
Chile	14.3	22	6	1.7	41	49
Colombia	37.7	24	6	1.8	39	94
Cuba	11.2	14	7	0.7	102	263
Mexico	93.7	27	5	2.2	34	127
Nicaragua	4.4	33	6	2.7	26	97
Peru	24.0	29	7	2.1	33	49
Venezuela	21.8	30	5	2.6	27	64
NORTH AMERICA	293	15	9	0.7	105	—
Canada	29.6	14	7	0.7	102	8
United States	263.2	15	9	0.7	105	74
EUROPE	729	11	12	−0.1	—	—
Denmark	5.2	13	12	0.1	770	318
France	58.1	12	9	0.3	217	274
Germany	81.9	10	11	−0.1	—	606
Hungary	10.2	12	14	−0.3	—	287
Italy	57.7	9	10	−0.0	—	508
Poland	38.6	12	10	0.2	301	328
Spain	39.1	10	9	0.1	578	203
Sweden	8.9	13	12	0.1	990	56
United Kingdom	58.6	13	11	0.2	385	628
CARIBBEAN	36	23	8	1.5	46	—
Bahamas	0.3	20	5	1.5	47	71
Barbados	0.3	16	9	0.7	98	1,578
Grenada	0.1	29	6	2.4	29	716
Jamaica	2.4	25	6	2.0	35	585
Puerto Rico	3.7	18	8	1.0	67	1,074

Source: Population Reference Bureau, Inc.

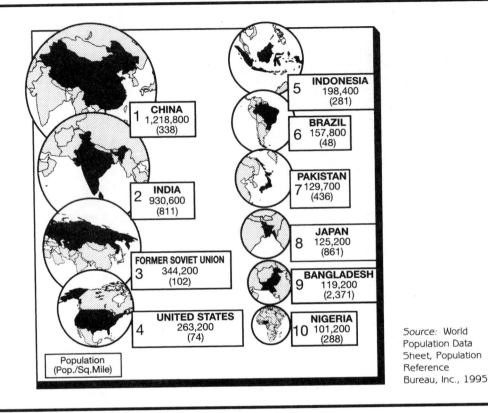

FIGURE 1.3 Most populous nations.

Source: World Population Data Sheet, Population Reference Bureau, Inc., 1995

In some cultures having large families is socially desirable. The reasons vary. Some want children for working in agriculture, some for military advantage, and some for political influence. Some religions advocate large families and teach that the higher being will provide for the children.

EFFECTS OF OVERPOPULATION

In 1791, Thomas Malthus predicted that the population would grow faster than the ability to feed it. This was before automation of farm life, tractors, synthetic fertilizer, mass transport, freeze-drying, and so forth. He suggested that populations grow geometrically (2–4–8) while food production increases arithmetically (1–2–3–4). Malthus' claim may have an unsettling amount of truth.

Despite several decades of agricultural research aimed at increasing the worldwide food supply, one of every three persons living in poor, underdeveloped countries is unable to find enough to eat. These people suffer from starvation and from diseases such as kwashiorkor, which results from a lack of protein. In many cases large families cannot provide for the children properly and do not receive much-needed health, social, and agriculture services from their government.

Approximately 12 million people die of starvation each year. Thirty million more people each year suffer from diseases made worse by hunger. More disturbing perhaps is that in the

Environmental Health

areas hit hardest by hunger, the population doubles every 17 to 30 years.

pollution, water pollution, land pollution, ozone depletion, and crowded, dirty cities.

EFFORTS TO CONTROL OVERPOPULATION

Over the years some effort has been made to address the problem of the large family. Slogans such as "zero population growth" (**ZPG**), "Stop at two," "How dense can we get?" and others have brought attention to the need for controlling family size.

Until about 1984, the United States encouraged worldwide population planning and control activities. It gave financial support for family planning programs and research groups such as the International Planned Parenthood Federation and the United Nations Fund for Population Activities (UNFPA). In 1985, however, the U.S. government, as a result of pressure from anti-abortion groups, cut off its contributions to UNFPA.

To combat the problem of overpopulation, some countries have legalized abortion and others have offered free sterilization. Many countries have offered educational programs explaining the need for family planning and discussing the undesirable effect of having too many children. These programs, along with other factors, have been somewhat effective in stabilizing the population in developed countries, but not in less developed countries where parents are less able to support the children.

Overpopulation causes the majority of undesirable environmental, social, economic, educational, and political problems. Many of the problems discussed in this book are the result, either directly or indirectly, of overpopulation. Improved technology and a desire for affluence, linked with an ever increasing population, are factors in causing environmental degradation. The denser the population, the more severe are the potential environmental problems. Many of these have occurred because of refusal to manage the effluent from the affluent society, resulting in noise pollution, hazardous waste, air

URBANIZATION

In 1800, approximately 6% of the U.S. population lived in urban areas. By 1900, 45% resided in cities. Presently, 73% of the U.S. population lives in urban areas. Worldwide, approximately 28% of the population lived in cities in 1950. By A.D. 2020, more than 66% is expected to live in cities, as shown in Figure 1.4. Around the world, as families continue to produce more children than they can support, the children

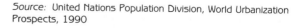

City	Population (millions)
Leningrad, USSR	2.8
Naples, Italy	2.8
Detroit, USA	2.8
Rio de Janeiro, Brazil	2.9
Bombay, India	2.9
Philadelphia, USA	2.9
Mexico City, Mexico	3.1
Milan, Italy	3.8
Osaka, Japan	3.8
Tianjin, China	3.9
Los Angeles, USA	4.0
Calcutta, India	4.4
Moscow, USSR	4.8
Chicago, USA	4.9
Buenos Aires, Argentina	5.0
Shanghai, China	5.3
Paris, France	5.4
Tokyo, Japan	6.7
London, United Kingdom	8.7
New York, USA	12.3

Population in Millions

Source: United Nations Population Division, World Urbanization Prospects, 1990

FIGURE 1.4 Approximate population for major cities in year 1950.

flock to the cities in search of work, where they find that computer-operated machinery and other modern technology reduce the need for manpower. This leads to unemployment, and unemployment leads to problems such as drug addiction, alcoholism, crime, and homelessness. In some cities in developing countries, babies are born in the streets, live there, and die there, with little potential for advancement.

Much of the population growth is the result of unplanned and unwanted pregnancies. Many cities do not provide shanty towns and slums with adequate drinking water, sanitation, food, health care, housing, schools, and jobs because of a lack of money and the fear that improvements will attract even more of the rural poor. In 1994, a report indicated the world's biggest cities were growing by one million a week. Figure 1.5 shows the largest urban agglomerations in the world.

THE NEED FOR FAMILY PLANNING

If we could determine what percent of the babies born in the world each year are not wanted by the parents, the result no doubt would be embarrassingly high. Further, if we could determine how many of the children are not wanted in large families that cannot provide a good quality of life for the children, we probably would be shocked at the high percentage. The point is that each day many of the children born throughout the world in developed and undeveloped countries alike are not planned and are unwanted. In many of these families each new baby adds to the misery of the family. I believe that unwanted babies are a fundamental problem because overpopulation is the underlying cause of so many of the economic, social, and environmental problems.

John D. Rockefeller, III, an authority on population and family planning, remarked in a speech to the U. S. House of Representatives that in the long run no substantial benefits will result from further growth of the nation's population.

Rather, population growth is an intensifier and multiplier of many problems: environmental, social, political, economic. The nation has nothing to fear, he said, from a gradual approach to population stabilization.

He further explained that a strong moral consensus is fundamental to any consideration of the population problem. The realization is increasingly widespread that the motivation behind population control is not negative and restrictive but, rather, positive and constructive. The concern is not merely about numbers and fertility; it is about human values and the quality of human life.

Thus, one real need is to prevent unwanted pregnancies around the world. The developed

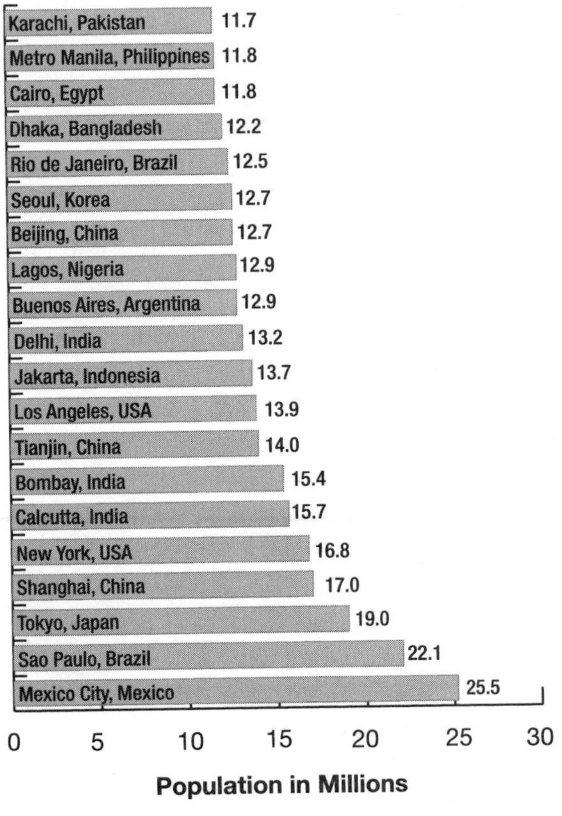

City	Population in Millions
Karachi, Pakistan	11.7
Metro Manila, Philippines	11.8
Cairo, Egypt	11.8
Dhaka, Bangladesh	12.2
Rio de Janeiro, Brazil	12.5
Seoul, Korea	12.7
Beijing, China	12.7
Lagos, Nigeria	12.9
Buenos Aires, Argentina	12.9
Delhi, India	13.2
Jakarta, Indonesia	13.7
Los Angeles, USA	13.9
Tianjin, China	14.0
Bombay, India	15.4
Calcutta, India	15.7
New York, USA	16.8
Shanghai, China	17.0
Tokyo, Japan	19.0
Sao Paulo, Brazil	22.1
Mexico City, Mexico	25.5

Population in Millions

Source: United Nations Population Division, World Urbanization Prospects, 1990

FIGURE 1.5 Expected population for major cities by year 2000.

Environmental Health

nations need to help their own people and those in less developed countries to prevent unwanted babies by providing parent education programs. If the number of unwanted babies could be reduced around the world, overcrowding no longer would be a problem and many of the ensuing environmental, political, social, and economic problems would be greatly reduced. A family planning program should be available worldwide to everyone who wants it. Parents should be able to have only the number of children they want.

In Planned Parenthood programs, the two general approaches to decreasing birthrates are family planning and economic growth. Planned Parenthood programs are offered in many developed nations and in some developing countries. Throughout the world, lowering the birthrate is the focus of most of these efforts to control population growth. By 1986, programs to reduce birthrate were available to 91% of the population of less developed countries (LCDs). The effectiveness and sources of funding for these programs vary from country to country.

President Lyndon B. Johnson once said: "Let's act on the fact that five dollars spent on population control is equivalent to one hundred dollars in economic growth." Economic development may reduce the number of children parents want by enhancing education, providing economic security, and reducing the need to consider children a substitute for old-age social security. In developed parts of the world such as in North America, Europe, and Japan, family planning services help to reduce the population growth rate by providing guidance to parents in regulating family size and health.

Family planning clinics vary as to the method of preventing pregnancies (progestational agents). However, the methods listed and described in Table 1.4, page 10, are the most common methods.

IDEAL POPULATION LEVELS

Dr. Theodore Morgan and other ecologists believe that the world population will continue to grow until the quality of life has been degraded for all. Some ecologists believe the growth will continue until it becomes necessary to create a "super" world agency to set and enforce ideal population for the various countries. Some believe that the ideal population level will be determined by factors such as each country's per-capita income, quality of life, length of growing season, topography, quality of waste disposal facilities, size, technology level, and quality of air and water. Even if optimum population levels are determined, though, the difficulty will be in enforcing the population levels.

Something will keep the population in check. What will it be? Will it be the aforementioned "super agency?" Will it be that the air becomes so polluted as to cause population control? Will the 1% of fresh water become so polluted that it spreads diseases and keeps the population in check? Or will the population control agent be toxic materials? Will it be the lack of food? Will it be the lack of sufficient space? Will it be that the lack of space and resources causes war? Or will it be that nations share and support family planning programs and prevent unwanted pregnancies? Let us hope that the population is controlled by family planning rather than by starvation.

MANAGING HUMAN ENVIRONMENTS

The **biosphere** (atmosphere, hydrosphere, and lithosphere) is the same size it was thousands of years ago. The population and its desire for affluence, however, have greatly increased over those thousands of years. With more people living longer and demanding more resources, and consequently producing more effluent, a greater demand is being placed on the environment each year. That demand is divided into two primary areas:

1. The environment must provide food, water, air, fuel, building materials, and other resources for a rapidly expanding population.

TABLE 1.4   Summary of Birth Control/Contraceptives

Type	Male Condom	Female Condom	Spermicides Used Alone	Diaphragm with Spermicide	Cervical Cap with Spermicide
Estimated Effectiveness	About 85%	An estimated 74%–79%	70%–80%	82%–94%	At least 82%
Risks	Rarely, irritation and allergic reactions	Rarely, irritation and allergic reactions	Rarely, irritation and allergic reactions	Rarely, irritation and allergic reactions; bladder infection; very rarely, toxic shock syndrome	Abnormal Pap test; vaginal or cervical infections; very rarely, toxic shock syndrome
Protection Against Sexually Transmitted Diseases	Latex condoms help protect against sexually transmitted diseases, including herpes and AIDS	May give some protection against sexually transmitted diseases including herpes and AIDS; not as effective as male latex condom	Unknown	None	None
Convenience	Applied immediately before intercourse; used only once and discarded	Applied immediately before intercourse; used only once and discarded	Applied no more than 1 hour before intercourse	Inserted before intercourse; can be left in place 24 hours, but additional spermicide must be used if intercourse is repeated	Can remain in place 48 hours; not necessary to reapply spermicide upon repeated intercourse; may be difficult to insert
Availability	Non-prescription	Non-prescription	Non-prescription	Prescription	Prescription

Oral Contraceptive Pill	Implant Norplant	Injection (Depo-Provera)	IUD	Periodic Abstinence (NFP)	Surgical Sterilization
97%–99%	99%	99%	95%–96%	Highly variable, perhaps 53%–85%	Over 99%
Blood clots, heart attacks and strokes, gallbladder disease, liver tumors, water retention, hypertension, mood changes, dizziness and nausea; not for smokers	Menstrual cycle irregularity; headaches, nervousness, depression, nausea, dizziness, change of appetite, breast tenderness, weight gain, enlargement of ovaries and/or fallopian tubes, excessive growth of body and facial hair; may subside after first year	Amenorrhea, weight gain, and other side effects similar to those with Norplant	Cramps, bleeding, pelvic inflammatory disease, infertility; rarely, perforation of the uterus	None	Pain, infection, and, for female tubal ligation, possible surgical complications
None	None	None	None	None	None
Pill must be taken on daily schedule, regardless of frequency of intercourse	Effective 24 hours after implantation for approximately 5 years; can be removed by physician at any time	One injection every 3 months	After insertion, stays in place until physician removes it	Requires frequent monitoring of body functions and periods of abstinence	Vasectomy is a one-time procedure usually performed in a doctor's office. Tubal ligation is a one-time procedure performed in an operating room
Prescription	Prescription; minor outpatient surgical procedure	Prescription	Prescription	Instructions from physician or clinic	Surgery

2. The environment also must dispose of the effluent (sewage, refuse, hazardous waste, industrial waste, etc.) from the population.

Thus, the solutions might be found in two approaches:

1. Family planning services around the world may prevent unwanted babies.
2. Worldwide environmental management may enable humans and other animals to enjoy a good quality of life — thus a sustainable society.

The remainder of the book will explore the problems and their solutions.

SUMMARY

The earth's population is approximately 5.8 billion and increasing at a rate of about 78 million per year. This necessitates careful planning and management to ensure a healthy environment for the future. The developing countries have a greater potential for population growth coupled with more current health problems. For example, they are still dealing with epidemics of infectious diseases such as dengue, cholera, typhoid fever, malaria, yellow fever, typhus, and tuberculosis — diseases that have been largely eradicated in developed countries through proven sanitation and other environmental measures.

The two broad approaches to managing human environments are (a) family planning and (b) environmental management. The later encompasses means of controlling agents that cause disease, including, among others, water and wastewater treatment, insect and rodent control, and radiation control.

REFERENCES

Brown, Lester R., et al. 1997. *State of the World.* Norton & Company, New York.

Chiras, Daniel D. 1994. *Environmental Science — A Framework for Decision Making.* 4th ed. The Benjamin/Cummings Publishing Company.

"50% of Population to Live in Cities." *World Population News Service Popline.* 1995, Nov.–Dec. Vol. 17.

Miller, Tyler G., Jr., 1988. *Living in the Environment.* 5th ed. Wadsworth Publishing, Belmont, CA.

Morgan, Monroe T., "A World Fit To Live In." *World Health.* May 1989.

Nadakavukanen, Anne. 1994. *Man and Environment: A Health Prospective.* 3rd ed. Waveland Press.

Raven, R. H., Linda Berg, and George Johnson. 1995. *Environment.* Saunders College Publishers, Fort Worth, TX.

"World Population Data Sheet." *Population Reference Bureau, Inc.* 1995. Washington, DC.

Fundamentals of Environmental Health

Key Terms

Aerobic

Anaerobic

Causative agents

Disease

Environmental health practice

Epidermis

Facultative

Hypertonic

Hypotonic

Immunity

Isotonic

Mesophilic

Phagocytosis

Plasmolysis

Plasmoptysis

Psychrophilic

Resistance to disease

Thermophilic

Objectives

- Identify and discuss what determines our health.

- Enumerate the requirements for the growth of microorganisms.

- Name the causative agents of disease.

- Define environmental health and give a brief history of its evolution.

- Discuss the portals of entry for microorganisms.

- Determine the methods of spreading disease.

What determines the health of the approximately 6 billion people in the world? What determines the health of the 260 plus million individuals who currently inhabit the United States of America? The pressure of rising health care costs increases the need to understand the determinants of health and the role of environmental health in the health care system.

DETERMINANTS OF HEALTH

The four basic determinants of health are hereditary or biological factors, medical care, lifestyle, and environment.

Hereditary or Biological Factors

Major aspects of human biology are controlled by genetics. A person may be healthy in every other way but may have inherited conditions such as hemophilia, diabetes, mental retardation, various eye problems, lack of **resistance to disease**, or any number of other problems. Research now provides evidence that traits inherited from the mother and father can influence whether a person becomes addicted to alcohol or another drug.

Medical Care

The medical care we receive during our lifetime can determine our health. For example, if a child develops streptococcal infection and does not get medical care, he or she might develop a rheumatic heart condition. Or if a youngster breaks a limb and does not receive proper medical care, he or she might end up with a deformed arm or leg.

Two main aspects of health care affect everyone. One is *technology*, which has been in the limelight for several decades. Ever increasing technological advances have added productive years to thousands of lives. An example is the computerized axial tomograph or CAT scanner. Other technological devices include sophisticated equipment for kidney patients, artificial organs, monitoring instruments for the human fetus, and electrocardiograph devices worn by patients to detect an oncoming heart attack. These amazing instruments have captured the fancy of society and added to the cost of health care. The second trend in health care is a heightened interest in medical self-help. This trend is illustrated by self-examination of the skin, breasts, mouth, eyes, and nails, for example.

Lifestyle

Lifestyle has a lot to do with one's health. Lack of sleep and rest reduces our resistance to infections and leads to bodily degeneration. A person who has an excellent body but eats poorly, does not exercise enough, and smokes and drinks heavily may develop health problems rather quickly. Many Americans indulge in high-fat, high-sugar, high-salt, low-fiber diets. Moving sidewalks, escalators, elevators, cars, buses, and other means of transportation may be leading people to an early demise. Like all muscles, the heart muscle will waste away if it is not used vigorously. Considering these factors, it is rather easy to understand why heart disease is the number-one killer in the United States.

In contrast to the overindulgence and sedentariness that characterize modern American life, the lifestyle in underdeveloped countries has its own health problems. People in some areas of the world suffer malnutrition and other diseases caused by the lack of proper nutrition. Overall, infectious diseases dominate the health problems of underdeveloped countries.

Of all the health determinants, lifestyle may be the easiest to control. Even so, it will require much effort.

Environment

Considering the world's population as a whole, the environment affects people's health more strongly than any of the other determinants. The environment encompasses the water we drink, the food we eat, the air we breathe. In the past, because of poor environmental management, many people died from environmentally related diseases such as typhoid fever. Some estimates, based on morbidity and mortality statistics, indicate that the impact of the environment on health status is as high as 80%.

Human evolution has been selective. People have adapted to the environment in which they found themselves by, for example, producing biological defenses against disease. People also have acquired intelligence, knowledge, and expertise that have allowed them to make significant changes in the environment, thereby creating conditions that lessen the likelihood of disease. This is accomplished mainly by controlling the causative agents of disease while they are still in the environment, before they reach people, so the body does not have to produce defenses and therapeutic measures are not required.

Environmental health practice, as the name suggests, refers to the relationship between environment and health. Some important elements of environmental health practice — the first line of defense against disease — include:

- Water quality management — ensuring that potable water is available through treatment of water supplies.

- Human waste disposal — disposing of human wastes in septic tank systems and sewage treatment plants.
- Solid and hazardous waste management — treating and disposing of solid and hazardous wastes.
- Rodent control — removing potential harborage and sources of food.
- Insect control — utilizing natural, biological and other methods to reduce insect populations.
- Milk sanitation — ensuring that all milk for human consumption is produced under sanitary conditions and is pasteurized.
- Food quality management — maintaining surveillance over food from the farm to the consumer so as to prevent contamination.
- Occupational health practice — assuring a healthy and safe work environment.
- Interstate and international travel sanitation — preventing the spread of communicable diseases between states and nations.
- Air pollution control — reducing the emissions of pollutants into the atmosphere.
- Water pollution control — reducing the effects of industrial and other waste on water supplies and recreational areas by the pretreatment of industrial and domestic waste.
- Environmental safety and accident prevention — designing into the environment features, such as pedestrian ramps, that promote safety or compensate for people's inadequacies.
- Noise control — abating high noise levels in industrial settings and in the community to avoid health degradation.
- Housing hygiene — promoting housing conditions necessary for the physiological and psychological well-being of inhabitants.
- Radiological health control — controlling radiation sources such as X-ray equipment, nuclear fission plants, and radioactive waste.
- Recreational sanitation — monitoring the environment to prevent unsafe conditions at swimming pools and other recreational facilities.
- Institutional environmental management — preventing the spread of nosocomial infections.
- Land use management — zoning to direct land use to desirable purposes.
- Product safety and consumer protection — ensuring that drugs, toys, appliances, and the like are safe for human use.
- Environmental planning — applying environmental design to minimize human stress and accidents.

Throughout history, reduction of disease and discomfort have been accomplished largely by altering the environment. Therapeutic programs are glamorous and tend to be successful in obtaining funding and publicity. Prevention programs — the preferable approach — many times are taken for granted and are not funded properly.

REQUIREMENTS FOR THE GROWTH OF MICROORGANISMS

We live in a world that harbors countless microorganisms that are both beneficial and detrimental to humans. The disease-causing, or pathogenic, microbes are of particular concern. By better understanding what specific elements are necessary for these biological causative agents of disease to live and reproduce, one also learns ways of controlling their populations. The following eight elements are required for the growth of microorganisms:

1. Favorable oxygen supply.
2. Favorable temperatures.
3. Food.
4. Moisture.
5. Favorable pH.
6. Favorable osmotic pressure.
7. Absence of toxic materials.
8. Space.

Many microorganism need free *oxygen* from the atmosphere to survive. These organisms are termed **aerobic**. Other microorganisms live in environments void of free oxygen. These are **anaerobic** organisms. You may have been in a swampy area where a sulfur or "rotten egg" odor was prevalent. Often these odors can be attributed partly to the presence of anaerobic bacteria degrading organic matter. Some bacteria are **facultative**. They have the ability to exist either aerobically or anaerobically, depending on their surrounding environment. For instance, if we were to place an aerobic microbe in an environment without free oxygen, it would not survive. A facultative organism, however, would tolerate a range of oxygen levels.

Growth of microorganisms can be controlled by manipulating their oxygen requirements. For example, because aerobes may hasten the spoilage of perishable products, many foods are vacuum-packed to prevent the growth of aerobic organisms. This oxygen-free environment, however, is desirable for anaerobic organisms such as *Clostridium botulinum*, which produces a toxin that causes botulism.

Microorganisms also have specific *temperature* requirements for growth. At optimal temperature, a cell multiplies most rapidly. At temperature extremes — both very hot and very cold — the cell may stop growing and reproducing or simply die.

Three groups of microorganisms — thermophilic, mesophilic, and psychrophilic — grow in various temperature ranges:

1. **Thermophilic**, or "heat-loving" **microbes,** grow from roughly 113°F to 167°F.

2. **Mesophilic** organisms prefer a medium range roughly from 69°F to 113°F.

3. **Psychrophilic**, or "cold-loving" organisms, grow in a range of roughly 19°F to 68°F.

The psychrophilic organism spoils foods under refrigeration. The bacteria most important from a public health standpoint are the mesophilic because they thrive and reproduce at approximately 98.6°F and thereby are able to exist within the human body.

Temperature affects all of us. At room temperature (68°F to 70°F) we feel comfortable and active. If we lower the temperature to 38°F or below, however, our bodies are stressed and we shiver in an attempt to raise the body's temperature. Because the body is exothermic (must emit heat), we also feel stressed when the surrounding temperature is 98°F or above and the body perspires to cool itself. If the temperature is sufficiently hot or cold for an extended time, the human body becomes overstressed, possibly leading to death.

The same principle applies to bacterial microbial populations, although they are less adaptive to temperature changes than humans are because they lack control of their own cell temperature. By controlling the temperature around the organisms, we can control their activity or induce their death. Through refrigeration or heating of foods, we control many of the pathogens responsible for foodborne illness. This can be accomplished by adjusting the temperature out of the mesophilic range — preferably colder than 45°F or hotter than 140°F. An adage concerning food is "Keep it hot, keep it cold, or don't keep it long."

Food is another growth requirement for microorganisms. Microbes consume many of the foods we eat. Just as with humans, limiting the amount of food available to a microbial population limits growth. By thoroughly cleaning and sanitizing eating utensils and equipment, we can greatly control the growth of many disease-causing microorganisms in restaurants, institutions, and homes.

Just as humans require water, microorganisms require some degree of *moisture*. Removing moisture from an environment inhibits the growth of microorganisms. Freeze-drying, or desiccating, is a good example of such a measure used to protect food. Commercially, the process involves removing moisture from a food product and then sealing the product in a moisture-proof container. The waxed paper surrounding the dried corn flakes you may have eaten for breakfast is a product of this principle. Once you open a package of dried food, the moisture in the air may spark the growth of microorganisms that can spoil the product.

Microorganisms also require a *favorable pH* in order to reproduce. Pathogenic organisms generally prefer a neutral pH, around 7.0. A sudden change in pH, either above or below 7.0, will kill the organisms. Many foods are potentially hazardous to humans because their neutral pH readily supports the growth of pathogens. We can reduce the potential hazard of foods such as cream-filled pastries and mayonnaise by adding vinegar or an acid to reduce the pH. But who likes vinegar in cream-filled pies? Therefore one refrigerates them to create an unfavorable environment for pathogens.

Favorable osmotic pressure is a requirement for growth of microorganisms. Living microbes have a certain saline, or salt, concentration within their cells. Placing these organisms in a surrounding environment that contains either more or less salt than in the organism (cell) itself inhibits their growth. A saline solution surrounding a cell that has a salt concentration equal to that within the cell is **isotonic**, and provides optimum growth potential. The condition in which the saline content within the cell is greater than that of the surrounding environment is called **hypotonic**. A hypotonic environment allows moisture to enter the cell by the process of osmosis. This results in the cell expanding to the extent that it may rupture in a process called **plasmoptysis**. In a third condition, termed **hypertonic**, the environment surrounding the organism contains a greater saline concentration than that within the organism. When a food is surrounded by a high concentration of salt, the moisture within the cells escapes, by the process of an attempt to dilute the surrounding salt solution. This loss of water is called **plasmolysis**. Removing the moisture from food by creating a hypertonic environment produces conditions unfavorable for microbial growth within a food, such as with salt-cured ham.

Another requirement for microbial growth is the *absence of toxic materials*. Many commonly used household products limit the growth of microorganisms because they introduce some form of toxin to the organisms' surrounding environment. Common bleach, spray disinfectants, and various phenol-based compounds are examples. Most municipal water treatment facilities use chlorine as a disinfectant. Chlorine, or a "bleach solution," also is used in food service establishments to sanitize equipment and utensils that may harbor pathogens. Further examples of materials used to kill microorganisms are antibiotics, Mercurochrome, and iodine.

Finally, *space* is a requirement for growth of microorganisms. Microbes multiply exponentially and will heavily populate an area within a short time (several hours for some species if all requirements for growth are favorable). Imagine what would happen if the entire population of a small city of 30,000 people were forced to live in an area no larger than a football field! They would have no means of human waste disposal and only a limited food supply. Within a short time, starvation would occur and disease would spread, causing the population to die out. A similar condition exists within a colony of microorganisms. Without enough space, concentrations toxic enough to kill the vast majority of the colony occur.

Optimal Growth Curve

Altering any of the above growth requirements can result in effectively controlling the growth of microorganisms detrimental to humans. If all requirements for microbial growth exist, the individual organisms will multiply as shown in Figure 2.1. As this figure shows, a phase of acclimation first occurs when a small group of organisms is introduced to a new environment. The stresses of new surroundings may induce death of a few organisms. The remaining microbes, however adjust and reproduce. This brings the microbes to the next phase, the logarithmic growth phase.

In the logarithmic, or log, growth phase the organisms reproduce exponentially. One cell divides and becomes two, two then divide and become four, four cells divide and become eight, and so on until the numbers reach the billions. As the numbers of organisms increase, the

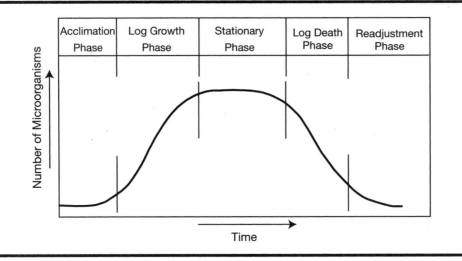

FIGURE 2.1 Optimal growth curve.

amount of their toxic waste products also increases. This, coupled with a reduced amount of nutrients available, slowly kills the organisms. The stage in the cycle when the death of the organisms (death rate) equals that of new organisms being produced (birthrate) is called the stationary phase. In this phase the number of organisms reaches equilibrium and remains stationary until onset of the logarithmic death phase.

When the microbes have consumed most or all nutrients and the microbial waste products reach a concentration high enough to destroy the majority of the population, they find themselves in the logarithmic death phase. The overcrowded environment is unfavorable for growth because of lack of food, changes in pH, waste buildup, crowding, and other factors. A few organisms may remain after the log death phase. These organisms proceed into the readjustment phase, as the few surviving organisms of the log death phase attempt to reproduce. Enough nutrients may be available to allow some cell division; however, the death rate will equal or slightly surpass the reproduction rate for a time. Eventually new nutrients may be introduced into the environment and the existing toxins may be diluted. Upon creation of new, favorable environmental conditions, the

organisms enter once more into the phase of acclimation. This optimal growth curve cycle can continue time and time again if favorable growth conditions allow.

Controlling Microbial Growth

Communicable diseases pose major public health problems around the world. If a society is to control communicable disease, people must know what is necessary for microbial growth so it can be limited or stopped by creating an unfavorable environment. Much of environmental health practice involves creating an unfavorable environment for the causative agents of disease and thereby creating a favorable environment for humans. In other areas of public and environmental health, such as wastewater treatment, cheese processing, and others, we need to create a favorable environment for microorganisms so they will degrade the waste or produce the food.

CAUSATIVE AGENTS OF DISEASE

Now let's take a look at the etiology or causative agents of disease. Specifically, what can

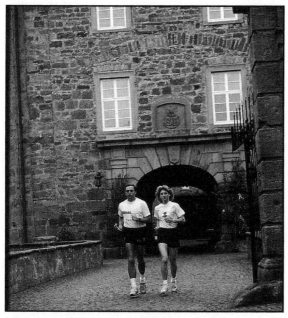

Lifetime participation in aerobic activities is one of the most important factors in preventing cardiovascular disease.

make humans sick? The major **causative agents** of disease may be classified as:

1. Biological agents
2. Chemical agents
3. Physical agents
4. Too little of something
5. Too much of something
6. Hereditary disease
7. Stress
8. Diseases of unknown cause

Biological agents of disease are living things that cause disease because of their effect on characteristics associated with life. These agents are living cells that induce a wide range of illnesses. Nearly every year an individual is overcome by some type of *virus*, of which the common cold is an example. Pathogenic *bacteria* can cause diseases such as salmonellosis, typhoid, and strep throat. Other biological disease-causing classifications are fungi (yeasts, and molds) and protozoa, such as those that produce some sexually transmitted diseases.

Metazoa, such as tapeworms, form the final class. These are illustrated in Figure 2.2.

Chemical agents of disease are substances that cause disease because of their mass or ability to engage in chemical reactions with molecules in the body. Most living quarters contain chemicals that can cause disease. Commonly found items include cleansing agents, pesticides, petroleum products, and chemical drain openers. On crowded interstate highways, too, we view hazardous chemicals in transport. Consequently, the proper treatment, storage, and disposal of these chemicals is of critical concern to human health.

Physical agents of disease do their damage by transferring energy to the body, damaging body cells. For example, ionizing radiation, at high doses, can endanger life, whether its source is X-ray equipment or a nuclear power plant. Noise-producing physical agents also may harm health. Excessive noise can lead to hearing loss, hypertension, heart disease, strokes, and other problems. The sun's ultraviolet radiation is another disease-causing physical agent. In America, a dark tan often is associated with physical beauty. The skin tans as a defense against the sun's rays. Overexposure to these rays can damage the skin and cause severe illness or death.

Too little of, or a lack of, certain life supporting materials can cause disease. For example, if a person takes no food or water into the body, the body weakens and eventually dies. The body requires specific nutrients, without which illness occurs. For example, a lack of Vitamin D will cause rickets, and a lack of niacin in the diet (protein-calorie deficiency) causes kwashiorkor.

Just as too little of certain substances can cause disease, so can *too much of* something. For instance, an individual who eats improperly and excessively may become obese. Even overconsumption of a life-supporting chemical such as water can be fatal. Likewise, a high concentration of carbon dioxide, a natural respiratory waste product, can cause illness.

Heredity can be a disease agent. Poor eyesight, hemophilia, and baldness are examples of inherited genetic traits.

Pathogen	Examples

Viruses

Poliovirus
0.03 micrometers
in diameter

Common cold
Influenza
Poliomyelitis
Hepatitis B
Herpes
HIV/AIDS
Chicken pox
Mononucleosis
(Epstein-Barr)

Bacteria

Tuberculosis bacilli:
3 micrometers long

Syphilis spirochetes:
10 micrometers long

Tuberculosis
Strep throat
Gonorrhea
Syphilis

Fungi

Yeast: causes vagi-
nal infections; 5–30
micrometers long

Mold: causes
athlete's foot, ring-
worm, and jock itch

Candidiasis
(yeast infection)
Ringworm
Athlete's foot

Protozoa

Trichomonas: causes
genital tract infections;
50–100 micrometers long

Amoeba: causes
amoebic
dysentery

Trichomoniasis
(STD)

Metazoa (Helminths or parasitic worms)

Tapeworm
up to several meters long

Pubic lice
Tapeworm

FIGURE 2.2 Classes of pathogens with examples of each.

Stress may cause ill health. From time to time, everyone comes under stress. Demands and expectations placed upon a person sometimes are so great that the body becomes overstressed. This may result in emotional disorders, hypertension, stroke, and even heart attack, all of which may lead to death. Stress also can contribute to alcoholism and other drug abuses when individuals prefer to intoxicate their system to "cope" with stressful situations. We would do well to consider the effects of stress upon us and learn to manage it so that we can live healthier lives.

A final causative agent of disease is the *unknown*. Many people die each year because of environmental pollutants working synergistically with other factors. Cancer is a serious problem in today's society. Because it is caused by exposure or a series of exposures to carcinogens in the environment years before the onset of disease, in many cases the exact cause of illness may never be known.

The main three causative agents of disease — biological, chemical, and physical agents — can be spread in several ways — by air, water, food, insects, fomites (inanimate objects such as forks and door knobs) and animals. In environmental health, many programs address the need to control the causative agent while it is in the environment before it gets to the public and causes disease.

HUMAN DEFENSE AGAINST DISEASE

Throughout recorded history, people have tried to reduce suffering and disease. The first attempts consisted of treating the symptoms of disease. Common practice to treat a fever was to put on more quilts and blankets (*after* the causative agent had entered the body) and raise the temperature until the fever "broke." (We now know that the microorganism causing the fever was killed by the high temperature.) In the next era, we administered a medicine such as penicillin to kill the organism *after* it had entered the body. The third era is characterized by immunization. Doctors give people an antigen to cause the body to produce antibodies against specific biological agents. This provides **immunity** so *after* that agent enters the body, the antibodies will kill it. In each of the cases mentioned above, except immunization, the treatment is administered *after* the causative agent had entered the body.

In the mid-19th century, Edwin Chadwick of England and Lemmuel Shattuck of Boston, Massachusetts, wrote reports on the sanitary condition of the environment. They emphasized the environment's role in spreading germs and other causative agents of disease. Thus, they recommended sanitation programs to control the causative agents of disease while they are in the environment, *before* they get inside humans. They also in essence recommended the basis for the fourth era and the first line of defense — environmental health practice. Figure 2.3 lists the four lines of defense through the health care system.

First Line of Defense

Humans have adapted to the environment in which they live by producing biological defenses against disease. As a direct result of this evolution, humans also have acquired knowledge that allows them to make significant changes in the environment. Some changes, such as pollution, may make conditions less suitable to humans. Controlling both manmade and naturally occurring environmental conditions through environmental health practices provides people's first line of defense against disease. Thus, environmental health practice is people's first line of defense against disease, by applying environmental technology and the arts and sciences to control the causative agents of disease in the environment before they reach humans.

Second Line of Defense

Humans' second line of defense against disease is the body's adaptation to prevent the agents of

I. *Humans' First Line of Defense Against Disease (Environmental Management)*
   A. Water quality management
   B. Proper human waste disposal
   C. Solid and hazardous waste management
   D. Rodent control
   E. Insect control
   F. Milk sanitation
   G. Food quality management
   H. Occupational health practice
   I. Interstate and international travel sanitation
   J. Air pollution control
   K. Water pollution control
   L. Environmental safety and accident prevention
   M. Noise control
   N. Housing hygiene
   O. Radiation control
   P. Recreational sanitation
   Q. Institutional environmental management
   R. Land use management
   S. Product safety and consumer protection
   T. Environmental planning

II. *Humans' Second Line of Defense Against Disease (Public Health and Preventive Medicine)*
   A. Proper nutrition
   B. Good personal health practice
   C. The body's reflexes, chemicals, and barriers
   D. Routine health and dental check-up
   E. Application of health education
   F. Other

III. *Humans' Third Line of Defense Against Disease (Public Health and Preventive Medicine)*
   A. Phagocytosis (a natural process)
   B. Immunity (active and passive)

IV. *Humans' Fourth Line of Defense Against Disease (Curative Medicine)*
   A. Surgery
   B. Administering of medication and radiation
   C. Diagnosing by means of various lab methods
   D. Corrective Dentistry
   E. Corrective therapy (i.e., speech, hearing, respiratory)

FIGURE 2.3 The role of environmental health in the health care system.

disease from becoming established within it. The human body possesses mechanisms that deter disease-causing agents from entering. The first of these is the *skin* covering the body. Because the skin is relatively impermeable, it provides a barrier to many pathogenic agents. Another protective mechanism consists of the *mucous membranes*, which secrete a protective fluid that traps undesirable particles, microorganisms, and so forth. In addition, *cilia* — tiny, hairlike projections — sweep mucus and other debris from the respiratory tract. The body also has *secretions of various fluids*, such as saliva, gastric juice, and perspiration, containing protective substances. For eye protection, tears contain lysozyme, a chemical that dissolves the cell walls of certain bacteria. Ears secrete wax that keeps out undesirable particles. Reflexes (involuntary movements in response to stimuli) also play a role in protecting the body from disease.

Nutrition is an important defense because an adequately nourished body is able to better resist disease. An individual's *condition of health* also plays a major role in preventing disease. Individuals who are ill are more susceptible to infection by other disease-inducing agents than are persons who are in a good state of health.

Third Line of Defense

If the aforementioned defense mechanisms are insufficient and do not destroy or prevent the entrance of the causative agent, humans have a third line of defense consisting of phagocytosis and immunity.

Phagocytosis is the primary *cellular* defense against disease. In this defense, cells show an adaptive response to the presence of pathogenic agents. Shortly after pathogens invade host cells, the *inflammation response* occurs. This is characterized by reddening of the affected area because of capillary dilation; swelling from the leakage of plasma through the capillary walls, which increases the fluid content of the tissue; heat/fever, which aids the destruction of some pathogens by increasing the action of white blood cells; and pain, indicating to the body that a problem is present.

During inflammation, phagocytes destroy the pathogens. In the blood system these phagocytes are leukocytes, or white blood cells. In the lymphatic system microphages and macrophages carry out the process. If phagocytosis fails to destroy the pathogens — possibly because the number and character of the invading organism — the body has to depend on its own **immunity**. There are many diseases for which one cannot be immune. Immunity results from the presence of an antibody that attacks the specific microorganism (causative agent). The substance that stimulates the production of antibodies in the body is known as the antigen.

Immunity is divided into categories according to how the body acquires it.

1. *Active immunity*, in which the body of the user produces the antibodies. Active immunity can be acquired either naturally or artificially. To possess naturally acquired active immunity, the individual first must have an infection for which the body produces antibodies, with or without symptoms. To possess artificially acquired active immunity, the body must be vaccinated with weak or attenuated germs, which stimulate antibody production without causing observable signs of disease, or be vaccinated with toxoids. Treatment of the body with a toxoid stimulates the production of antibodies without producing the signs and symptoms of the disease.

2. *Passive immunity*, in which the required antibodies are not produced within the body that needs them but are produced within some other body. Passive immunity can be either naturally or artificially acquired also. Naturally acquired passive immunity results from the transfer of antibodies across the placenta from the immune mother to the fetus or via the mother's colostrum to her breast-fed infant. Artificially acquired passive immunity is acquired from antibodies or antitoxin received from the blood serum of immune human beings or animals. Figure 2.4 depicts the forms of immunity.

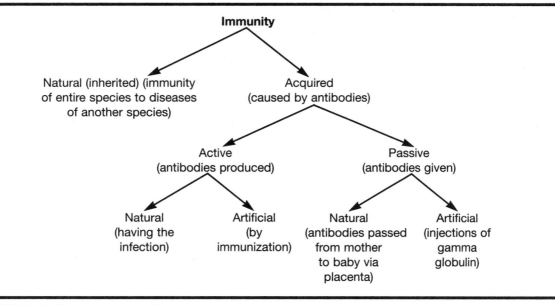

FIGURE 2.4 Types of immunity.

Fourth Line of Defense

Admittedly, when one is in pain, sick, or needs surgery, the curative medicine professionals — doctor, dentist, nurse — are the professionals one wants to see. Whenever possible, however, people would rather the pain or sickness be prevented by the environmental health, public health, or preventive medicine specialist. Thus, because of high cost of curative medicine, there is greater need for environmental health practice, public health, and preventive medicine than ever before. The public would rather pay for prevention than the fourth line of defense — curative medicine. *To help the public better understand the role of environmental heath practice in the health maintenance system, this book emphasizes the need to prevent disease rather than have to utilize curative medicine.*

PORTALS OF ENTRY

If microorganisms are to have an optimum chance to establish themselves, they must enter a host through an appropriate portal. They must enter the body where they can obtain nutrients, reproduce, and ultimately cause disease. As examples, organisms such as salmonella enter the body through the host's digestive tract, whereas the virus of yellow fever enters via an insect (mosquito) bite. The major portals of entry to the human body are the skin, the reproductive organs, the respiratory tract, and the digestive tract.

The Skin

About two square meters of skin, on average, insulate the human body — obviously providing a large surface area for the potential ingress of chemicals and microorganisms. The outermost layer of skin, the **epidermis**, provides the defense against the entry of causative agents of disease. The epidermis is essentially a layer of dead skin in the process of being shed, much like an insect molts or sheds its outer protective layer — although with humans the process is much more gradual. Cuts or breaks in the epidermis weaken this protective layer, allowing microorganisms to enter. This can occur, for example, when a blood-sucking insect feeds by puncturing the epidermis and, in the process of taking blood, introduces contaminated materials or pathogens into the body.

Hair follicles originate in the dermis. They are spread throughout the epidermis, concentrating on the arms, legs, and head. Oils and sweat are secreted through pores of the epidermis. When the ducts becomes clogged, as with acne, the sweat and oils are retained and the area becomes swollen or festered. Bacteria and other microorganisms colonize the affected area, resulting in increased blood flow to the area, elevated body temperature, and more white blood cells to fight the infection. The infection may become widespread, causing severe and possibly permanent damage to the affected areas.

The Reproductive Organs

Human reproductive organs — in males, the penis and testicles; in females, the uterus and ovaries — require direct bodily contact to transmit disease. Sexually transmitted diseases — syphilis, gonorrhea, AIDS, and others — rely on intimate contact because the infecting organisms are incapable of survival outside the body. Preventive measures include prophylactics or abstention from sex.

The Respiratory Tract

The human respiratory tract consists of the nose, trachea, left and right bronchi, bronchioles, alveolar ducts, and alveoli. Microbes such as *Mycobacterium tuberculosis*, which causes tuberculosis, enter the body through the nose (or mouth) during breathing and progress into the lung tissues. Eventually they reach the bloodstream, where infection may spread throughout the body. Often, foreign materials (smoke, dust) precipitate lung diseases as they, too, irritate sensitive lung tissue. Black lung disease, common to coal miners and others who inhale large quantities of dust or dirt, is a good example.

The human respiratory tract is not totally defenseless against disease. The nose and lungs have a number of protective devices. Nose hair filters inhaled air, removing large particulate matter that otherwise might become imbedded in the lungs. The mucus of the nose and throughout the respiratory tract traps various other foreign matter, both macroscopic (visible to the naked eye) and microscopic. The cough reflex is yet another protective device, triggered when the nasal sinus passages are irritated. Cilia — short, fingerlike projections that line the inner wall of the lungs and have a constant and coordinated motion — trap fine particles that escape the nasal filter.

The Digestive Tract

The human digestive tract consists of the mouth, esophagus, stomach, small intestine, and large intestine. Harmful microorganisms can enter the digestive tract in food or liquids. Many foodborne and liquid-borne diseases such as botulism and salmonellosis, respectively, are quite severe.

The digestive tract has two basic protective mechanisms. The mucous membrane that lines the digestive tract is hard for pathogens to penetrate and entraps many particles. Also, the digestive tract secretes chemicals, the most important of which are:

- HCi, secreted by the stomach, which kills some germs and incapacitates others;
- bile, secreted by the liver into the intestinal tract, which has an antiseptic power because of its high pH.

If the built-in defenses against disease fail, modern medicine has developed to such an extent that the disease can be treated successfully in many cases. The body, however, is not people's first line of defense. Environmental health practice — controlling the causative agent before it can reach a person — precludes a challenge to the body's defenses and renders the advances of modern medicine unnecessary. Environmental health practice, therefore, arguably is the most important consideration in preventing disease in the future.

SUMMARY

The four basic determinants of health are: hereditary (biological) factors, medical care, lifestyle, and environment. Examples of biologically inherited diseases are hemophilia and juvenile diabetes. Medical care now includes advanced technologies such as electrocardiographs, CAT scans, kidney dialysis, artificial organs, and many others.

Among lifestyle contributors to disease are inadequate rest and sleep, smoking, heavy drinking, high-fat, high-sugar, high-salt, low-fiber diet, sedentariness, and stress. Conversely, sound nutrition, regular exercise, adequate rest and sleep contribute to a healthy life.

The causative agents of disease can be classified as biological, chemical, and physical agents. These enter the body via the skin, reproductive organs, respiratory tract, and digestive tract. Thus, diseases can be spread by air, water, food, insects and other animals, and fomites. Environmental measures concentrate on controlling these factors while they are still in the environment and before they enter the human body. Leading environmental practices that promote health include water quality management, sanitary waste disposal, rodent and insect control, milk sanitation, air and water pollution control, and others.

REFERENCES

Floyd, P. A., S. E. Mimms, and C. Yelding-Howard. 1995. *Personal Health: A Multicultural Approach.* Morton Publishing, Englewood, CO.

Morgan, M. T. May/June 1975. "Environmental Health Practice and Medicine." *Journal of Environmental Health.* Vol. 37, No. 6.

____. 1988. "The Role of Environmental Health in the Health Care System." Proceedings, Inaugural World Congress of Environmental Health, Sidney, Australia.

Ng, Lorenz, and D. L. Davis. 1981. *Strategies for Public Health: Promoting Health and Preventing Disease.* Van Nostrand Reinhold, New York.

Prescott, P. M., J. P. Harvey, and D. A. Klein. 1996. *Microbiology.* Wm. C. Brown. Dubuque, IA.

Chronic and Communicable Diseases

Key Terms

Acute

Carrier

Chronic

Communicable

Endemic

Epidemic

Fomites

Incubation period

Pandemic

Sporadic diseases

Vehicle of infection

Zoonoses

Objectives

- Discuss and give examples of chronic diseases.

- Define communicable diseases and explain their significance.

- Discuss disease transmission.

- Explain how communicable disease is transmitted by intestinal discharges.

- Explain how diseases are spread by nose and throat discharges.

- Define zoonoses and explain them.

- Discuss the diseases spread by vectors.

Until about 1950, infectious diseases — typhoid fever, cholera, the dysenteries, bubonic plague, the typhus fevers, and tuberculosis — were major killers in the United States and throughout the world. As a result of advances in public health, environmental health, and medicine in developed countries, these diseases have come under control. Yesterday's success, however, often brings tomorrow's challenge. As we enjoy a longer life span — a mark of progress — we also face another group of basic health problems, the chronic degenerative diseases.

CHRONIC DISEASES

Chronic diseases are those that linger. They are degenerative because they cause progressive destruction of human tissue. Whereas many of the communicable diseases have a sudden onset, chronic diseases usually have a poorly defined beginning. Many times their causes are unclear, and often they develop over a long time. Usually they reduce the body's function for a long time and their treatment is costly because those afflicted require long-term care.

COMMUNICABLE DISEASES

Throughout history communicable diseases have caused much suffering and millions of deaths. They still comprise the leading causes of death in most underdeveloped countries of the world. **Communicable diseases** are those that are contagious. An individual with cancer is not a threat to others because the population will not catch the causative agent of cancer directly from the afflicted individual. Cancer is not communicable. In contrast, an individual with a communicable disease can transmit the causative agent to the surrounding population via the respiratory tract. The cold virus, for example, exits the body of one individual and another can contract it. The disease is communicable. We can avoid the transmission of many communicable diseases by understanding their modes of transmission and by controlling the causative agents in the environment before they reach humans. Figure 3.1 illustrates the conditions necessary for infectious or communicable diseases.

COMPARING CHRONIC AND COMMUNICABLE DISEASE

Chronic and infectious diseases may be differentiated along at least three dimensions. One consists of their *causes*. Although some causes can be shared — for instance, genetic, nutritional, economic, and social factors — they more often are different. The onset of infectious diseases requires exposure to a biological agent such as a virus. In contrast, the major causes of chronic diseases are related to lifestyle. These factors include exercise level, nutritional intake, and use of tobacco and alcohol. In recent years we have learned that the environment, particularly the occupational environment, plays a major role in the initiation and aggravation of certain chronic diseases.

A second dimension is the timeline associated with chronic and infectious diseases. Infectious diseases usually are **acute**. They have sudden onset and last for a relatively brief time. Chronic diseases, on the other hand, often have a slow and insidious onset and last for a long time. Sometimes the person never recovers.

A third dimension consists of the *outcomes* associated with chronic and infectious diseases. Given proper treatment, most persons with infectious diseases recover within a relatively brief time. In contrast, people with chronic diseases usually remain ill for a long time — often the remainder of their lives. Because getting people to change their lifestyles is difficult, chronic diseases associated with lifestyle are more difficult to control than communicable diseases, for which the person may be administered medication to control the causative agent. Table 3.1 gives a comparison of chronic and communicable diseases.

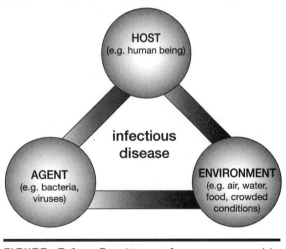

FIGURE 3.1 Conditions for communicable diseases.

TABLE 3.1 Comparison of Chronic and Communicable Diseases

	Chronic Diseases	Communicable Diseases
Causes	Often lifestyle- or environmentally related	Exposure to a biological agent
Timeline	Slow, insidious onset; long-lasting	Usually acute; sudden onset
Outcome	Often no recovery, gradual deterioration or degeneration	Relatively rapid recovery in most cases

Health professionals, particularly health educators, strive to motivate people to alter their lifestyles so as to enhance their health. They stress the benefits of walking, running, biking, hiking, stress control, stopping smoking, and reducing alcohol consumption.

ENVIRONMENTAL INFLUENCES

The chronic diseases for which the causative agent is environmentally induced by outdoor pollution or in the occupational setting, along with the "lifestyles diseases," are a particular challenge in the United States and other developed nations today. In 1964 the World Health Organization first stated that, on the basis of the available evidence, 60% to 80% of all cancer was caused, at least in part, by natural and manmade carcinogens in the environment (Higginson and Muire, 1976). More recent research has supported the accuracy of that conclusion.

Most experts agree that human health and longevity are determined to a great extent by the "health" of the environment in which we live. Russell Train, former administrator of the Environmental Protection Agency, commented:

> Today we are plagued with chronic diseases that an increasing number of health experts believe are largely caused by environmental factors — where we work or live, our habits, diets, or lifestyles. The more sophisticated and sensitive our monitoring devices become, the more data we accumulate on health effects of pollutants and other agents in the environment, the worse things look. The battle against disease must increasingly be fought, not simply in the hospitals and doctors offices, but in our streets, homes, and work places; in our air and water; in our food and products; and in our habits and lifestyles. Such a shift in emphasis will require a searching re-examination, and radical revision of popular understanding of, and public approach to, health care and disease. If environmental disease is becoming "the disease of the century," as it appears to be, then environmental protection must become the most important ingredient in our national health programs. (Willgoose, 1979, p. 1)

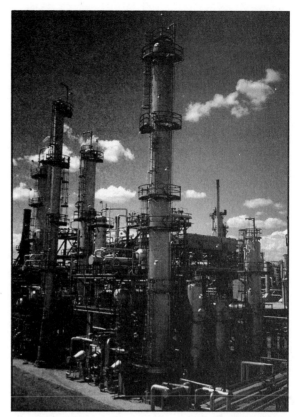

Industries follow guidelines of the Environmental Protection Agency (EPA) to prevent air and water pollution.

Individuals do not have as much control over environmental influences on health as they do on lifestyle. Instead, environmental control is the responsibility of everyone, but environmental agencies such as the Environmental Protection Agency (EPA) and state health and environmental departments. The chapters in this book address environmental management as it relates to the prevention and control of infectious diseases as well as the chronic and degenerative diseases.

METHODS OF DISEASE TRANSMISSION

Let's look at some methods of spreading diseases, the foremost of which are via air, water, food, fomites, animals, and insects (see Chapter 8). We have been taught to cover our mouth whenever we cough, to reduce the transmission of disease (such as the common cold) through the *air*. Nature provides its own defense against airborne diseases. Ultraviolet radiation from sunlight physically destroys some causative agents. Lack of humidity reduces the amount of moisture required for some organisms to reproduce.

Humans always have deposited many of their waste products in surface *water* as a means of sweeping the waste "out of sight and out of mind." Over time the concentration of wastes has increased and overloaded the ability of many water bodies to cleanse themselves, and epidemics of cholera, typhoid, and others have been the result. Today, virtually all surface water supplies used for human consumption require some form of treatment for removing disease-causing agents prior to consumption.

Some *foods* provide excellent growth media for biological causative agents. Salmonellosis is a good example. By controlling the factors required for growth, one can limit food's ability to transmit foodborne diseases. Food also can transport chemical and physical agents such as arsenic and radioactive materials.

Fomites are any inanimate objects that provide a "resting place" for causative agents of disease. We often observe people with a pencil or ink pen in the mouth. Transferring such objects between people can transmit infectious agents of disease like tuberculosis. Common examples of fomites are money, paper, counter tops, and doorknobs, among any number of others.

Animals also can transmit disease to humans. The rabies virus and the bacillus of bovine tuberculosis are examples. A few of the many other diseases transmitted by animals are tularemia, brucellosis, anthrax, and psittacosis.

Because these organisms spread in the variety of ways listed above, they are difficult to control. In some cases the same agent may be spread in a combination of ways. For example, cholera can be spread via water, food, flies, or feces. Thus, environmental control has to be a multiple-defense control effort — covering the spectrum of water, food, air, insects, personal hygiene, and sewage disposal. In the remainder of the chapter we will group communicable diseases by causative agent, mode of transmission, how they affect the body, incubation period, and desired environment (chain of infection), with emphasis on methods of control.

COMMUNICABLE DISEASES TRANSMITTED BY INTESTINAL DISCHARGES

Some diseases spread by the intestinal discharge of humans are typhoid, paratyphoid, cholera, dysentery (amoebic), polio, bacillary dysentery (Shigellosis), and infectious hepatitis, campylobacteriosis, and Giardiasis.

Typhoid Fever

Causative agent: *Salmonella typhi* (about 106 types)

Methods of spreading:

- direct and indirect contact with patient or carrier
- contaminated water or food
- raw fruit and vegetables
- milk and milk products
- shellfish (especially oysters)
- other foods and liquids contaminated by carriers of the diseases
- under certain conditions, flies and other vectors

Effects on the body: Systemic bacterial infection characterized by insidious onset of fever, headache, malaise, anorexia, enlarged spleen, rose spots on the trunk, nonproductive cough, constipation, involvement of lymph system.

Incubation period: 1 to 3 weeks (2 weeks average).

Chain of infection: Susceptible animal → causative agent → water, food, flies, roaches.

Control measures:
- sanitary disposal of human excrement
- control of flies
- pasteurization of milk
- chlorination of water supplies
- shellfish sanitation
- education of public concerning personal cleanliness
- prevention of overcrowded living conditions
- proper handling of food, water, and human waste

Paratyphoid Fever

Causative agent: *Salmonella paratyphi, S. Schottmuelleri, S. hinschfeldi*

Methods of spreading: Same as typhoid.

Effects on the body: Bacterial enteric infection, abrupt onset of fever, malaise, headache, enlarged spleen, rose spots on trunk, diarrhea, involvement of lymphoid tissue.

Incubation period: 1 to 10 days for gastroenteritis; 1 to 3 weeks for enteric fever.

Chain of infection: Susceptible animal → causative agent → water, food, fomites, flies, roaches.

Control measures: Same as for typhoid.

Cholera

Causative agent: *Vibrio cholera,* including El Tor strain

Methods of spreading:
- ingestion of fecal-contaminated water
- sometimes food contaminated by carriers
- direct contact
- contaminated soiled hands and utensils
- flies
- raw uncooked seafood from polluted water

Effects on the body: Sudden onset, profuse watery stools, occasional vomiting, rapid dehydration, acidosis, circulatory collapse.

Incubation period: Few hours to 5 days (usually 2 to 3 days).

Chain of infection: Susceptible animal → causative agent → water, food, flies, roaches.

Control measures: Same as for typhoid.

Shigellosis (Bacillary dysentery)

Causative agent: *Genus Shigella* (27 types), a rod-shaped organism

Methods of spreading:
- direct contact, fecal-oral transmission
- indirect by objects soiled by feces
- consumption of contaminated foods, water, milk
- flies

Effects on the body: Diarrhea, fever, nausea, vomiting, cramps, tenesmus, convulsions (in children); stools may contain blood, mucus, pus.

Incubation period: 1 to 7 days (usually 1 to 3 days).

Chain of infection: Susceptible animal → causative agent → water, food, flies, roaches.

Control measures:
- sanitary disposal of human feces
- public health education
- protection of water and food supplies and shellfish
- surveillance of food
- control of flies and roaches

Amoebic Dysentery

Causative agent: *Entamoeba histolytic* (protozoan)

Methods of spreading:
- direct contact with water
- mouth-to-mouth transfer of feces
- contaminated vegetables (especially raw vegetables)
- flies
- contaminated hands of food handlers

Effects on the body: Acute fever, chills, bloody or mucoid diarrhea, mild abdominal discomfort, diarrhea containing blood or mucus.

Incubation period: Varies, few days to several months or years (usually 2 to 4 weeks).

Chain of infection: Susceptible animal → causative agent → water, food, flies, roaches.

Control measures:
- sanitary disposal of human feces
- protection of public water supplies
- public health education
- personal hygiene
- fly and roach control
- food quality management

Poliomyelitis (polio)

Causative agent: polio viruses Types 1, 11, and 111 (Type 1 is most common)

Methods of spreading:
- direct contact through association with infected persons
- sometimes milk
- water suspected at times
- fecal-oral route (major route of transmission)
- nasal discharges

Effects on the body: Fever, malaise, headache, nausea, vomiting, excruciating muscle pain and spasms, stiffness of neck and back with or without flaccid paralysis (hallmark of the disease).

Incubation period: 7 to 14 days (range of 3 to 35 days).

Chain of infection: Susceptible animal → causative agent → humans → water, or food.

Control measures:
- active immunization (successful in U. S.)
- health education
- prevention of crowded conditions
- isolation in some cases

Infectious Hepatitis

Causative agent: Hepatitis A virus (a filtering agent has not been demonstrated)

Methods of spreading:
- intimate person-to-person contact by fecal or oral route with respiratory spread possible
- blood transfusions
- contaminated syringes
- contaminated water, milk, or food (including oysters and clams)

Effects on the body: Fever, malaise, anorexia, nausea, abdominal discomfort followed in a few days by jaundice.

Incubation period: 15 to 20 days, depending on dose (average 8 to 21 days).

Chain of infection: Susceptible animal → causative agent → humans, food, water, fomites.

Control measures:
- health education
- management of water and food (especially shellfish)
- monitoring of blood and blood products
- proper disposal of syringes
- sanitary disposal of feces, urine, blood
- hand washing to minimize fecal-oral transmission

Campylobacteriosis

Causative agent: *Campylobacter jejuni, Campylobacter fetus, Campylobacter coli* (rarely), *C. cinaedi, C. fennelliae*

Methods of spreading:
- found in human excreta and reservoirs
- found in cattle and poultry; puppies, kittens, other pets; swine, sheep, rodents, and birds
- transmitted by ingesting organisms in food, unpasteurized milk, and water
- contact with infected pets, wild animals, infected infants; infected children may

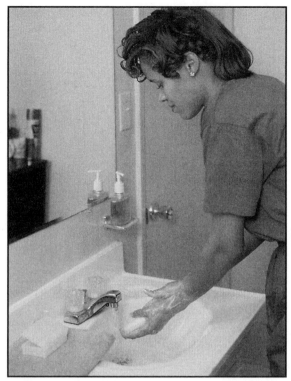
Washing the hands is one of the most effective means of preventing infectious diseases.

transmit to puppies and kittens, which then may expose other children

Effects on the body: Acute bacterial disease of variable severity characterized by diarrhea, abdominal pain, malaise, fever, nausea, and vomiting; illness may be prolonged in adults; relapses may occur. Many infections are asymptomatic.

Incubation period: Usually 3 to 5 days (range of 1 to 10 days possible).

Occurrence: These organisms cause diarrheal illnesses in all parts of the world of all age groups (5% to 14% of diarrhea world-wide). In developed countries, children and young adults have the highest incidence of illness; in developing countries, illness is confined largely to children under age 2. Common sources of outbreak include chicken, unpasteurized milk, and unchlorinated water. Most cases occur in temperate

areas in warmer months. This is an important cause of travelers' diarrhea.

Control measures:

- thoroughly cooking all foodstuffs derived from animal sources, especially poultry
- pasteurizing milk, chlorinating all water supplies
- recognizing, preventing, controlling campylobacter infections in domestic animals, pets (i.e., separate puppies, kittens with diarrhea)
- washing hands after contact with animals
- minimizing contact with poultry and their feces; washing hands as needed when this cannot be avoided
- avoiding mass feeding and poor sanitation

Giardiasis

Causative agent: *Giardia lamblia* (G. intestinalis), a flagellate protozoan

Methods of spreading: Human excreta, duodenal fluid, and small-intestine mucosa; hand-to-mouth transfer of cysts from feces of infected individual (especially in day-care centers, institutions, and the like); also occurs by ingesting fecally contaminated water. Contaminated food is less often implicated. Humans are the most common reservoirs, with beaver and other wild and domesticated animals implicated.

Effects on the body: May include chronic diarrhea, nausea, abdominal cramps, vomiting, weight loss, and fatigue lasting from a few days to several weeks; more often asymptomatic. Infection usually occurs in the upper small intestine. In severe cases duodenal and jejunal mucosal cells may be damaged.

Incubation period: 5 to 25 days or longer (average 7 to 10 days).

Occurrence: Worldwide, with children affected more frequently than adults; more prevalent in areas of poor sanitation, and where children are not toilet-trained (e.g., day care centers). U. S. outbreaks (waterborne) occur mostly in mountain communities where streams or rivers are sources of drinking water without a water filtration system. It is also prevalent in certain temperate and tropical countries and often is associated with tour groups infected after drinking inadequately treated water.

Control measures:

- education of families, personnel, and inmates of institutions, especially day care personnel, personal hygiene
- filtration of public water supplies that may be contaminated with human or animal feces (routine chlorination of water will not kill the giardia cysts, especially if the water is cold)
- protection of public water supplies from human and animal fecal contamination
- sanitary disposal of feces
- boiling of emergency water supplies

DISEASES SPREAD BY NOSE AND THROAT DISCHARGES

Tuberculosis

Causative agent: *Mycobacterium tuberculosis hominis* (human); *Mycobacterium bovis* (cattle)

Methods of spreading:

- exposure to bacilli in airborne droplet — sputum of infected persons
- indirect contact through contaminated articles or dust
- nasal secretions of infected cow
- consumption of unpasteurized milk from infected cow

Effects on the body: Primary infection usually goes unnoticed clinically, lesions commonly become inactive, leaving no residual changes except pulmonary or tracheobronchial lymph node calcification. Tuberculin sensitivity appears within a few weeks.

Incubation period: From infection to demonstrable primary lesion, about 4 to 12 weeks; to progressive pulmonary or extrapulmonary tuberculosis may be years.

Chain of infection: Susceptible person → causative agent → humans or cattle.

Control measures:

- improvement of poor social conditions that increase the risk of infection, such as overcrowding
- education of the public in mode of spread and method of control
- availability of medical, laboratory, and X-ray facilities for examinations of patients, contacts, and suspects; early treatment of cases
- pasteurization of milk
- TB control in cattle

Diphtheria

Causative agent: *Corynebacterium diphtheriae*

Methods of spreading:

- contact with a patient or carrier; or, rarely, with articles soiled with lesion discharges of infected persons
- raw milk (occasionally)

Occurrence: Diphtheria does not occur much any more in the United States because of DPT immunization given to children. (In the past, diphtheria killed many.)

Effects on the body: Acute infectious disease of tonsils, pharynx, larynx, nose, and, occasionally other mucous membranes or skin; sore throat; enlarged cervical lymph nodes.

Incubation period: Usually 2 to 5 days.

Chain of infection: Susceptible person → causative agent → humans → food.

Control measures:

- active immunization with diphtheria toxoid on a population basis, including an adequate program to maintain immunity

- immunization of adults subject to unusual risk, such as physicians, teachers, nurses, and other hospital personnel
- educational measures to inform the public, and particularly the parents of young children, of the hazards of diphtheria and the necessity and advantages of active immunization
- milk sanitation

Measles

Causative agent: Measles virus.

Methods of spreading: By droplet spread or direct contact with nasal or throat secretions or urine of infected persons by children who are not immunized.

Effects on the body: Fever, conjunctivitis, coryza bronchitis, Koplik spots on the buccal mucosa, dusky red blotchy rash appearing on the third to seventh day. A high percentage of children with the disease suffer brain damage.

Incubation period: About 10 days (varying from 8 to 13 days) after exposure to onset of fever; about 14 days until rash appears; uncommonly longer or shorter.

Chain of infection: Susceptible person → causative agent → humans.

Control measures:
- vaccination
- isolation
- education

Scarlet Fever

Causative agent: *Streptococcus pyogenes*

Methods of spreading:
- direct or intimate contact with patient or carrier
- indirect contact with patient or through transfer by objects or hands

Effects on the body: Fever, sore throat, tonsillitis, pharyngitis, leucocytosis. Can cause a heart murmur if the infection becomes systemic.

Incubation period: 1 to 3 days.

Chain of infection: Susceptible person → causative agent → humans → fomites → food or milk.

Control measures:
- lab tests for recognition of group A hemolytic streptococci
- education of the public in modes of transmission
- boiling or pasteurization of milk likely to be contaminated
- disinfection of soiled handkerchiefs, bed clothing

Whooping Cough

Causative agent: *Bondetella Pertussis*

Methods of spreading: Primarily by direct contact with discharges from respiratory mucous membranes of infected persons, airborne by droplets, and indirect contact. (Whooping cough once was prevalent, but incidences have dropped since introduction of DPT vaccine).

Effects on the body: Irritating cough, sore throat.

Incubation period: Commonly 7 days; almost always uniformly within 10 days.

Chain of infection: Susceptible person → causative agent → humans → air or fomites.

Control measures:
- active immunization with vaccine
- education of the public, particularly parents of children and infants
- control of fomites and indoor air

Smallpox

Smallpox was a worldwide problem until the 1960s. It is one of the first diseases eradicated using medical and public health technology.

Pneumonia

Causative agent: *Diplococcus pneumoniae*

Methods of spreading: Droplet; by direct oral contact; or indirectly, through articles freshly soiled with respiratory discharges. It is a major problem in hospitals and nursing homes, where it kills older persons.

Effects on the body: Chills, fever, pain in chest; cough productive of "rusty" sputum.

Incubation period: Believed to be 1 to 3 days.

Chain of infection: Susceptible person → causative agent → humans → air or fomites.

Control measures:
- avoidance of crowding in living quarters whenever practical, particularly in institutions, barracks, and on ships
- control of patient's respiratory discharges
- good personal and institutional hygiene

Influenza

Causative agents: Viruses.

Methods of spreading: Direct contact, through droplet infection; also spread by nose and throat discharges and doorknobs infected people have touched.

Effects on the body: Fever, chills, headache, myalgia, prostration.

Incubation period: 24 to 72 hours.

Chain of infection: Susceptible person → causative agent → humans → air → fomites.

Control measures:
- active immunization when vaccine is potent
- avoidance of discharges from infected persons
- good personal and institutional hygiene
- education of the public in basic personal hygiene
- disinfection of eating and drinking utensils

Common Cold

Causative agent: A variety of viruses.

Methods of spreading:
- by direct oral contact or by droplet
- indirectly by articles freshly soiled by discharges from nose and mouth

Effects on the body: Lacrimation (secrete tears), irritated nasopharynx, chilliness, malaise, fever.

Incubation period: 12 to 72 hours.

Chain of infection: Susceptible person → causative agent → humans → air or fomites.

Control measures:
- good personal health and hygiene
- disinfection of eating and drinking utensils and articles soiled by secretions and excretions of patients
- avoidance of articles and areas where infections are or have been

DISEASES OF ANIMALS TRANSMITTABLE TO HUMANS (*Zoonoses*)

Rabies

Causative agent: Lyssavirus type I (a neurotropic virus of family *rhabdoviridae*)

Methods of spreading:
- bite of rabid animal; rarely, by saliva of rabid animals entering a scratch or other fresh break in skin
- airborne transmission from bats to humans (possible in caves where bats are roosting)

Effects on the body: Onset with a sense of apprehension, headache, fever, malaise, and indefinite sensory changes. Disease progresses to paresis or paralysis, with muscle spasms or deglution (thickening of saliva cavity, choking) on attempt to swallow. Delirium and convulsions follow. Death is from respiratory paralysis. Rabies is almost invariably fatal by acute encephalitis.

Incubation period: Usually 4 to 6 weeks; occasionally shorter or longer, depending upon the extent and site of laceration or wound and other factors.

Chain of infection: Susceptible agent → causative agent → bite of dog, or other rapid animal.

Control measures:

- specific prevention by vaccination. Protection depends upon how quickly vaccination is started after injury. Vaccine is usually given for 14 consecutive days. Vaccination often is supplemented by passive immune serum

- prevention measures include the following

  a. If the animal is apprehended, confined, and observed for 10 days, vaccination is started in affected person at the first physical sign or laboratory evidence of rabies in the observed animal

  b. If the animal is not apprehended and rabies is known to be present in the area, vaccination in the affected person is started immediately.

  c. In severe bites, particularly in the region of head, face, and neck, with any likelihood that the animal is rabid, a dose of hyperimmune serum is given immediately, followed promptly by a full course of vaccine.

  d. Rabies vaccine is not given unless the skin is broken, as it may cause post-vaccinal encephalitis.

- prompt cleansing of wounds caused by bite or scratch of rabid or suspected rabid animal with soap or detergent solution. Hyperimmune serum may be infiltrated beneath the bite wound

- education of people regarding pet vaccinations, seeking immediate medical attention for any bites, confinement and observation of animals that have inflicted bites, reporting incidents promptly

- observation of dogs or other animals known to have bitten a person and knowing signs of rabies (change in behavior, with excitability and paralysis, followed by death)

- laboratory examination of brain from iced intact heads of animals dying of suspected rabies to search for Negri bodies, demonstration of which confirms rabies

- immediate destruction or detention of unvaccinated dogs or cats bitten by animals known to be rabid

- registration/licensing/vaccination of dogs and cats; destruction of stray animals

Brucellosis (Undulant Fever)

Causative agent: *Brucella melitensis*; *Brucella abortus*; *Brucella suis*

Methods of spreading: Contact with infected animals' tissues and secretions; by ingestion of milk and dairy products from infected animals.

Effects on the body:

- may have acute or insidious onset; continued, intermittent, or irregular fever of variable duration; headache, weakness, profuse sweating, chills or chilliness, generalized aching.

- disease may last several days, months, occasionally even years; recovery is usual, with a fatality rate of 2% or less of all cases

Incubation period: Highly variable; usually 5 to 21 days, occasionally several months.

Chain of infection: Susceptible agent → causative agent → fluid or tissue of diseased animal.

Control measures:

- education of farmers and workers in slaughter houses, packing plants, and butcher shops about the nature of the disease and the dangers in handling carcasses and products of infected animals

- search for infection among animals by agglutination reaction and elimination of infected animals by segregation and slaughter

- calf immunization in enzootic areas

- pasteurization of milk and dairy products from cows, sheep, and goats; boiling of milk when pasteurization is impossible or unavailable

Bovine Tuberculosis

Causative agent: *Mycobacterium tuberculosis*

Methods of spreading: Ingestion of unpasteurized milk or dairy products from tuberculous cows, by airborne infection in barns, and from handling contaminated animal products.

Effects on the body: Fatigue, fever, weight loss; infection may spread to any part of the body through lymph and bloodstream and then cause manifestations in the specific locality.

Incubation period: Variable, from a few weeks to even years.

Chain of infection: Susceptible agent → causative agent → fluids and/or tissue of diseased animal.

Control measures:
- health education of the public regarding the importance of pasteurized milk
- BCG vaccination of uninfected persons
- elimination of tuberculosis among dairy cattle by tuberculin testing and slaughter of diseased animals
- pasteurization of milk and milk products

Q-fever

Causative agent: *Rickettsia burnetti* (*Coxiella burnetti*)

Methods of spreading: Commonly by airborne dissemination of rickettsiae in or near contaminated premises, in establishments processing infected animals or their by-products, and at necropsy (post mortem examination); also, raw milk from cows or direct contact with infected animals or other contaminated materials.

Effects on the body: Sudden onset of chilly sensation, headache, weakness, malaise, severe sweats; also, in most cases, pneumonitis with mild cough, scanty expectoration, chest pain, minimal physical findings and little or no upper respiratory involvement.

Incubation period: 2 to 3 weeks.

Chain of infection: Susceptible agent → causative agent → tissue fluid or hair of diseased animal or ticks.

Control measures:
- immunization of laboratory workers and others in exposing occupations
- pasteurization of milk from cows, goats, sheep, to inactivate rickettsiae
- public health education on sources of infection and the importance of pasteurizing milk
- control of infection in animals by vaccination and by regulating movement of infected livestock

Anthrax

Causative agent: *Brucella anthracis* (a spore-forming organism)

Methods of spreading:
- infection of skin by contact with contaminated hair, wool hides, and manufactured products such as shaving brushes, or by direct contact with infected tissues
- inhalation anthrax (below) from aspiration of spores
- gastrointestinal anthrax (below) from ingestion of contaminated undercooked meat

Effects on the body:
- **Skin anthrax:** An initial papule or vesicle at the site of inoculation develops into a depressed black eschar (spot), often followed by hard, edematous (watery) swelling of deeper and adjacent tissues. Pain is unusual. Untreated infections may spread to regional lymph nodes and bloodstream, with overwhelming septicaemia (blood poisoning) and death.
- **Inhalation anthrax:** Initial symptoms are mild and nonspecific upper respiratory infections. Acute symptoms of respiratory distress, fever, and shock follow in 3 to 5 days, with death 7 to 25 hours thereafter. The fatality rate is very high.

Incubation period: Within 7 days, usually less than 4 days.

Chain of infection: Susceptible animal → causative agent → contact with tissue, wool, hair, etc., of diseased animal.

Control measures:

- immunization by cell-free vaccine, especially of veterinarians and persons handling potentially contaminated industrial raw materials
- for employees handling potentially contaminated articles, education in personal cleanliness, modes of transmission, and care of skin abrasions
- dust control and proper ventilation in hazardous industries; continuous medical supervision of employees, and prompt medical care of all suspicious skin lesions; adequate facilities for washing after work
- thorough washing, disinfection, or sterilization when possible, of hair, wool, or hides, and bone meal or other feed of animal origin, prior to processing
- ban on selling hides of animals infected with anthrax and carcasses used as food supplement
- postmortem examinations of animals dying of suspected anthrax
- non-contamination of soil or environment with blood and infected tissues
- incineration of carcasses or burial deeply with quicklime, preferably at the site of death
- prompt isolation and treatment of animals suspected of anthrax
- annual vaccination of animals when indicated

Leptospirosis (Weiel's Disease, hemorrhagic jaundice)

Causative agent: More than 80 serotypes of leptospira.

Methods of spreading:

- contact with water contaminated with urine of infected animals, as in swimming or accidental or occupational immersions
- direct contact with infected animals (infection presumably results from penetration of abraded skin or mucous membrane, or possibly through ingestion)

Effects on the body: Acute fever, headache, chills, severe malaise, vomiting, muscular aches, meningeal irritations, conjunctivitis; infrequently, jaundice, renal insufficiency, hemolytic anemia, hemorrhage in skin and mucous membrane. Clinical illness lasts 1 to 3 weeks; fatality is low.

Incubation period: 4 to 19 days.

Chain of infection: Susceptible animal → causative agent → animal urine.

Control measures:

- protection of workers in hazardous occupations with boots and gloves
- education of the public on mode of transmission and the need to avoid swimming or wading in potentially contaminated waters
- rodent control in rural and recreational human habitations
- segregation of domestic animals and prevention of contamination of living and working areas of people by urine of infected animals
- same as Campylobacteriosis and Giardiasis — see earlier listings

Salmonellosis

Causative Agents: *Salmonella typhimurium, S. heidelberg, S. newport, S. oranienburg, S. infantis, S. enteritidis, S. derby*

Methods of spreading: Foods including meat pies, poultry products, raw sausages, lightly cooked foods containing egg or egg products, unpasteurized milk or dairy products, foods contaminated with rodent feces or by an infected food handler, or even through utensils, working surfaces, or tables used previously for contaminated foods such as egg products.

Effects on the body: Sudden onset of abdominal pain, diarrhea, and vomiting; fever nearly always. Deaths are uncommon, though anorexia and bowel looseness may continue for several days.

Incubation period: 6 to 48 hours; usually 12 to 24 hours.

Chain of infection: Susceptible person → causative agent → animals, eggs, meat, etc.

Control measures:

- thorough cooking of all foodstuffs derived from animal sources
- prevention of recontamination within kitchen after cooking turkey and other poultry
- not eating raw eggs
- refrigeration of prepared food before use
- education of food handlers and cooks in the necessity of protecting prepared food against rodent and insect contamination, in refrigeration of foods, and in hand washing before and after food preparation
- control of salmonella infection among domestic animals

ARTHROPOD-BORNE DISEASES

Typhus fever (epidemic typhus, louse-borne typhus)

Causative agent: *Rickettsia prowazeki*

Methods of spreading: body louse *Pediculus humanus* is infected by feeding on the blood of a patient with acute typhus fever. Infected lice excrete rickettsia in their feces and usually defecate at the time of feeding. Humans are infected by rubbing feces or crushed lice into the bite or into superficial abrasions. Inhaling infective louse feces as dust may account for some infection.

Effects on the body: Variable onset; often sudden and marked by headache, chills, prostration, fever, general pains. A macular (spot) eruption appears on the fifth to sixth day, initially on the upper trunk.

Incubation period: 1 to 2 weeks; commonly 12 days.

Chain of infection: Susceptible person → causative agent → body louse → poor hygiene.

Control measures:

- at appropriate intervals, application of an effective residual insecticide powder to clothes and persons living under conditions favoring lice.
- improved living conditions with provisions for bathing and washing clothes.

Murine Typhus Fever (endemic typhus fever, flea-borne typhus)

Causative agent: *Rickettsia typhi* (Rickettsia mooseri)

Methods of spreading: Infective rat fleas (usually *Xenophylla cheopsis*) defecate rickettsia while sucking blood, contaminating the bite site and other fresh skin wounds.

Effects on the body: Similar to louse-borne typhus, but milder.

Incubation period: Usually 10 to 12 days (varies from 6 to 21 days).

Chain of infection: Susceptible person → causative agent → fleas.

Control measures:

- preventing contact with infected mites by personal prophylaxis against the mite vector, by impregnating clothes and blankets with miticidal chemicals (benzyl benzoate) and applying mite repellents
- spraying with lindane or malathion.

MOSQUITOES

Yellow Fever Mosquito
(Aedes aegypti)

Diseases spread by: Urban yellow fever, dengue fever, encephalitis, filariasis, dog heartworm.

Biological characteristics: The life cycle of all mosquitoes has four stages: egg, pupa, larva, and adult, with the first three stages occurring in water. Semidomesticated, mosquitoes can breed in artificial containers in and around human habitations. Eggs are laid singly on the side of containers at or above the waterline and are able to withstand drying for several months. When containers are filled with water again they hatch quickly. If temperatures are high, hatching can take place in 2 or 3 days. Under favorable conditions the larvae can complete development in 6 to 10 days. The pupal period lasts about 2 days. The entire life cycle can be completed in 10 days, or it may vary as long as 3 weeks or more.

Identification: Small dark species with lyre-shaped, silver-white lines on the thorax and white bands on the torsal segments.

Desired environment: Prefers warm temperatures; susceptible to cold and usually does not survive the winter in northern U.S. Found in artificial containers in and around human habitations, such as: flower vases, tin cans, jars, discarded automobile tires, unused privies, cisterns, rain barrels, sagging roof gutters, and tree holes. *Aedes aegypti* prefers to live near human habitats.

Control measures: Keeping the habitat clean and free of objects that serve as breeding places for the mosquito (artificial containers such as cans, bottles, birdbaths, stopped-up gutters, old tires, automobiles, catch basins, watering containers, old appliances) to prevent mosquitoes from having a place to lay their eggs.

Malaria Mosquito
(Anopheles quadrimaculatus)

Diseases spread by: Malaria; have been found infected with encephalitis viruses and may have a role in the transmission of filariasis as well. This species was the most important vector of malaria in the United States.

Biological characteristics: The eggs of *anophelines* are always laid singly on the water surface and are supported by lateral floats. The female lays her eggs in batches of 100 or more. The eggs hatch in 2 to 6 days; the larval stages last 6 to 7 days to several weeks, depending on the species and environmental conditions, especially the water temperature. Most *anopheles* need a blood meal before they can produce fertile eggs. They usually winter as hibernating, fertilized females. A single female may deposit more than 3,000 eggs in as many as 12 batches. Hibernating females may survive 4 to 5 months.

Identification: Fairly large, dark brown with four dark spots near center of each wing. Palpi and tarsi are entirely dark.

Desired environment: Breeds chiefly in permanent freshwater pools, ponds and swamps that contain aquatic vegetation or floating debris. It is most abundant in shallow waters. This species shows a preference for clear, quiet waters neutral to alkaline. Common habitats are lime-sink ponds, burrow pits, sloughs, bayous, sluggish streams, shallow margins, and backwater areas of reservoirs and lakes. Production is greatest in waters with aquatic vegetation or flotage of twigs, bark, and leaves. The most favorable temperature for development is between 85° and 90°F. An improperly constructed farm pond could be the desired environment for *Anopheles quadrimaculatus*.

Control measures: Altering the favorable environment described and creating an unfavorable environment for breeding: filling potholes, depressions, swamps, and marshes with soil or other media; deepening trenches to remove standing water; placing tile under the ground for drainage; fluctuating the water level of farm ponds, reservoirs and other water impoundments (used to control mosquitoes in TVA lakes).

Northern House Mosquito (*Culex pipiens pipiens*) and Southern House Mosquito (*Culex pipiens quinquefasciatus*)

Diseases spread by: St. Louis encephalitis, filariasis.

Biological characteristics: These species lay eggs in clusters of 50 to 400. These clusters, known as egg rafts, float on the water surface. In warm weather the eggs hatch within a day or two. Eight to 10 days are required to complete of the larval and pupal stages. These mosquitoes can survive and produce fertile eggs without a blood meal. They are active only at night.

Identification: Brown mosquitoes of medium size with cross bands of white scales on the abdominal segments but without other prominent markings.

Desired environment: Develop prolifically in rain barrels, tires, tanks, tin cans, and practically all types of artificial containers; also live in storm-sewer catch basins, poorly drained street gutters, polluted ground pools, and cesspools. Heavy production is found in water with high organic content. Faster development occurs in warm environment.

Control measures: Same as those listed for *Aedes*.

TICKS

American Dog Tick (*Dermacentor variabilis*) and Wood Tick (*Dermacentor andersoni*)

Diseases spread by: Rocky Mountain spotted fever (tick-borne typhus), tularemia, Colorado tick fever, possibly Q-fever, anaplasmosis, tick paralysis.

Biological characteristics: The life history has four stages: egg, six-legged larva, eight-legged nymph, adult. "Hard" ticks usually mate while they are on the host animal. The female drops to the ground and, after a brief pre-oviposition period (usually 3 to 10 days), begins to deposit eggs on or near the earth. The female feeds once and lays one large batch of eggs, sometimes numbering in the thousands. The eggs hatch in 2 weeks to several months depending on temperature, humidity, and other environmental factors. The larvae, or "seed ticks," possess only six legs and are not distinguishable as to sex. Their chance of attaching to a host is precarious, sometimes making prolonged fasts obligatory. After a blood meal, the engorged larvae usually drop to the soil and molt to the eight-legged nymph stage. This stage also requires a critical waiting period for a suitable host. After engorgement, the nymph drops from the host, molts, and becomes an adult. Although the life cycle of some species of hard ticks is completed in less than 1 year, it may require 2 years or longer.

Both male and female hard ticks are blood suckers, and both require several days feeding before copulation. After the male hard tick becomes engorged, he usually copulates with one or more females and then dies. Following copulation, the female tick drops to the ground. The eggs require several days to develop. She then begins oviposition. After a few more days, the female hard tick also dies.

Identification: Dorsal shield; tapered anteriorly.

Desired environment: Climatic factors, particularly temperature, important. The several tick species are extremely variable in their ability to withstand temperature extremes, some surviving frigid winters as hibernating adults, nymphs, or larvae, and others surviving high temperatures and arid conditions. In most species the higher temperatures of spring and summer accelerate tick development and activity.

Control measures (for humans):

- buttoned clothing, trouser legs tucked into socks, shirttail tucked into trousers
- no sitting on ground or logs in brushy areas.
- clearing or burning brush along paths and keeping weeds and grass cut in recreation areas
- in residential areas, closely cut lawns and well-kept yards
- tick repellents to the skin impractical but the military treats clothing with repellents.

Control measures (for animals):

- dusting the animal
- using flea and tick collars (may be ineffective on large dogs)
- Ronnel, an organic phosphorus insecticide (in pill form), prescribed by veterinarian
- insecticides (dust or spray) in vegetated areas
- removing the hosts (dogs can be put outside)
- for cattle tick infestation, rotation of pastures

Deer tick (Borrelia burgdonferi)

Disease spread by: Lyme disease.

Method of spreading: Bite from tick belonging to Genus *Ixodes: Ixodes dammini* or *Ixodes ricinus*.

Effects on the body: Lyme disease; clinical manifestations vary, mimicking several disorders, but affecting primarily the skin, nervous system, heart, and joints. The disease typically occurs in three stages. A patient can have one or all of the stages, and the infection may not become symptomatic until Stage 2 or 3.

- **Stage 1:** The first stage is characterized by localized erythema chronicum migrans, a rapidly expanding skin lesion, usually occurring in a circular radiating pattern. This lesion occurs in 60% to 80% of the patients and may be accompanied by flu-like symptoms and/or regional lympadenopathy. Secondary lesions may develop within several days of the initial lesion, but they are smaller, less radiating, and are not indurated or in the area of the tick bite. Other clinical manifestations at this stage can be conjunctivitis (eye infection), hives, and a malar (spot) rash.

- **Stage 2:** The second stage consists of disseminated infections including neurologic and/or cardiac abnormalities. The most common neurological problem is Bell's palsy, which can be unilateral or bilateral and sometimes occurs in conjunction with radiculopathic syndrome, a condition of the small nerves caused by the disease. Aseptic meningitis often occurs without fever and may begin as recurring headaches, stiff neck, photophobia, nausea, and vomiting. Various encephalitic symptoms may include lethargy, fatigue, poor memory, dementia, personality changes, and psychoses with auditory hallucination. Less commonly reported are neurologic syndromes including pseudotumor cerebri and chorea — jerky movement.

  Carditis, which occurs in 4% to 10% of Lyme disease cases, manifests with varying degrees of atrioventricular block. This transient myocarditis usually occurs 3 to 6 weeks after the initial illness and generally resolves completely with antibiotic therapy. Complete heart block rarely persists more than a week, and the long-term prognosis is excellent. In more severe cases, hospitalization with continuous monitoring and temporary cardiac pacing may be required, as death is a possibility. Lyme carditis usually affects otherwise healthy young men. Prompt recognition and treatment is crucial to avoid unnecessary, permanent pacemaker implantation or death.

- **Stage 3:** This stage is rheumatologic, lasting months rather than weeks. Symptoms may arise within weeks of the secondary stage or within a gap of several years. Symptoms begin as migratory musculoskeletal discomforts that involve the joints, bursae, and tendons. The knee, the most commonly affected joint, usually is more swollen than painful. In severe cases, chronic Lyme disease may lead to erosion of cartilage and bone, and rarely to permanent joint disability.

Congenital infection through transplacental transmission of *B. burgdorferi* can cause adverse fetal outcomes, but this is not usually the case.

Incubation period: Anywhere from 3 to 30 days from the time of the bite, in some cases may be much longer.

Chain of infection: Susceptible animal → causative agent → *Ixodes* tick.

Control measures (for humans):

- buttoned clothing, trouser legs tucked into socks, shirttail tucked into trousers
- no sitting on ground or logs in brushy areas.
- clearing or burning brush along paths and keeping weeds and grass cut in recreation areas
- in residential areas, closely cut lawns and well-kept yards
- tick repellents to the skin impractical but the military treats clothing with repellents.

Control measures (for animals):

- dusting the animal
- using flea and tick collars (may be ineffective on large dogs)
- Ronnel, an organic phosphorus insecticide (in pill form), prescribed by veterinarian
- insecticides (dust or spray) in vegetated areas
- removing the hosts (dogs can be put outside)
- for cattle tick infestation, rotation of pastures

Treatment: Causative agent is susceptible to several antibiotics including penicillin, tetracycline, ampicillin, ceftriaxone, and imipenem. Erythromycin is effective against the spirochete in vitro but not as effective in vivo. Amoxicillin is the drug of choice for children. No appropriate treatment for pregnant women has been developed. In the past, high doses of penicillin have been introduced intravenously. Corticosteroids, which were used to treat the disease before antibiotics came into use, have been used with success in treating carditis in patients not responding to antibiotic therapy. Prophylactic antibiotic therapy remains unresolved, and no vaccine is yet available.

MITES

Scabies or itch mite (*Sarcoptes scabiel*)

Diseases spread by: Sarcoptes scabial causes scabies. Other mites spread sheep scab, Texas itch of cattle, mange in dogs and horses, scrub typhus (not found in U.S.), rickettsial pox, encephalitis virus, dermatitis; infestation of the lungs, intestines, urinary passages.

Biological characteristics: Mites lay eggs that hatch into larvae that pass through two or more nymphal stages to finally become adults. Larvae have two pairs of legs, and the nymphal stages have four pairs. The females burrow beneath the outer layer of skin and lay their eggs in the sinuous tunnels that they excavate. The eggs hatch into larvae. Some believe that males have only one nymphal stage and complete their life cycle in 9 to 11 days, and that the females have two nymphal stages and take 14 to 17 days — perhaps longer in cold weather — to complete their life cycle. The adults live about a month.

Identification: No well-defined segmentation of the body. Females average 0.2 to 0.4 mm in length, and males are somewhat smaller.

Oval sac-like body; body surface is finely wrinkled; long body hairs.

Desired environment: Most commonly in tiny papules, particularly in the webbing between fingers, and folds of the skin at wrist.

Control measures:

- trapping or poisoning rodents to eliminate the source of the blood meal essential for nourishment and reproduction of mites
- starving out rodents by storing garbage and food in rat-proof containers, rooms, buildings.
- keeping rodents out of buildings
- removing vegetation near houses; pruning shrubs so they are at least one yard from buildings
- chigger (mite) control depends on modifying the environment to permit sunlight and air to circulate freely, drying out its usual damp habitat
- sulfur has been used for years as a chigger (mite) repellent

FLIES

House fly (*Musca domestica*)

Diseases spread by: Bacillary dysentery, infantile diarrhea, typhoid fever, paratyphoid fever, cholera, amoebic dysentery, giardiasis and pinworm, roundworm and tapeworm infections.

Biological characteristics: The developmental stages of the house fly are: the egg, larva, pupa, and adult. This cycle requires 8 to 20 days under average conditions. The female begins laying eggs within 4 to 20 days after emergence as an adult. The small, white oval eggs are about 1 mm long and are deposited in batches of 75 to 150. The average female lays five or six batches her lifetime. Eggs usually are placed in cracks and crevices in the breeding material, away from direct light. Hatching occurs in 12 to 24 hours during the summer months. The larval stage lasts from 4 to 7 days in warm weather. When ready to pupate, the larva contracts until the skin forms a case about 6 mm in length. The pupal stage ordinarily lasts 4 or 5 days. When the pupal period is complete, the fly breaks open the end of the puparium and works its way out. The wings unfold and the body expands, dries, and hardens. This requires about 1 hour under summer conditions. Adulthood is reached in about 15 hours. Mating then may take place. Two or more generations per month may be produced during warm weather.

Identification: Small species, 6 mm to 9 mm long with dull thorax and abdomen. The thorax has four longitudinal dark stripes, sides of the abdomen usually are pale basally, and the fourth wing vein is angled sharply, ending before the wingtip. The arista of the antenna has many fine hairs like a feather.

Desired environment:

- almost any type of warm, moist organic material, such as animal manure and garbage. Flies are inactive at temperatures below 45°F and are killed by temperatures slightly below 32°F.
- flight begins when air temperature is about 53°F and complete activity occurs at 70°F. Maximum activity is reached at 90°F, with a rapid decline at higher temperatures until 112°F, which produces paralysis and death. Flies are phototropic.

Control measures:

- sanitary refuse storage and regular collection
- control of feces of warm-blooded animals
- elimination of open dumps and littering
- sanitary landfill (refuse is compacted and covered with dirt daily)
- garbage grinders and compactors
- incinerators
- proper sewage and industrial waste disposal

- elimination of any organic material accumulation that remains moist long enough to produce flies
- elimination of weeds
- screening, electrocution (very expensive)
- release of sterile flies
- chemical methods (such as larviciding, fly baits, space sprays, fly cords and resin strips, residual sprays, fly repellents, fly attractants)

Black horse fly (*Tabanus atratus*)

Diseases spread by: Several diseases of humans and animals caused by viruses (equine infectious anemia, vesicular stomatitis, hog cholera, and California encephalitis), bacteria (anthrax and tularemia), rickettsia-like organisms (Q-fever and anaplasmosis), trypanosomas (surra), and filarial worms (loiasis and elaephorosis). Black horse fly is a major pest of cattle and horses.

Biological characteristics: Many species deposit their eggs on vegetation near water, and their larvae develop in damp soil or water. Biting flies may take 2 to 3 years for development. Horse flies are vicious biters, inflicting wounds that can itch for days. Only the females suck blood; the males feed on plant nectar.

Identification: Large fly; five posterior cells on the wing and three-segmented antenna.

Desired environment: Moist soil in the shade of trees under dry or sparse grass, where standing water seldom or never occurs. Some larvae develop in dry pasture land.

Control measures: Difficult, though repellents are somewhat effective.

Stable Fly (*Stomoxys calcitrans*)

Diseases spread by: Probably a vector of surra (a disease of horses and mules) and infectious anemia (a viral disease of horses). Stable fly larvae have been reported as causing myiasis in humans and domestic animals.

Because of its blood-sucking habits, it is suspected of transmitting a number of diseases.

Biological characteristics: Stable flies do not breed in human excrement and usually are not attracted to feces or garbage. Therefore, they are less likely to pick up germs of diarrhea and other intestinal diseases. Larval development takes 8 to 30 days or more, depending on temperature.

Identification: 5 mm to 6 mm long, dull thorax with four dark longitudinal stripes and a pale spot behind the head, dull-colored abdomen with dark spots. Both male and female are vicious biters. Distinguished from all other common domestic flies by its piercing proboscis that protrudes bayonet-like in front of the head.

Desired environment: For laying eggs — plant waste more so than manure, and in old straw stacks, piles of fermenting weeds, grass, peanut hay, or stable manure well mixed with straw or hay.

Control measures:
- careful disposal of plant waste
- control of piles of fermenting weeds, peanut hay waste
- control area where manure is mixed with straw
- good environmental sanitation

Black Fly (*Simulium venustum*)

Diseases spread by: Tularemia in North America, human onchocerciasis in Africa and Central American, and bovine onchocerciasis in Europe and Australia. Some black fly species transmit deadly protozoa to ducks and turkeys.

Biological characteristics: Both sexes suck nectar from flowers, and most females suck blood. The eggs are laid in or near flowing water, and the larvae and pupae are found attached to submerged rocks, sticks, and vegetation. The adult emerges from the pupa in a submerged cocoon and floats to the surface of the water in a bubble of air. Many species mate soon after emergence. Black fly bites are painless at first but later become swollen, hard, and painful, and sometimes infected from scratching. They swarm around exposed parts of the body, particularly the head, and get into the nose, eyes, ears, and mouth. Heavy attacks may be fatal to humans, cattle, horses, and poultry, possibly from toxemia, anaphylactic shock, or suffocation brought about by inhalation of large numbers of swarming insects.

Identification: 2 mm to 5 mm long, stout-bodied with short antennae, wings with well developed anterior veins, and a "humped" thorax, bestowing the common name "buffalo gnats."

Desired environment: Flowing water with rock and vegetation to which they may attach eggs, larvae.

Control measures:
- creation of unfavorable environment
- application of insecticides into breeding area
- encouragement of natural predators, such as the rainbow eating crabs

Deer Fly (*Chrysops discalis*)

Diseases spread by: In the United States tularemia, known locally as deer fly fever; particularly in the southern United States, mechanical carriers of anthrax bacteria from domestic animals to humans,

Identification: Average 6 mm to 12 mm long, spotted wings, two spurs on hind tibiae. Similar to horse fly characteristics.

Desired environment: Moist soil in the shade of trees under dry to sparse grass where standing water seldom or never occurs. Some larvae develop in dry pasture land.

Control measures: Difficult, though repellents are somewhat effective.

LICE

Body Louse ("cooties") (*Pediculus humanus humanus*)

Diseases spread by: Louseborne typhus, trench fever, relapsing fever, pediculosis

Biological characteristics: Life cycle has three stages: eggs, nymphs, adults. Eggs are yellowish and about 0.8 mm long by 0.3 mm wide. The egg (called a "nit") is cemented to fibers of underclothing. The eggs are incubated by heat from the body and hatch in about a week. Hatching of eggs is greatly reduced or completely prevented by exposure to temperatures above 100° F or lower than 75° F. Thus, the body louse is controlled readily when the same articles or apparel are worn intermittently. If clothing were stored for a month, even without treatment, all eggs would hatch or die, and any young that hatch would die. After emerging from the egg, the louse nymph molts three times before becoming a sexually mature adult. The nymphal stages require 8 to 9 days for lice remaining in contact with the human body but may require 2 to 4 weeks when the clothing is removed at night. The total life cycle of body lice may be completed in about 18 days. The adult body louse differs little from the nymph except in size and sexual maturity. The male is smaller than the female. Mating occurs frequently and at any time in the adult's life, from the first 10 hours until senescence. Eggs are laid 24 to 48 hours later, depending upon temperature conditions. Body lice may deposit 9 to 10 eggs each day and a total of 270 to 300 eggs in a lifetime. See Figure 3.2.

Body lice can move fairly rapidly and will pass from host to host, or from one host to bedding, by simple contact.

Identification: 2 mm to 4 mm long; elongated abdomen, without hairy lateral processes; legs are three pair approximately equal; grayish-white in color; legs have hook-like claw for grasping. (Body louse rests on clothing except when feeding.)

Desired environment: Inner surface of the clothing, next to the skin — their blood meal. Hatching of eggs is greatly reduced or prevented by exposure to temperatures above 100° F and below 75° F. These lice depend upon human blood for sustenance. It is difficult to find human lice away from humans.

Control measures:

- examination of clothing along seams and folds
- ordinary laundering with hot water
- dry cleaning to destroy lice on wool garments
- treated shampoos and lotions
- insecticide powders for dusting
- bathing with emulsifiable concentrates (requires a physician's prescription)

Head Lice (*Pediculus humanus capitis*)

Diseases spread by: Pediculosis.

Biological characteristics: Metamorphosis same as body lice. Head lice live on head and neck region. Eggs are cemented to hairs of the scalp, where they incubate. Head lice

are less prolific than body lice, depositing about four eggs per day, for a total of about 88 in a lifetime.

Identification: 1 mm to 2 mm; elongated abdomen without hairy lateral processes; three pairs of legs and approximately equal; grayish-white with dark margins (see Figure 3.2).

Desired environment: Most prevalent on back of neck and behind ears; head and neck region. Preferred temperatures same as body. Most abundant in children.

Control measures:

- very close haircut
- shampoo with emulsions
- not sharing personal belongings such as brushes or combs
- dusting of applications with DDT where permitted, or 1% lindane (kwell)
- preschool examination of children

Crab Lice (*Pthirus pubis*)

Diseases spread by: pediculosis

Biological characteristics: Life cycle is similar to that of head and body lice; eggs are glued to hairs. It is not known definitely how many eggs are laid in nature, but one female confined under a stocking laid 26 eggs,

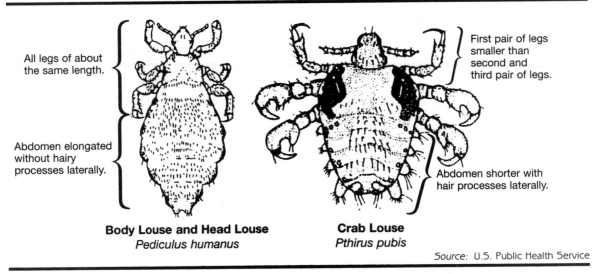

All legs of about the same length.

Abdomen elongated without hairy processes laterally.

Body Louse and Head Louse
Pediculus humanus

First pair of legs smaller than second and third pair of legs.

Abdomen shorter with hair processes laterally.

Crab Louse
Pthirus pubis

Source: U.S. Public Health Service

Figure 3.2 Lice commonly found on humans.

averaging three per day. There are three nymphal stages. In a few specimens that have been studied, it took 13 to 17 days for them to become adults. Adult life apparently lasts less than a month. Legs are adapted for grasping large hairs, and adult prefers widely spaced hairs. These insects survive only a short time away from hosts because they are blood-sucking lice.

Identification: small, 0.8 mm to 1.2 mm, grayish-white with short abdomen bearing hairy lateral tufts and large second and third pairs of legs (Figure 3.2).

Desired environment: Most commonly on hair in pubic and anal areas. May be found on hairy areas of chest and armpits. Infestations of eyebrows and eyelashes have been reported frequently. Crab lice are spread chiefly by sexual contact but may be acquired by other means such as infested toilet seats and beds, and by close personal contact.

Control measures:

• shaving or cutting infested hair to remove adults, immature stages, and eggs glued to hairs.
• dusting with 1% lindane or malathion
• ophthalmic ointment for eyelashes and brows
• sanitization of restrooms, beds, self

ROACHES

American Cockroach (sometimes called "water bug") (*Periplaneta americana*)

Diseases spread by: Organisms causing enteric diseases (diarrhea, dysentery, typhoid fever, food poisoning, cholera). American cockroaches may carry many strains of salmonella and staphylococcus bacteria that can cause food poisoning. They often visit sewers, garbage cans, then people's food.

Biological characteristics: The life cycle has three stages: egg, nymph, adult. The eggs are deposited in an egg capsule shaped like a clam shell. Tiny wingless nymphs emerge. Growth occurs during a succession of molts in which the body covering and some interior body linings are cast away. New characters, such as wing buds and eventually wings, appear after these molts. Males mature more rapidly than females and have fewer molts during their development. Average about a year developing from egg to adult. Females lay 14 to 16 eggs per case.

Identification: Largest species, 35 mm to 40 mm in length, reddish or dark brown with variable amount of yellowish color on pronotum.

Desired environment: Almost worldwide in distribution, preferring a warm, humid environment, as in sewers, boiler rooms, basements, kitchens, and cracks of homes. Also be found in tree hollows, wood piles, and accumulations of trash. Has an appetite for beer and sweets but will eat starch and glue, damaging books and pictures.

Control measures:

• basic sanitation (deprives them of food, water, harborage)
• proper refuse storage (trash bags) and litter control (clean up litter)
• proper food storage
• insecticides

German cockroach (Blattella germanica) (most common pest in homes and restaurants)

Diseases spread by: Organisms causing enteric diseases (diarrhea, dysentery, typhoid fever, food poisoning, cholera). They often visit sewers, garbage cans, then people's food.

Biological characteristics: Life cycle has three stages: egg, nymph, adult. Develops from egg to adult in 2 to 3 months. Female differs from females of most other species by carrying the egg case (ootheca) protruding from the abdomen until shortly before the young emerge. The young may emerge from the egg case even before the female drops it.

The adults can fly but rarely do. Females lay 37 to 44 eggs per case.

Identification: Small, 10 mm to 15 mm long, grayish color with two blackish bars on pronotum covering the head.

Desired environment: Most abundant in kitchen and pantry; also bathroom and sometimes throughout buildings.

Control measures: Same as American cockroach.

REFERENCES

Altman, Lawrence K. 1996, April 2. "Mad Cow Epidemic Puts Spotlight on Puzzling Human Brain Disease (research into the causes of Creutzfeldt-Jakob disease) (Medical Science Pages)." *New York Times*. v. 145 p. B8 (N) p. C3 (L) col 4.

Barbour, Alan G. 1989, April 1. "The Diagnosis of Lyme Disease: Rewards and Perils." *Annals of Internal Medicine*. v. 110 n. 7. pp. 501–502.

Benenson, Abram. 1995. *Control of Communicable Diseases in Man*. 16th ed. American Public Health Association, Washington, DC.

Benenson, Abram S. 1989, Jan. "The Continuing Saga of Lyme Disease." *American Journal of Public Health*. v. 79 n. l. pp. 9–10.

"Changes in National Notifiable Diseases Data Presentation." 1996, Jan 19. *Morbidity and Mortality Weekly Report*. v. 45 n. 2. p. 41.

"Diagnosis of Lyme Disease." 1989, July 22. *Lancet*. v. 2 n. 8656 pp. 198–199.

Falco, Richard C., and Darland Fish. 1989, Jan. "Potential for Exposure to Tick Bites in Recreational Parks in a Lyme Disease Endemic Area." *American Journal of Public Health*. v. 79 n. l. pp. 12–14.

Finkel, Michael F. 1988, Jan. "Lyme Disease and Its Neurologic Complications." *Archives of Neurology*. v. 45 n. l. pp. 99–104.

Garrett, Laurie. 1996, Jan-Feb. "The Return of Infectious Disease." *Foreign Affairs*. v. 74 n. l. pp. 66 (14).

Grimes, Deanna. 1991. *Infectious Diseases*. Mosby Year Book, St. Louis.

Katzmann, Jerry A., et al. 1985, June. "Ticks, Spirochetes, and New Diagnostic Tests for Lyme Disease." *Mayo Clinical Procedures*. v. 60. pp. 402–405.

Lederberg, Joshua. "Infection Emergent." 1996, Jan 17. *Journal of the American Medical Association*. v. 275 n. 3. pp. 243.

Lugkin, llene. l991. *Chronic Illness*. Jones and Bartlett Publishers, Boston.

McAlister, Hugh F., et al. 1989, March 1. "Lyme Carditis: An Important Cause of Reversible Heart Block." *Annals of Internal Medicine*. v. 110 n. 5. pp. 339–345.

McNabb, Paul. 1986, Aug 15. "Nouveau Maladies: Coagulase Negative Staphylococci Capnocytophaga, Lyme Disease, Cat Scratch Fever." *New Pathogens and the Clinical Microbiology Laboratory — The Challenge of the 80's*. pp. 402–927.

Morse, Stephen S. 1995, Oct. "Controlling Infectious Diseases." *Technology Review*. v. 98 n. 7. pp. 54.

"National Surveillance for Infectious Diseases, 1995." 1995, Oct 6. *Morbidity and Mortality Weekly Report*. v. 44 n. 39. pp. 737.

Patlak, Margie. 1996, April. "Book Reopened on Infectious Diseases." *FDA Consumer*. v. 30 n. 3. pp. 19.

Patz, Johnathan A., Paul R. Epstein, Thomas A. Burke, and John M. Balbus. 1996, Jan 17. "Global Climate Change and Emerging Infectious Diseases." *Journal of the American Medical Association*. v. 275 n. 3. pp. 217.

Prescott, P. M., J. P. Harvey, and D. A. Klein. 1996. *Microbiology*. Wm. C. Brown, Dubuque, IA.

"Rising Toll from Infectious Diseases." 1996, April. *American Journal*. v. 96 n. 4. pp. 11.

Seachrist, Lisa. 1996, Jan 20. "Infections Make Deadly Comeback." *Science News*. v. 149 n. 3. pp. 38.

Steere, Allan C. 1989, Aug. 31. "Lyme Disease." *New England Journal of Medicine*. v. 321 n. 9. pp. 586–596.

Willgoose, Carl E. 1979. *Environmental Health: Commitment for Survival*. W. C. Saunders, Philadelphia.

Winker, Margaret A., and Annette Flanagin. 1996, Jan 17. "Infectious Diseases: A Global Approach to a Global Problem." *Journal of the American Medical Association*. v. 275 n. 3. pp. 245.

Water Supplies

Key Terms

Aquifer
Bored well
Cistern
Coliform group
Drilled well

Driven well
Dug well
Floc
Maximum contaminants levels (MCLs)

Potable
Safe Drinking Water Act of 1974
Spring
Turbidity

Objectives

- Explain the hydrologic cycle.
- Identify the various types of wells.
- Discuss water quality.
- Explain water distribution.
- Discuss municipal water supplies.
- Explain the importance of the municipal groundwater supply and treatment.

Water may well be the most valuable natural resource. There could be no life on earth without water. Humans can live only a few days without it. Civilizations, therefore, always have located their communities close to water sources. The water supply, however, is limited because only a fraction of 1% of all water is fresh surface water and groundwater. Figure 4.1 shows the earth's distribution of water.

The water we consume can transport disease agents responsible for cholera (from which approximately 500 people in Peru died in 1991), shigellosis, amebic dysentery, helminth infections, typhoid fever, paratyphoid, and many others. Table 4.1 gives a synopsis of reported cases in the United States over three decades.

In addition, many harmful chemicals — arsenic, pesticides, fertilizers, lead from pipes — are dissolved in and conveyed to humans by water. Physical agents such as the radionuclides Iodine-131, Phosphorus-32, and Strontium-90 may concentrate in surface waters after nuclear bomb testing. Radioactivity also is found naturally in some waters.

The availability of water can have a great impact on an area's economy and health. The presence of an abundant water supply can increase property values and provide incentives for agricultural, industrial, and overall community growth. **Potable** (of good taste, odor, and microbiological quality) water helps prevent economic strain resulting from water-related illnesses affecting individual and community health. The critical importance of a potable drinking water supply cannot be over emphasized.

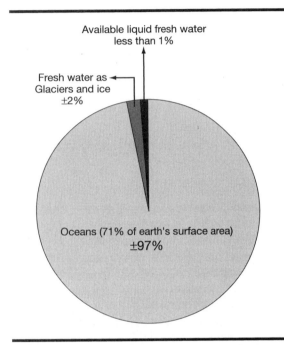

FIGURE 4.1 Water distribution on earth.

THE HYDROLOGIC CYCLE

The amount of available water is finite. There is essentially the same amount of water today as there was after the formation of the earth. The water may be altered in form and distribution, but the quantity always stays the same. Just think — the last water you consumed was as old as the earth!

Water is recycling continuously through what is called the hydrologic cycle (Figure 4.2). Atmospheric moisture — rain, snow, sleet, and the like — contain water that has been drawn from the earth by evaporation. Water evaporates from oceans, streams, ponds, soil, moisture on leaves, transpiration of plants, and while falling. This is a natural process. As the sun draws the moisture into the atmosphere, any existing pollutants are left behind.

Many students have done a simple experiment in science class in which salt is placed into a dish of water. The water is heated and evaporates. The salt remains behind in the dish. A similar process occurs in nature on a much larger scale. This natural cleansing of water allows atmospheric moisture to be water in its purest, most natural state. The atmospheric moisture then condenses and falls back to the earth as some form of precipitation.

As the precipitation falls toward earth, the water's naturally pure quality is influenced by

TABLE 4.1 Summary of Reported Cases, United States, 1960–1989

Disease	1960–1969	1970–1979	1980–1989
U.S. resident population (in thousands)	1,915,709	2,121,804	2,374,749
Amebiasis	30,278	30,586	48,282
Cholera	2	18	71
*Hepatitis	462,673	421,787	258,112
Leptospirosis	815	716	656
Shigellosis	124,009	180,859	207,801
Typhoid Fever Cases	5,292**	4,493	4,476
Carriers			424

*Reported cases include both infectious hepatitis and serum hepatitis in one combined figure.
**1960–1979 data for typhoid include one combined figure, cases and carriers.

Environmental Health

FEBRUARY 15, 1991
PERU'S CHOLERA EPIDEMIC SPREADING

LIMA, Peru — A deadly cholera epidemic in Peru continues to spread despite government assurances that it is being controlled, threatening thousands of people in Lima's filthy shantytowns.

Fear of the highly contagious disease has also prompted dramatic actions by countries in Latin America and Europe to try to prevent its spread.

At least 500 people have died in Peru of cholera since the end of January and more than 70,000 cases have been reported, Peruvian health officials said. But the actual number of victims is expected to be higher because the figures do not include cases reported in the remote highland and jungle regions.

Officials of the Geneva-based World Health Organization warned earlier this week that cholera could spread quickly throughout Latin America if not controlled.

"There is panic abroad," Health Ministry spokesman Raul Fernandez said. "In the twenty-four hours it takes the symptoms to develop, a carrier could board a plane to Miami and spread the disease there."

"We've been declared a 'fourth-world country' because of this epidemic," he added.

The epidemic is the first cholera outbreak in the Western Hemisphere since early this century. It is transmitted mainly by food and water contaminated by the feces of cholera victims, and its symptoms include diarrhea, vomiting, severe cramps, and dehydration.

Lima's shantytowns, which frequently lack sewage or running water, are home to 4 million of the city's 7 million people.

At the health clinic in Huaycan, a shantytown ten miles outside Lima, flies swarmed through the consulting room and open piles of refuse rotted outside.

Huaycan, a collection of ramshackle huts crowded onto a parched desert hill, has no water or sewage system, no electricity and no telephone service. Water, which is often contaminated, is brought in by truck.

"Terrifyingly, health conditions in 19th century London were similar to those of Lima today," the news magazine *Caretas* said this week. In the mid-19th century, 30,000 Londoners died over a seventeen-year period in one of the worst cholera epidemics on record.

News reports Wednesday said the disease had spread into the highland Mantaro Valley, a main source of food for the capital, Lima. At least three people have died of cholera in the valley, 120 miles east of Lima.

The rapid spread of the disease has led Bolivia, Ecuador, and Chile to increase health precautions at border crossings and to ban imports of Peruvian perishable foods. But officials from Chile and Ecuador refused to confirm news reports that cholera had spread to frontier towns in their countries.

Argentina, which does not share a border with Peru, has banned Peruvian fish imports and suspended upcoming soccer matches between the two countries' teams in Peru.

In Europe, Peruvian air passengers were sent back from Spain, and the French government banned Peruvian seafood imports, according to news reports. A spokesman for the Spanish Embassy said the travelers were turned back because they had not complied with visa requirements.

In Lima, the government has closed beaches and unhygienic street food stalls. But sewage pipes still discharge into the sea.

Health standards in Peru are among the lowest in South America because the government has neglected to invest in archaic water, sewage, and health services for years, due to an economic crisis marked by hyperinflation and a huge foreign debt.

Claudio Lanata, a Peruvian epidemiologist, predicts as many as 440,000 Peruvians could come down with cholera. The Housing Minister of Lima announced that laboratory analysis indicated that Lima's drinking water contained human feces.

Associated Press

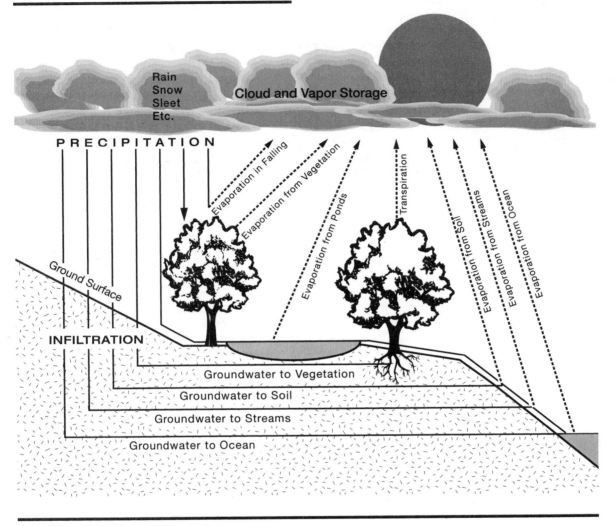

Rain
Snow
Sleet
Etc.

Cloud and Vapor Storage

PRECIPITATION

Evaporation in Falling

Evaporation from Vegetation

Evaporation from Ponds

Transpiration

Evaporation from Soil

Evaporation from Streams

Evaporation from Ocean

Ground Surface

INFILTRATION

Groundwater to Vegetation

Groundwater to Soil

Groundwater to Streams

Groundwater to Ocean

FIGURE 4.2 The hydrologic cycle.

the atmosphere through which it passes. Air pollutants, such as carbon dioxide and the oxides of nitrogen and sulfur from industrial processes, change the qualities of falling water. Acid rain is one direct result.

Once the precipitation reaches the earth, several situations may occur. Some water may land in an existing reservoir; some will run over the surface of the ground toward lakes, streams, rivers, and oceans; and some water may be absorbed into the soil. In short, when water hits the ground, it will become either surface water or groundwater. The ground surface, topography,

soil type, and the like influence whether it will become surface water or groundwater.

Surface water picks up the characteristics of the surface over which it passes. If water flows across a parking lot, gasoline, oil, and other contaminants may be carried by or dissolved into the water. Water may pick up fertilizers, road salts, radioactivity from fallout, and biological contamination from farms, as well as countless other biological, physical, and chemical pollutants.

The same principle holds true for groundwater. As the water enters the ground, it picks

Environmental Health

up the characteristics of the formation through which it passes. Water may pick up pathogens from subsurface sewage systems, and many minerals from the soil dissolve in the water. As the water moves through the ground, the soil often filters out biological contaminants. The soil type and geological structures can have a great effect on the extent of biological filtration. For example, water moving slowly through a fine, sandy, clay soil will be filtered much better than water moving through a fractured rock formation. Water can move for miles through cracks in a limestone formation with very little filtration. For this reason, stabilization ponds are not permitted in limestone areas.

Usually, the deeper an underground water source is located, the better is the biological quality, because of filtration. On the other hand, theoretically, the deeper the water source is located, the poorer the chemical quality. Generally, deep water has been in the ground for a longer time, allowing prolonged contact with the underground strata. The increased contact time may cause additional minerals to dissolve into the water, changing the chemical quality. Examples are calcium and magnesium compounds, which dissolve in groundwater and cause hardness.

Once above ground, spring water may flow directly to lakes, rivers, or oceans, or may evaporate directly. Then the hydrologic cycle starts all over again.

SURFACE WATER SUPPLIES

Water supplies come either from the surface or below the ground. If the water comes to the surface naturally, it constitutes a surface water supply. Examples of this are water in cisterns, ponds, lakes, and rivers.

A **cistern** is a tank for storing rainwater from a catchment area, such as the ground's surface or a rooftop, or for storing water that has been hauled in from some outside source. Now used in the United States rarely, cisterns still find application in developing nations. The

cistern as a water source is limited greatly by the amount of rainfall an area receives. The catchment area and the size of the storage tank for a cistern should be large enough to hold enough water to provide for even the driest periods of the year.

As mentioned earlier, water picks up the characteristics of the surface over which it flows. Therefore, the type of material used for the catchment area can alter the quality of the water that is collected for storage and consumption. When using a rooftop for a catchment area, the type of roofing materials and roof coating are important. The most suitable roofing materials for catchment are galvanized steel and aluminum.

Imagine the amount of pollutants on a rooftop in an area where no rain has fallen for an extended time. Raindrops flowing across such a surface introduce bird droppings, decaying leaves, soot, and many other contaminants into the water. Thus, the first flow of water off a roof's surface should be prevented from entering the cistern. This can be accomplished by using a flow diversion valve at the downspout of the gutter prior to the cistern entrance. Once the rooftop has had an adequate rinse, the operator diverts the water toward the cistern (see Figure 4.3).

The influent is filtered to remove any suspended particles prior to entering the cistern. The cistern should be constructed solidly to prevent entrance of any surface water that has not been filtered. A screened drain and manhole allow draining, entering, and cleaning of the cistern. The manhole should extend beyond the surface of the ground and be covered with a shoebox-type lid or another type of lid to prevent surface water from entering. Because water does not run upward, the shoebox lid prevents surface water from entering.

A **spring** appears where a water table or some water-bearing strata discharges at the surface. Before using a spring as a drinking water source:

1. Note whether the spring has a relatively constant flow throughout the year. The

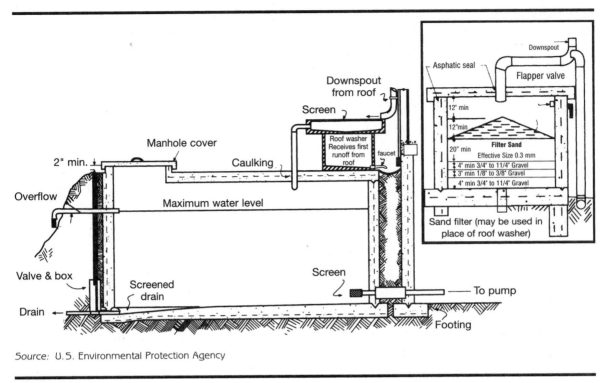

Source: U.S. Environmental Protection Agency

FIGURE 4.3 Cistern.

spring should provide enough water to supply needs even during the driest time of the year. The flow rate should not be affected by slight precipitation.

2. Observe the effluent from the spring after rainfalls and note whether the water supply is more turbid or "muddy" at that time.

A substantial variation in the rate of flow coupled with increasing turbidity could indicate surface water or shallow groundwater intrusion. Springs often are located in low areas and get contaminated from pollution sources at higher elevations. For instance, a spring located directly down slope from a farmyard, septic tank system, or parking lot, or one that becomes muddy or has increased flow after a rain, is not a desirable water source.

If the spring has an adequate flow rate to meet consumption needs and is not affected greatly by precipitation, it may be considered as a water source. Special care must be taken when

developing a spring. The overall objective is to collect the water flowing from the water table and at the same time prevent any surface water intrusion. This is achieved by various construction techniques (Figure 4.4).

Like a cistern, a spring storage tank should have some means of access for cleaning. A manhole extended above the surface of the ground with a shoebox lid is suitable.

GROUNDWATER SUPPLIES

Many areas of the world do not have access to adequate springs, cannot rely on precipitation to fill a cistern, or do not have available surface water. If surface water is not accessible naturally, we may dig into the earth physically in an attempt to locate underground water-bearing strata. This is achieved by the construction of a water well.

Underground water can be found below the surface of most of the earth. The location of this water may vary from a few feet to thousands of feet below the ground. In some areas the groundwater is ponded and has almost no "new water" entering from the hydrologic cycle. Other areas have free-flowing underground streams that are recharged from water entering through the earth's surface miles away. A porous stratum that stores water underground and yields the water is called an **aquifer**.

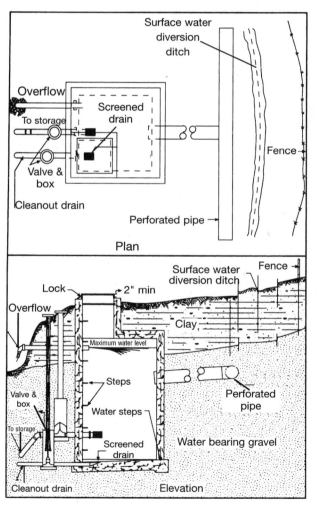

Source: U.S. Environmental Protection Agency

FIGURE 4.4 Spring protection.

Before constructing a well, the builders must conduct a survey of the proposed construction area to determine the presence of any pollution sources. In particular, these include feedlots, underground on-site sewage disposal systems, and sewage stabilization ponds. Also, they are on the alert for any chemical contamination of the soil, which may consist of materials used in treating termites, spraying of herbicides near overhead power lines, leaks in underground storage tanks, and others. Future uses of an area also must be considered. It would not be desirable to construct a well and later have to confront the construction of a new house requiring termite treatment.

The local health department imposes minimum separation distances (in many cases this is 100 feet, or 30.4 meters) between drinking water wells and pollution sources. Also, a well should be located in an area that receives a minimum amount of surface water runoff. Low areas and natural drainageways are not desirable locations for a well. Surface waters should flow away from, rather than toward, a well.

The four major types of wells are: dug, bored, driven, and drilled. The type of well to be constructed is often dependent upon the geological formations in an area.

Dug Wells

In many cases groundwater collects over the surface of the bedrock or some other dense formation, which creates a water source over the top of the rock. If this condition exists and enough water is available, the site may be appropriate for a dug well (see Figure 4.5). A **dug well** is constructed by digging straight down into the earth until reaching water. The depth of a dug well can be limited by the depth of dense bedrock. With conventional tools it is difficult for workers to dig manually into the bedrock. Also, dug wells have particular potential for contamination.

Bored Wells

A **bored well** is similar to a dug well. The difference between a dug well and a bored well lies in the methodology used to reach the water. Whereas a dug well is constructed by hand, a mechanical device such as a power-operated auger is used to dig a bored well. A bored well has the same limitations as a dug well in that its depth usually is no deeper than the underlying consolidated bedrock or impervious strata. Like a dug well, the water collected from a bored well has moved down from the surface and has ponded on some confining layers. The depth of the well has to be adequate to allow for soil filtration of any microorganisms that may have collected in the air or on the surface. Bored wells may also be subjected to reduced flow rates from the water table in times of drought, because of their dependency on precipitation for recharge.

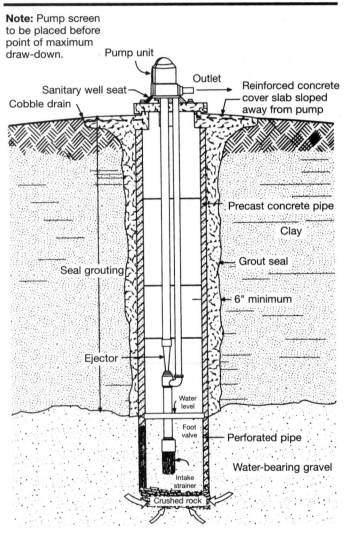

Note: Pump screen to be placed before point of maximum draw-down.

- Pump unit
- Outlet
- Sanitary well seat
- Cobble drain
- Reinforced concrete cover slab sloped away from pump
- Precast concrete pipe
- Clay
- Grout seal
- 6" minimum
- Seal grouting
- Ejector
- Water level
- Foot valve
- Perforated pipe
- Water-bearing gravel
- Intake strainer
- Crushed rock

Source: U.S. Environmental Protection Agency

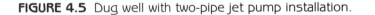

FIGURE 4.5 Dug well with two-pipe jet pump installation.

Driven Wells

In a **driven well**, a pipe with a special screened point drives into the ground until locating water. Driven wells are limited to areas where soil particles are large, such as sands, sandy loams, and dense layers where rock and compacted soils do not exist.

They often are found in coastal regions with shallow water tables. Operators drive the pipe into the ground manually or with a machine. The pipe driven into the ground has a diameter too small to allow a submersible pump to be lowered to the water table. For that reason, operators place a pump at the top of the well that cannot draw water from more than approximately 25 feet (7.6 m) of pipe, thus limiting the depth of the well. The shallow depth of the driven well, along with its location in sandy soils, may make its water undesirable for human consumption.

Drilled Wells

A **drilled well** (Figure 4.6) may be the most versatile in that it is not limited by depth to rock. Operators construct drilled wells to thousands of feet in depth by mechanically drilling through rock and compacted areas. The water collected from a deep-drilled well is often less subject to reduced flows in times of drought and not as prone to biological contamination.

Protecting the Water Supply

One point all of these wells have in common is that a hole is constructed from the earth's surface down to the aquifer. Without some means of protection, surface water could simply flow across the top of the ground, picking up contaminants, and flow directly into the well.

Well drillers prevent surface water from entering the well with casing, grout, and an adequate cap (seal) at the top. Casing consists of watertight pipe, or sections of pipe, inserted directly down into the well until some restrictive barrier is reached. The casing should extend high enough above the ground to prevent intrusion from flood water. The grout is neat cement (cement and water) that is either poured into or forced under pressure into the space between the casing and the original hole. This will seal any spaces between the casing and earth that may allow surface water to enter. The depth of the grout depends upon local regulations and type of well. A cap, whether it be a shoebox lid

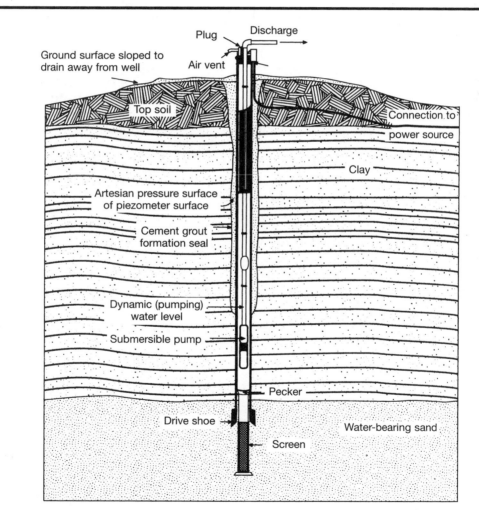

Source: U.S. Environmental Protection Agency

FIGURE 4.6 Drilled well submersible pump.

or a sanitary seal, must be placed over the top of the casing to prevent any surface water from entering. This lid for a dug well should have some overhang beyond the outside of the casing to allow precipitation and contaminants to drop on the exterior rather than the interior of the casing. Figure 4.5 shows an example of casing, grout, and protective lid.

The sanitary seal for a drilled well should have a vent to permit air to enter the well shaft; the well pump creates a negative pressure, allowing atmospheric pressure to push the water out of the well. This vent (Figure 4.6) should be screened to prevent the entrance of insects.

Using the proper casing, grout, and well cap, surface pollution can be "built out," preventing it from entering the well. After completing the well's construction, a water sample is collected to determine the quality of water in the well. In most cases a bacteriological analysis should be done, using the coliform group as an indicator. The **coliform group** consists of two different gram-negative bacillus species: *Escherichia coli* and *Aerobacter aerogenes*. *E. coli* is found widely in the intestinal tract of all warm-blooded animals. *A. aerogenes* is found widely in the soil, on our hands, and in the air. Presence of the coliform group indicates that contamination is entering the water supply. The contamination or pollution may not be limited to just coliform organisms. Many types of pollutants including pathogens may be present. The coliform group merely indicates the presence of pollution.

After construction of a new well, collection of a positive (contaminated) coliform sample is almost inevitable. The mere handling of the well's piping and pump is enough to introduce pollutants into the water supply. The pipes also may have been stored in an area subject to surface contamination prior to installation. For this reason, the well should be disinfected prior to use, using a chemical to kill any organisms present. This consists of placing at least 50 mg/l* (ppm) of chlorine into the water. Then the water is introduced through the plumbing fixtures in the building that the well supplies. (A chlorine

*milligrams per liter

odor will be present once the disinfectant reaches the plumbing fixtures.) The chlorine is left in the well at least overnight. The water is flowed until it removes all the disinfectant from the system. After disinfection, the sterile sampling bottle should contain sodium thiosulfate to chemically reduce any chlorine that still may be present.

After collecting the sample, a laboratory analyzes the water. Lab technicians commonly use two techniques when conducting a coliform analysis: (a) the multiple-tube fermentation test and, (b) the membrane filtration technique, which is the usual choice today. If the results of either of these techniques is positive, the well is disinfected once more and another sample collected. If the results continue to be positive and a physical area where pollutants may be entering the well is not found, the water source may require more extensive treatment. A common procedure is to chlorinate the well continuously. Unlike the disinfection described previously, this chlorination is the continuous mechanical application of chlorine in proportion to flow for the purpose of killing any pathogens that may be present.

WATER QUALITY

As discussed earlier, the ground's surface and the ground through which water flows can influence its quality. The characteristics of water easily can be changed biologically, physically, or chemically. Biological quality is altered any time living organisms enter the water. Some organisms cause illnesses in humans. Removing all disease-producing organisms in water enhances its quality and reduces the chance of illness.

Water has many physical parameters. One of these is **pH**. When the pH of water becomes too alkaline (far above neutral pH 7), many dissolved materials settle out of the water. Sometimes the resulting incrustations completely clog pipes, requiring total replacement of plumbing systems. Of the combination of factors that lead to encrusted pipes, the foremost is excessive dissolved minerals.

Water with very low pH, on the other hand, can dissolve the metal of which many pipes are constructed. Water that is too acidic (below pH 7) has the capability of "eating away" plumbing systems.

Another physical parameter is the *color* of water. Imagine drawing a glass of water from a faucet and having it appear the color of tea. The water may be safe to drink (although this is unlikely), but the color makes it unappealing. In laundering, water color also can stain clothing. The color of water is altered by the natural breakdown of organics within it. These organics (such as tannin) produce a yellowish-brown color if untreated. Iron in water causes a reddish color, and manganese a black color. Copper produces green stains. Other materials may affect a water's color as well.

Turbidity is another physical parameter. Whereas water color often results from substances dissolved into the water, turbidity is a result of particles suspended in the water. Turbid waters, too, may stain clothes. If allowed to stand in a sink or tub, turbid water often produces sediments. Much turbidity, however, comes from a colloid, which will not settle easily.

Taste and *odor* also can affect a water's physical quality. Even though water with taste and odor irregularities may be safe for human consumption, its palatability might be prohibitive. Foul taste and odor can come from tannic acid produced by decaying vegetation. Dissolved gases such as hydrogen sulfide are other contributors. Salts also produce objectionable taste, especially if present in high concentrations.

Many *chemicals* have the capability to alter water quality greatly. For example, nitrites and nitrates can cause methemoglobinemia, commonly known as "blue baby syndrome." The list of chemicals detrimental to human health is long. Only a chemical laboratory can detect their presence in most cases.

Hardness is a chemical quality that affects a water's ability to lather soap, as hardness precipitates soap. Hardness is caused predominantly by the presence of calcium, magnesium, strontium, and iron dissolved into the water. Iron in water can stain porcelain fixtures a reddish color. Manganese can leave black flakes in the water. Copper can leak from pipes, because of low pH, leaving behind a green stain.

WATER DISTRIBUTION

If one were to trace a drop of water pumped from a well, it would follow the path outlined in Figure 4.7. First the water in the aquifer passes through a well screen. The screen allows water to flow while keeping sand and gravel out. The water passes through a foot valve, which keeps water from flowing back into the aquifer when the pump is not in operation, to a jet pump, which is a device to help the surface pump obtain a negative pressure, and then into the surface pump itself. From the pump the water flows through a check valve and into a hydropneumatic pressure tank, which is a sealed tank full of air. As the pump pushes the water into the tank, it compresses the air. This column of compressed air is what forces water into the building.

The check valve between the pump and pressure tank takes pressure off the pump when it is not in operation. The check valve is on the entrance, or influent side, of the pressure tank. On the exit, or effluent side, is a main cutoff valve, designed to stop all water flow into the building if necessary. From the pressure tank the water flows directly into the dwelling and to the plumbing fixture where a person can draw water when desired.

In water supplies, it is necessary to prevent cross-connections. A cross connection is a physical connection between a potable water line and a line that contains a source of contamination. An example is a common garden hose attached to a faucet with the end of the hose lying in overflowing septic tank discharge. Other examples are a garden hose attached to a mop sink, with the open end of the hose submerged in the sink; and a wash basin with the hot and cold water lines below the flood-level rim.

The wash basin cross-connections can be corrected, as shown in Figure 4.8 by providing an air gap twice the diameter of the service

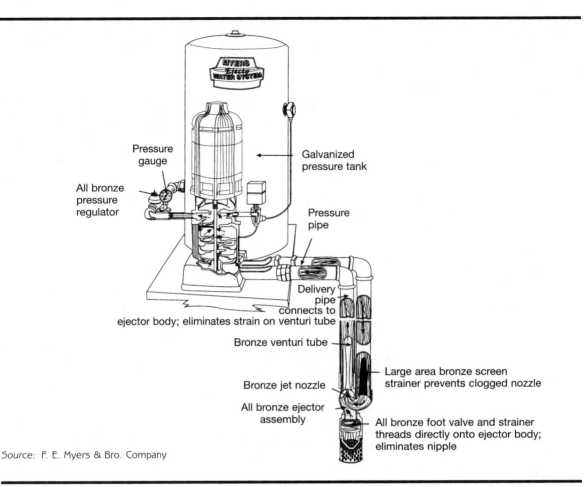

Pressure gauge

All bronze pressure regulator

Galvanized pressure tank

Pressure pipe

Delivery pipe connects to ejector body; eliminates strain on venturi tube

Bronze venturi tube

Bronze jet nozzle

All bronze ejector assembly

Large area bronze screen strainer prevents clogged nozzle

All bronze foot valve and strainer threads directly onto ejector body; eliminates nipple

Source: F. E. Myers & Bro. Company

FIGURE 4.7 Deep well jet pump system.

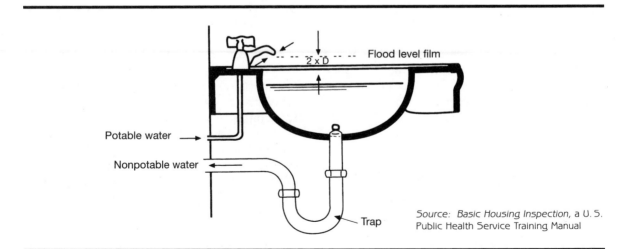

Flood level film

2 x D

Potable water

Nonpotable water

Trap

Source: Basic Housing Inspection, a U.S. Public Health Service Training Manual

FIGURE 4.8 Details of an air gap at a wash basin.

opening. Other cross-connections can be prevented by providing a vacuum breaker as shown in Figure 4.9. Another method of preventing back siphonage is the reduced pressure backflow preventer.

MUNICIPAL WATER DISTRIBUTION

Thus far we have concentrated on individual water supplies obtained from wells, springs, and cisterns. Now we will discuss water supplies serving large populations, with a focus upon the principles of standard municipal water treatment, based on a surface water supply.

Chances are great that if one lives in a city or town within the United States, the water he or she drinks has passed through a water treatment plant. Let's consider a city whose primary water source is a river and trace a drop of water from the river to a traditional water treatment plant to the home. The pattern of flow here is:

River → pumps → pretreatment → rapid-mix basin → flocculation basin → settling basin → filters → clear well → disinfection → storage tanks → city

Rivers usually are in low areas. Therefore, pumps get the water from the river to the treatment plant. Auxiliary pumps provide a backup in the event the main pump fails. After arrival, water enters the treatment plant at the rapid-mix basin. Workers add aluminum sulfate, or alum (a traditional coagulant), although polyelectrolytes and polymers now have become common. In some areas lime and furic chloride are used as coagulants. The coagulant helps draw the suspended solids together, allowing them to settle out of the water.

After leaving the rapid-mix basin, the water flows into flocculation basins. These basins gently stir the water, allowing the alum or other coagulant to mix thoroughly with the suspended solids. These solids, which cause turbidity, clump together with the aid of the alum, forming large particles that are heavy enough to settle from the water.

Once the particles of small solids have combined and formed larger particles, or **floc**, the water flows into a settling basin. The water flows very slowly through the settling basins, allowing the floc to settle from the water. Most of the removable turbidity should be settled from the water before it reaches its next treatment step — filtration. Activated carbon often is added to the water after sedimentation and prior to filtration. The activated carbon absorbs color and some radioactivity and removes taste and odor. The water then passes through filters that remove most of the remaining suspended solids and the added activated carbon. The filters are important in that they filter out bacteria and turbidity as the water passes through.

After flowing through the filters, the water enters a clear well. At this point, approximately 1 milligram per liter of additional chlorine is introduced to kill pathogens if present. In water supplies requiring adequate sanitary protection throughout their entire distribution system, it is recommended that a minimum free-chlorine residual of not less than 0.2 ppm* be maintained in all vital parts of the system, regardless of the added amount of chlorine necessary. This varies from state to state and locality to locality.

Housing

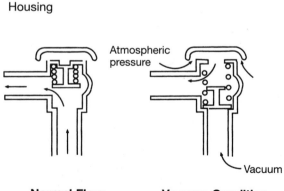

Normal Flow   **Vacuum Condition**

Source: Water Supply and Plumbing Crossconnections, U.S. Public Health Service

FIGURE 4.9 Operational details of a pressure-type vacuum breaker.

*ppm = parts per million which equals milligrams per liter

Next, approximately 1 milligram per liter of fluoride is added in water supplies that are fluoridated, and pH adjustments will take place if necessary. The water is now potable, palatable, and ready for distribution to the consumer. Pumps take the water from the plant into large, elevated tanks that store it and provide gravity flow pressure. From these tanks the water simply flows downhill through the distribution system and into your home.

Water treatment plants have a quality control laboratory in which technicians perform bacteriological, physical, and chemical tests on the raw and finished water to see if the water meets standards. In the lab, a pH meter determines the pH, a colorimeter determines the color, a turbidimeter determines the amount of turbidity, and so on. The tests done on the finished product are critical to the public health.

Before 1974 the United States had no enforceable national standard for drinking water. The **Safe Drinking Water Act of 1974** required the EPA to establish national drinking water standards, called **maximum contaminants levels (MCLs)**, for any pollutants that may have adverse effects on human health. The standards apply to all public water supplies that have at least 15 service connections or regularly serve an average of 25 or more people daily at least 60 days during the year. Each state sets its own standards that can be no lower than the U.S. Public Health Service's recommended standards. These vary from state to state. Generally, these standards are not enforced for private wells because of the cost of water quality determination. Table 4.2 presents additional water standards.

MUNICIPAL GROUNDWATER SUPPLIES

Groundwater is a major water source for homes served by private wells (as discussed earlier) as well as for many municipalities. For example, Memphis, Tennessee, though located on the Mississippi River, obtains most of its water from wells of varying depths. The quality of its groundwater depends upon many factors, such as depth of the well, existing geological formations, distance from sources of pollution, and demand for groundwater in the vicinity.

The extent of treatment required for municipalities using groundwater varies greatly depending almost exclusively upon the quality of the water. In some areas, the water needs only chlorination before use. In other areas, where water is of poor chemical, physical, and biological quality, the water must undergo complete treatment like that for the surface supplies, discussed previously. For example, if the water contains hydrogen sulfide (H_2S), aeration and chlorination are the basic treatments.

When a municipal water supply uses wells, the wells must be grouted the total depth to prevent surface and other polluted water from entering. In addition, well water must meet the same drinking water standards that surface water supplies must meet.

Tables 4.3 and 4.4 contain information that is helpful in planning water supplies and water use.

SUMMARY

In the hydrologic cycle, water evaporates from surface water into the atmosphere, where it falls to the earth again in some form of precipitation. Some impurities enter the water while it is in the atmosphere — called air pollution — and others contaminate the surface water or groundwater. Surface water supplies are obtained from cisterns, ponds, lakes, and rivers. Water quality is tested by measuring its pH, color, turbidity, taste, and odor. In addition, chemicals such as nitrites and nitrates are considered contaminants if they are present in specified quantities. The Environmental Protection Agency has set forth national drinking water standards that municipal water supplies must meet.

Groundwater is obtained through wells that tap into underground streams or aquifers. Health departments stipulate minimum separation distances between drinking water wells and pollution sources.

TABLE 4.2 EPA Fact Sheet: National Primary Drinking Water Standards

Contaminants	Health Effects	MCL*	MCLG	Sources
Microbiological				
Total Coliforms (Coliform bacteria, fecal coliform, streptococcal, and other bacteria)	Not necessarily disease-producing themselves, but coliforms can be indicators of organisms that cause assorted gastroenteric infections, dysentery, hepatitis, typhoid fever, cholera, and others; also interfere with disinfection process	1 per 100 milliliters	0	human and animal fecal waste
Turbidity	Interferes with disinfection	1–5tu***	0	erosion, runoff, discharges
Inorganic Chemicals				
Arsenic	Dermal and nervous system toxicity effects	.05	.05	natural deposits; smelters, glass, electronics wastes; orchards residues, industrial waste and smelter operations
Barium	Circulatory system effects	1	2	natural deposits; pigments, epoxy sealants, spent coal
Cadmium	Kidney effects	.005	.005	galvanized pipe corrosion; batteries, paints
Chromium	Liver/kidney/ circulatory effects	.1	.1	natural deposits; mining, electroplating, pigments
Lead	Central and peripheral nervous system damage; kidney effects; highly toxic to infants and pregnant women	.05**	0	natural/industrial deposits; plumbing, solder, brass alloy faucets
Mercury	Central nervous system disorders; kidney effects	.002	.002	crop runoff; natural deposits, batteries, electrical switches
Nitrate	Methemoglobinemia ("blue-baby syndrome")	10	10	animal waste, fertilizer, natural deposits; septic tanks, sewage
Selenium	Liver damage	.05	.05	natural deposits; mining, smelting, coal/oil combustion
Silver	Skin discoloration (Argyria)	.05		geological, mining
Fluoride	Skeletal damage	4		geological, additive to drinking water, toothpaste, foods processed with fluorinated water
Organic Chemicals				
Endrin	Liver, kidney, heart damage	.002	.002	pesticide used on insects, rodents, birds; restricted since 1980
Lindane	Liver, kidney, nerve immune, circulation	.0002	.0002	insecticide used on cattle, lumber, gardens; restricted 1983

(Continued)

TABLE 4.2 EPA Fact Sheet: National Primary Drinking Water Standards *(Continued)*

Contaminants	Health Effects	MCL*	MCLG	Sources
Methoxychlor	Growth, liver, kidney nerve	.04	.04	insecticide for fruits, vege-tables, alfalfa, livestock, pets
2,4-D	Liver and kidney damage	.07	.07	herbicide used to control broad-leaf weeds in agriculture; used on wheat, corn, rangelands, lawns
2,4,5-TP Silvex	Liver/kidney effects	.05	05	herbicide, on crops, right-of-way, golf courses; canceled in 1983
Toxaphene	Cancer	.003	0	insecticide used on cattle, cotton, corn, grain; cancelled in 1982
Benzene	Cancer	.005	0	some foods; gas, drugs, pesticide, paint, plastic industries
Carbon tetrachloride	Cancer	.005	0	solvent and their degradation products
p-Dichlorobenzene	Cancer	.075	.075	room and water deodorants, aand "mothballs"
1,2-Dichloroethane	Cancer	.005	0	leaded gas, fumigants, paints
1,1-Dichloroethylene	Liver/kidney effects, cancer	.007	.007	plastics, dyes, perfumes, paints
1,1,1-Trichloroethane	Liver/nervous system effects	.2	.2	adhesives, serosols, textiles, paints, inks, metal degreasers
Trichloroethylene (TCE)	Cancer	.005	0	Improper disposal of dry cleaning and ther solvents
Vinyl chloride	Cancer	.002	0	may leach from PVC pipe; formed by solvent breakdown
Total trihalomethanes (TTHM) (chloroform, bromoform, bromodichloromethane, dibromochloromethane)	Cancer	.1	0	formed primarily when surface water containing organic matter is treated with chlorine
Radionuclides				
Gross alpha particle activity	Cancer	15pCi/L		decay of radionuclides in natural deposits
Gross beta particle activity deposits	Cancer	4 mrem/yr		decay of radionuclides in natural and manmade
Radium 226 & 228 (total)	Bone cancer	5 pCi/L	0	radioactive waste, natural deposits

*In milligrams per liter, unless otherwise noted
**Agency considering substantially lower number
***Turbidity units

Source: U.S. Environmental Protection Agency, Office of Water

Environmental Health

TABLE 4.3 Planning Guide for Water Use

Types of establishments	Gallons per day	Types of establishments	Gallons per day
Airports (per passenger)	3–5	Horse (drinking)	12
Apartments, multiple family (per resident)	60	Mule (drinking)	12
Bath houses (per bather)	10	Sheep (drinking)	2
Camps:		Steer (drinking)	12
Construction, semi-permanent (per worker)	50	**Motels:**	
Day with no meals served (per camper)	15	With bath, toilet, and kitchen facilities (per bed space)	50
Luxury (per camper)	100–150	With bed and toilet (per bed space)	40
Resorts, day and night, with limited plumbing (per camper)	50	**Parks:**	
Tourist with central bath and toilet facilities (per person)	35	Overnight with flush toilets (per camper)	25
Cottages with seasonal occupancy (per resident)	50	Trailers with individual bath units, no sewer connection (per trailer)	25
Courts, tourist with individual bath units (per person)	50	Trailers with individual baths, connected to sewer (per person)	50
Clubs:		**Picnic:**	
Country (per resident member)	100	With bathhouses, showers, and flush toilets (per picnicker)	20
Country (per non-resident member present)	25	With toilet facilities only (gallons per picnicker)	10
Dwellings:		**Poultry:**	
Boardinghouses (per boarder)	50	Chickens (per 100)	5–10
Additional kitchen requirements for nonresident boarders	10	Turkeys (per 100)	10–18
		Restaurants with toilet facilities (per patron)	7–10
Luxury (per person)	100–150	Without toilet facilities (per patron)	2½–3
Multiple-family apartments (per resident)	40	With bars and cocktail lounge (additional quantity per patron)	2
Rooming houses (per resident)	60		
Single family (per resident)	50–75	**Schools:**	
Estates (per resident)	100–150	Boarding (per pupil)	75–100
Factories (gallons per person per shift)	15–35	Day with cafeteria, gymnasiums, and showers (per pupil)	25
Highway rest area (per person)	5	Day with cafeteria but no gymnasiums or showers (per pupil)	20
Hotels with private baths (two persons per room)	60	Day without cafeteria, gymnasiums, or showers (per pupil)	15
Hotels without private baths (per person)	50	Service stations (per vehicle)	10
Institutions other than hospitals (per person)	75–125	Stores (per toilet room)	400
Hospitals (per bed)	250–400	Swimming pools (per swimmer)	10
Laundries, self-serviced (gallons per washing, i.e., per customer)	50	**Theaters:**	
Livestock (per animal):		Drive-in (per car space)	5
Cattle (drinking)	12	Movie (per auditorium seat)	5
Dairy (drinking and servicing)	35	**Workers:**	
Goat (drinking)	2	Construction (per person per shift)	50
Hog (drinking)	4	Day (school or offices per person per shift)	15

Source: Manual of Individual Water Supply Systems, EPA Water Supply Division, 1975, pp 15–17

TABLE 4.4 Rates of Flow for Certain Plumbing, Household, and Farm Fixtures

Location	Flow pressure[1] (pounds per square inch, psi)	Flow rate (gallons per minute, gpm)
Ordinary basin faucet	8	2.0
Self-closing basin faucet	8	2 5
Sink faucet, ⅜"	8	4.5
Sink faucet, ½"	8	4.5
Bathtub faucet	8	6.0
Laundry tub faucet, ½"	8	5.0
Shower	8	5.0
Ball-cock for closet	8	3.0
Flush valve for closet	15	[1]15 40
Flushometer valve for urinal	15	15.0
Garden hose (50', ¾" sill cock)	30	5. 0
Garden hose (50', ⅝" outlet)	15	3.33
Drinking fountains	15	75
Fire hose 1½", ½" nozzle	30	40.0

[1]Flow pressure is the pressure in the supply near the faucet or water outlet while the faucet or water outlet is wide open and flowing.

REFERENCES

"Cryptosporidium Infections Associated With Swimming Pools — Dane County, Wisconsin, 1993." 1994, September 28. *Journal of the American Medical Association.* v. 272 n. l2. pp. 914.

Droste, R. L. 1996. *Theory and Practice of Water and Wastewater Treatment.* John Wiley & Sons, New York.

Environmental Protection Agency. 1982. *Manual of Individual Water Supply Systems.* U. S. Government Printing Office, Washington, DC.

Friedman, Mel. 1996, March. "Troubled Waters." *Parents Magazine.* v. 71 n. 3. pp. 50.

Frost, Floyd J., Rebba L. Calderon, and Gunther F. Craun. 1995, Dec. "Waterborne Disease Surveillance." *Journal of Environmental Health.* v. 58 n. 5. pp. 6.

Grimes, Deanna E. 1991. *Infectious Diseases.* St. Louis, Mosby-Year Book.

Hammer, Mark. 1988. "Water and Wastewater." *Environmental Engineering.* Butterworth Publishers, Stoneham, MA.

Isaac-Renton, Judith. 1996, Jan. "Longitudinal Studies of Giardia Contamination in Two Community Drinking Water Supplies: Cyst Levels, Parasite Viability, and Health Impact." *Applied and Environmental Microbiology.* v. 62 n. l. pp. 47.

Jones, Keith. 1994, July 9. "Waterborne Diseases." *New Scientist.* v. 143 n. 1933. pp. A1.

New York State Dept. of Health. *Manual of Instruction for Water Treatment Plant Operators.* n.d., n.p.

Pickford, John. 1987. *Developing World Water.* Grosvenor Press International, Hong Kong.

Rhyner, Charles R., Leander J. Schwartz, Robert B. Wenger, and Mary Kohrell. 1995. "Waste Management and Resource Recovery." CRC, Boca Raton, FL.

Sawyer, Clair N., and Perry L. McCarty. 1994. *Chemistry for Environmental Engineering.* 4th ed. McGraw-Hill Book Company, New York.

Silverstein, Kenneth. 1994, March. "Everything in the Kitchen Sink (nonpoint pollution threatens city water supplies)." *American City & County.* v. 109 n. 3. pp. 26.

Smith, Richard A. 1994, Jan. "Water Quality and Health: A Global Perspective." *Geotimes.* v. 39 n. l. pp. 19.

Roizman, Bernard. 1995. *Infectious Diseases in an Age of Change: The Impact of Human Ecology and Behavior on Disease Transmission.* National Academy Press, Washington DC.

Vesiland, Aarne. 1997. *Environmental Engineering.* PWS Publishing Company, Boston.

Environmental Health in Recreational Areas

by Franklin B. Carver, Ph.D.
The Ohio University

Key Terms

Avalanche
Backsiphonage
Conduction
Convection
Evaporation
Frostbite

Hypochlorous acid
Hypothermia
Loose-snow avalanche
Mass gathering
Playground
Radiation

Recreation
Slab Avalanche
Snowmobile
Undertow
Wetlands
Winter white-out

Objectives

- 🌐 Identify health and safety issues common to most types of recreational areas.
- 🌐 Identify the major environmental concerns that should be addressed in the planning, development, operation, and maintenance of recreational areas.
- 🌐 Identify the environmental health concerns that must be addressed in planning and conducting a mass gathering.
- 🌐 Identify and discuss the safety issues and precautions specific to snowmobiling and snowskiing.
- 🌐 Discuss physical and biological safety in water-oriented recreation areas.
- 🌐 Understand the basics of swimming-pool construction, maintenance, and water quality.
- 🌐 Discuss the operation, maintenance, and safety of two specific types of special pools.
- 🌐 Discuss the most common playground equipment-related dangers.

Recreational activities come in all forms, shapes, and fashions. How Americans spend their leisure time has profound economic and environmental consequences on our society. As much as one fourth of the national income is based on recreational activities, and in many states it is the major source of income. American families spend anywhere from 5% to 25% of their household income in pursuit of recreational endeavors; lower-income families spend a larger percentage of their income on recreation than do middle or upper income families. With 4-day workweeks beginning to take hold in some industries, 3-day weekends and larger blocks of leisure time are expected to further increase the American family's appetite for recreational activities.

Recreation is a power-packed word with significant public health concerns. It is more than a game or a hobby or a hike through the woods. It is a term that has far-reaching implications into the physical, social, and mental well-being of a society. A golf match, a ski trip, a fishing expedition — all may sound like rewarding experiences. Depending on the participant's state of mind, physical well-being, and environmental factors, however, these activities may have stressful and physically debilitating results. Activities such as these are recreational only when they are perceived as really fun, relaxing, and rejuvenating, and do not present environmental health and safety concerns. With true diversion from the world of work and the stress of day-to-day activities to the world of leisure activities and enjoyment, the participant becomes "recreated" — made new again. This is the major role of recreation in the advancement and maintenance of physical, social, and mental health. The need for proper environmental health and safe surroundings to inspire and rejuvenate individuals as they pursue recreational activities is paramount.

This chapter provides a broad overview of the major aspects that should be considered when planning, developing, operating, and maintaining selected recreational environments. The recreational environments covered in this chapter were chosen because of their continually expanding and innovative use by the public, coupled with increased public health and safety concerns. They are: mass gatherings, winter recreation, water-oriented recreation, and playgrounds.

PROBLEMS ASSOCIATED WITH ALL RECREATIONAL AREAS

Recreational areas and activities have many problems in common. These problems often are related directly to the public's increased use and misuse of recreational areas. Therefore, public behavior in recreational settings is a growing concern. Problems caused by public behavior are attributed mainly to irresponsibility and a carefree attitude by consumers of all age groups. Lack of respect for rules and regulations in recreational areas has become all too common. Complaints about vandalism and other lawless

acts against people, property, and the environment have shown significant increases. Alcohol use and illegal drug use in recreational areas have been identified as major factors contributing to irrational public behavior. Most recreational areas by now have banned the use of alcohol and increased protection against illegal drugs.

Another growing concern for recreational areas is site selection. Sites selected for recreation areas should be well-drained, gently sloping, free from topographical, biological, chemical, and physical hazards. Marshes, swamps, and water containing domestic, industrial, or agricultural waste should not be near recreational areas. Swamps and marshes breed mosquitoes that spread diseases and annoy people with their bites. Agricultural waste (cattle urine and feces) in water can spread disease in addition to being unacceptable aesthetically.

Traffic and noise are additional considerations when selecting sites. Recreational facilities should be far enough away from main thoroughfares to minimize accidents. A facility's access road design should exclude sharp curves and other potential traffic hazards. The site should be away from railroads, airports, truck routes, factories, and other sources of noise and accidents. In addition, recreational sites should be as far removed as possible from sources of pollution such as manufacturing plants, refineries, oil and coal burning power plants, and industrial establishments that produce noise pollution plus smoke, fumes, dust, objectionable odors, and other forms of air pollution.

It stands to reason that a recreational site should not be located near a nuclear power plant, farmyard, swamp, wastewater treatment plant, or bombing range. With such extensive site selection criteria and the immense development of industrial and residential areas over the past decade, new recreational sites are difficult to locate. This has brought about intense scrutiny of environmental impact studies, including the preservation of **wetlands**, during the site selection process. Risk assessments commonly are done to determine the suitability of proposed sites.

Because of the seasonal nature of certain activities, various problems arise in relation to purchasing expensive equipment for use during short periods of time, hiring and maintaining trained personnel, and conducting inspection and enforcement procedures over a 3- to 4-month period. Managers of recreational areas have tried to compensate for seasonal economic losses by turning ski resorts into year-round vacation sites or extending prime months for skiing by using more sophisticated snow-making equipment. Others have opted to develop multi-use facilities that will accommodate indoor or outdoor recreational activities.

MASS GATHERINGS

Mass gatherings for recreational purposes are defined differently by individual states. Some states define a **mass gathering** as an assembly of 1,000 or more people. Other states consider it an assembly of 5,000 or more people, with or without overnight accommodations. Some states also define a mass gathering by the number of hours an activity will continue and whether it is sponsored by the government or any of its agencies, along with the proposed site of the activity. Regardless of the definition, when large numbers of people come together and interact closely, the likelihood for transmitting diseases increases.

Specific types of mass gatherings that require various permits from local and state enforcement and planning agencies, including health departments, are: rock concerts, fairs, carnivals, jamborees, auctions, and many other similar-type festive occasions. The planning stages for events such as these are important and should include all significant parties involved, especially promoters, local government officials, state and local police, public health officials, fire, transportation, and emergency medical personnel. All planning activities should be coordinated by one individual with distinct preparation for activities that are to occur before, during, and after the event. Some of the major environmental health concerns that have caused significant

public health problems at mass gatherings in the past are the lack of:

- potable water from approved sources
- adequate sewage disposal systems
- proper solid waste collection, storage, and disposal
- noise levels in excess of 70 dBA* at perimeter of site
- proper food sanitation practices

WINTER RECREATION

Winter recreational activities have extended outdoor recreation into a year-round industry and are growing faster than any other recreational activities. This activity has brought about major environmental health and safety concerns. Some of the most common and current winter recreational environmental health and safety concerns are discussed next.

Ice Safety

With every winter season come stories of accidents and deaths resulting from falls through breaking ice. These incidents could be prevented by taking a few basic precautions including supervising children, avoiding certain locations of icy areas, and knowing how to react in case of an ice emergency.

During the winter months when temperatures are near freezing, children never should be allowed to play outside without supervision if the area has bodies of water, no matter how large or small. The water body does not have to be a pond or lake for an accident to occur. A drainage ditch or even standing water in a field can be the site of a catastrophe.

A major principle of ice safety is respect for the ice. When ice is safe depends on the activity. The same ice could be safe for a person on skis but unsafe for someone on foot. Generally, a 2-inch depth of ice is considered safe for someone

---

* dBA = decibels in A scale.

on foot, and 4 inches to 6 inches will support groups of people or vehicles. Ice 8 inches thick is considered safe for loads up to 1,000 pounds per square foot.

Basic to all ice and water safety is the ability to swim. Beyond this, the two key rules are:

1. If something happens, do not panic. This alone has saved many lives.
2. If you feel you are breaking through an icy surface, throw yourself forward and out flat. If you fall through the ice and have your arms outstretched on the ice, use your feet as a propeller and edge yourself up onto the ice.

If an accident happens to a companion, a rope is the best means of rescue. If a rope is not available, a long branch or a pole can be used. Without these, and if several people are on hand, a "human chain" can be used for an effective rescue. To do this, individuals lie face down on the ice with another person holding their ankles and slowly propel across the ice to the victim.

Once rescued, frostbite precautions must be taken, along with seeking shelter and warmth immediately because the victim's clothes will quickly freeze.

Generally, activities on ice are relatively safe. One 25-year study found that recreation on ice is 20 times safer than other recreational sports on water and 50 times safer than highway travel. With the proper knowledge and precautions, ice can be a safe and enjoyable source of winter recreation.

Frostbite

James Wilkerson's book, *Hypothermia, Frostbite and Other Cold Injuries* (1988), defines frostbite as "a localized cold weather injury characterized by freezing with ice crystal formation." Frostbitten tissues typically are pale, firm or hard, and often lose sensation. Freezing of the body's fluids and soft tissue of the skin is a result of reduced blood flow. The two most common sites of frostbite are the toes and the fingers. The nose and ears also can be damaged. Hypothermia (see below) and restrictive clothing can invite frostbite. Either may restrict blood flow, leading to frostbite.

Frostbite can be prevented by wearing protective clothing to keep the skin warm and by not wearing restrictive clothing. Also, people should be aware that smoking restricts blood flow and that alcohol dulls the nervous system, providing a false sense of warmth and security.

Hypothermia

Hypothermia occurs mostly when the body is exposed to outside temperatures between 30° and 50°F. and the internal body temperature is reduced to 95°F or lower. The four major ways of reducing the body temperature are convection, conduction, evaporation, and radiation.

Convective and conductive loss of body heat both occur when air, water, or other elements around the body are cooler than the body and, by absorbing heat from the body, decrease the body's temperature. **Convection** can be defined as the transfer of heat from one location to another via movement in any "fluid," be it liquid (e.g., water) or gas (e.g., air). When convection takes place, the air or water around the body gains heat via transfer from the body, then the warmed fluid (air or water) circulates away from the body, loses the heat gained from the body, and is replaced next to the body by unheated fluid, which begins the convective process all over again. Although *convection* occurs in both air and water, water removes heat from the human body more readily than does air.

Conduction is defined as the transfer of heat from the body through substances with which the body may have direct contact. Unlike convection, conduction can occur with any solid substance, as well as any fluid, and the human body can gain heat through *conduction* from a warmer substance — for example, from hot water while bathing, or from contact with a heating pad.

Evaporation occurs when water escapes from the skin during respiration. It is responsible for 20% to 30% of heat loss in temperate climates.

Radiation is the largest source of heat loss. The human body gives off heat that cooler objects absorb. The body, too, absorbs radiant heat from the sun and from fires.

The human body is affected greatly by heat loss. The body's first defense against cold is shivering, which generates heat. As the body continues to lose heat, hypothermia decreases the brain's need for oxygen. This leads the victim into a disoriented and confused state. The circulatory system slows down, reducing the flow of blood, causing heat to leave areas of the body, notably the fingers and toes.

Protection from hypothermia is the same as for frostbite: wearing proper protective clothing. The best fabric is wool because of its insulating properties. Wool also is known to continue insulating even when fully saturated. Mittens, headgear, and footgear are the most significant protective clothing items. Mittens are better than gloves because they provide better insulation. Headgear is necessary because heat loss from the head can be great. For footgear, leather is the best material to use.

Snowmobiling

One of the fastest-growing winter recreational activities is snowmobiling. The State of Ohio defines a **snowmobile** as a self-propelled vehicle steered by skis, runners, or caterpillar treads, and designed to be used principally on snow or ice. Most state laws require the registration of snowmobiles every 3 years, and the annual registration of dealers who sell or furnish these vehicles for hire. An accurate account of the number of snowmobiles in use cannot be determined because many states do not require the registration of snowmobiles if used on private property. Snowmobilers must obey all operating regulations for motor vehicle traffic, with most state officials authorizing the use of snowmobiles for winter travel in the following situations: (a) to cross a highway other than a limited-access highway or freeway; and (b) on the berm or shoulder of any highway, other than a limited-access highway, or freeway when the terrain is such that the vehicle can be used safely.

When attempting to cross ice, the snowmobiler must be extra careful. It is best to stay off the ice unless local or state officials deem it safe. To support the weight of a driver as well as the snowmobile, the ice must be at least 4 to 6 inches thick. It also is necessary to watch out for areas between two or more big lakes or other bodies of water. This situation often indicates that fast-moving water is in the area, which can make the ice thinner in certain spots.

Most state officials enforce a law that allows the operation of snowmobiles only during specific hours of the day, usually between one-half hour before sunrise and one-half hour after sunset. Snowmobiles operating before sunrise and after sunset and during periods of poor visibility must be equipped with proper lighting. Officials also warn snowmobilers about operating their vehicles during **winter white-outs**, when an overcast sky or snow precludes shadows and thus causes the horizon to be indistinguishable from the terrain.

Over the last several years fatal and nonfatal injuries related to snowmobile use have increased. This, in part, reflects the rising popularity of the sport along with winter recreational activities in general. Most snowmobile accidents have involved operators between 20 and 30 years of age, and alcohol and excessive speed have played predominant roles. More than half of all fatal accidents have been attributed to head injuries, and a significant number of other fatalities have occurred as a result of operating on frozen bodies of water or hypothermia and drowning as a result of falling through the ice.

Snowmobile injuries range from hand trauma from engine belts to head injuries and open fractures caused by colliding with stationary objects. Data on snowmobile injuries are statistically irrelevant in comparison to other motor vehicle injuries mainly because most snowmobile accidents are not reported. Based on the analysis of fatalities, however, the following regulations would improve snowmobile safety if uniformly implemented:

- Increased and more accurate accident reporting by medical personnel, snowmobile operators, and winter-resort property owners.
- Registration of all snowmobiles for tags at the time of purchase.

- Requirement of a course in safety for owners and all prospective drivers. The course should involve training in handling the snowmobile and familiarization with the safety hazards before operation.
- Required licensure for snowmobile operation, including mandatory successful completion of a safety course, for individuals 16 years of age and older, regardless of a valid automobile driver's license.
- Application of the same alcohol-use penalties to snowmobile operators as are applied to drivers of automobiles who use alcohol.
- Strict prohibition of individuals under 16 years of age from operating snowmobiles.
- Requirement of safety-designed footwear for operation of snowmobiles.
- Mandatory use of safety helmets for all drivers and passengers.
- Yearly public awareness efforts, through the media, on safety requirements for the use of snowmobiles.
- Enforceable speed limits according to various terrain and conditions.

Skiing

Skiing has evolved through the years to become one of the favorite winter outdoor activities throughout the entire Northern Hemisphere. As a recreational sport, it can be enjoyed by most age groups and does not require special skills or elaborate training. Skiing, however, has earned the reputation of being a relatively dangerous activity.

For many years efforts have been made to improve ski safety by changes in boots, bindings, and skis, and in trail design, trail grooming, and crowd control. Many of the hazards of skiing never will be removed completely from the sport. To do so would be impossible and would take from skiing much of its aesthetic beauty as well as its appeal as a vigorous mountain or cross-country experience.

Some hazards at ski areas are operational necessities. For example, groups of trees strategically placed on specific trails can be hazardous, but these same trees provide necessary reference points to skiers when weather conditions cause poor visibility. Ski-lift towers are also essential, but when they stand alone in the middle of ski runs, they become serious hazards.

Many of the hazards once considered inherent in recreational skiing are no longer acceptable. As accidents and failures have pointed out flaws in systems, equipment, and machines, new technologies have been employed to remedy the problems. The result has been a steady improvement not only in equipment quality and performance but, more important, a reduction in the number and types of hazards and the resulting injuries they cause.

One of the most life-threatening natural environmental phenomena for skiers is a snow avalanche. No one can predict avalanche occurrence with certainty, and not even the experts fully understand their causation.

The two main types of snow **avalanches** are:

1. A **loose-snow avalanche,** which starts at the point or side of a slope when unattached snow crystals slide downward. It grows in size, and the quantity of snow increases as it

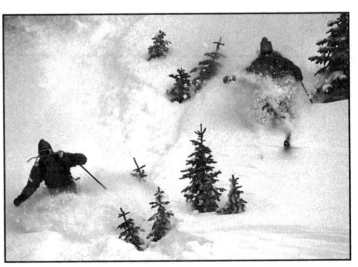

Snow skiing has become one of the most popular winter sports.

Environmental Health

descends. Loose snow moves as a formless mass with little internal cohesion.

2. **Slab avalanche,** which starts when a solid area of snow breaks away all at once. There is a well-defined fracture line where the moving snow breaks away from the stable snow. Slab avalanches are characterized by the tendency of snow crystals to stick together. The slide may contain angular blocks or chunks of snow. Slab avalanches often are triggered by the victims themselves. Their weight on the stressed snow slab is enough to break the often fragile bonds that hold it to the slope or to other snow layers. Loose-snow slides that trap victims usually are triggered naturally or by other members of the ski party.

Many other ski hazards are triggered by natural phenomena or environmental surroundings; however, most ski accidents and injuries have been directly correlated with the skier's behavior. Individual skiers have sole, personal, and final responsibility for knowing the range of their own abilities and skiing within the limits of those abilities. Each skier is responsible for judging whether he or she has the skills necessary to safely negotiate any slope or trail. Other responsibilities for which skiers are accountable, which commonly lead to accidents and injuries when disregarded are the following.

1. Each skier must maintain control of his or her speed and course at all times when skiing, and maintain a proper lookout so as to be able to avoid other skiers and objects.

2. The primary responsibility should be on the person skiing downhill to avoid colliding with any person or objects on the ski trail.

3. No skier should ski on any slope or trail that has been posted as "closed" or "off limits."

4. Skiers should stay clear of snow-grooming equipment, all vehicles, lift towers, signs, and any other equipment on the ski slopes and trails.

5. Skiers have the responsibility to heed all posted information and other warnings and to refrain from acting in a manner that may cause or contribute to the injury of the skier or others.

6. Skis used by downhill skiers while skiing should be equipped with a strap or other device capable of stopping the skis should they become detached from the skiers. (This requirement does not apply to cross-country skiers.)

7. Before beginning to ski from a stationary position, or before entering a ski slope or trail from the side, skiers are responsible for avoiding moving skiers already on the ski slope or trail.

8. Skiers should not move uphill on any passenger tramway or use any ski slope or trail while impaired by alcohol or by illicit drugs.

9. No skier should knowingly enter public or private lands from an adjoining ski area when the land has been posted as being closed by its owner or by the ski-area operator.

WATER-ORIENTED RECREATION

More than half of all outdoor recreation is related to water. This form of recreation ranges from sheer aesthetic appreciation to the excitement of jet skiing and includes activities in the water and along the shore. Examples are boating (rowing, sailing, canoeing, kayaking, float trips, scenic river trips), water skiing, swimming, diving, snorkeling, surfing, scuba diving, fishing, hunting, studying and observing water birds and aquatic life, sunbathing, camping on the shore, and collecting shells, driftwood and rocks. Theme parks featuring water-related activities such as water slides also have become extremely popular over the past few years.

Regardless of how water is used, the quality of the water historically has been the number-one concern in relation to recreational activities. Contamination from any substance that may pose a hazard to human health through ingestion, skin absorption, or entrance through body openings (such as the ear) is due cause for public health authorities to restrict a body of water to non-swimming recreation or, in severe cases, to prohibit the use of a body of water for recreation altogether.

Classification of Bathing Places and Water Quality

People swim in a variety of different settings. When swimming in any body of water, the person should be aware of the depth and quality of the water. Every swimming area should be free of debris such as glass, cans, logs, and rocks. The swimmer must know what kind of bottom is present, as slope and footing are important in preventing unintentional injuries and fatalities. Each specific bathing place requires unique safety knowledge and practices.

Natural Waters

One classification of bathing places consists of natural outdoor ponds, rivers, lakes, tidal waters, and beaches. These all depend on natural flow, temperature, and sunlight for sanitation, making this type of swimming area extremely difficult to manage from a public health standpoint. Usually there is a large volume of water per bather, which reduces the chances of water becoming contaminated. Nevertheless, one must be sure that no pollution from outside sources is present such as household waste piped to a stream, or a sewer outfall nearby, because of the possibility of contacting a pathogen. Natural bathing waters and their surroundings can be contaminated by waste from septic tanks, cesspools, privies, or sewage treatment plants entering the bathing water by any means. When polluted, the bathing area is condemned to protect the health of the people. This can be determined by a sanitary survey and coliform testing.

Studies have been made in an attempt to determine reasonable bacterial standards for this class of bathing place. Years ago, some states made extensive surveys of physical characteristics of saltwater beaches and correlated those with *E. coli* counts. Table 5.1 gives sample bacteriological standards.

Beaches where the coliform organism density exceeded 1,000 per 100 ml were considered unsafe.

Results of sanitary surveys were correlated with the bacteriological findings. The final classification of the bathing place is not made upon the basis of the bacterial test alone, but also upon sanitary-survey finding.

Whenever one swims in a river or at the seashore, dangers can arise from the various currents and tides. The current of a flowing stream or river can catch swimmers by surprise and pull them under the water or dash them against rocks before they have time to react.

In an **undertow**, the wave breaks over the beach and then recedes toward the lake or ocean. If the waves are large enough and the beach has

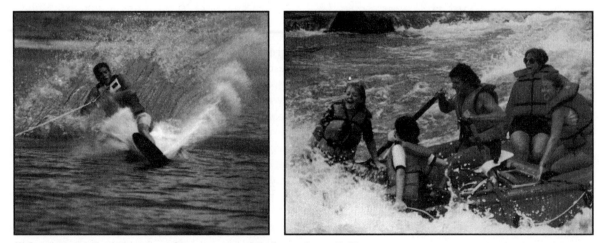

Waterskiing and whitewater rafting are very popular water activities.

TABLE 5.1 Average Coliform Index		
Class	per 100 ml	Standard
A	0 to 50	good
B	50 to 500	fair
C	500 to 1,000	doubtful
D	over 1,000	poor

a slope, the undertow has a force great enough to pull a person out into the water. A swimmer who is caught in such a current should not "fight" the water but, rather, be led by the current until reaching an object such as a tree limb that can be grasped or until the current recedes.

Outdoor Pools

Another classification of bathing consists of outdoor pools that are partly artificial and partly natural. These are found in camps where a stream is utilized for a constant flow and change of water. The stream often is widened with masonry but seldom is chlorinated. These pools are difficult to control from a sanitary standpoint because turnover of water depends on the flow of the stream. If no disinfectant, such as chlorine, is used to kill pathogens, it would not take long to transmit a pathogen from person to person. Also, a sanitary survey and bacteriological test should be made on the contributing stream.

Artificially Constructed Pools

A third classification of a bathing place encompasses indoor and outdoor pools that are entirely of artificial construction. These are of three types.

1. *Fill and draw pools,* which depend on frequent emptying and refilling to maintain sanitary conditions. If the water is not changed frequently, these pools can be as unsanitary as a communal bathtub. This type is rarely used today.

2. The *flow-through pool,* which gets its water from natural sources such as streams. In areas where water is cheap, water from the municipal supply or a private well may flow through the artificial pool; however, this latter type is rare, especially in arid regions.

3. *Recirculatory pools,* which are the most satisfactory from a public health standpoint. The water is recirculated through the filtering equipment by pumps, and chemicals are used to control the water quality. Disinfecting agents are added before the water reenters the pool. Some recirculating pools are filled only once a year, and the water is used, treated, filtered, and reused. The water should be recirculated at least every 8 hours, and preferably every 6 hours. If properly maintained, the recirculated water is relatively clear at all times to prevent accidents and to lower the amount of disinfectant needed. The water quality should be such that a 6-inch (15 cm) black disk painted on a white background is visible from the side of the pool at the deepest point.

pH

The pH of swimming-pool water is the single most important factor in maintaining pool water quality. Every other chemical balance in swimming pool water is affected by pH. Water with a low pH irritates the eyes, ears, and mucous membrane. Most state bathing codes require that pool water pH be maintained between 7.2 and 8.2, though the ideal range is between 7.4 and 7.6. If the pH is allowed to drop below 7.2, metal surfaces such as the filter tank, pipes, and heater coils can corrode. Skin irritation and excessive chlorine odor also may result.

High pH readings, above 7.6, also must be avoided. As readings approach 8.0, iron and calcium can form a precipitate (solid particles suspended in the water), causing turbidity or unclear water. In addition, scale can form on the filters and in the plumbing and heater. Precipitates also form from chemical conditions, such as hardness and alkalinity.

Another undesirable effect of high pH is that it reduces the efficiency of chlorine added to the water for disinfectant purposes. High pH impedes the formation of **hypochlorous acid,** the bactericide that is formed when chlorine is added to the water. At pH 7.2, approximately 60% of the chlorine dissolved in water will convert to hypochlorous acid. By comparison, at pH 8.5, the conversion is limited to approximately 10%. The remainder is converted to hypochlorite ion, a useless acid. If the pH exceeds the recommended maximum of 7.6, more chlorine will be required to maintain the desired level of disinfectant in the water, resulting in a higher operating cost.

Recirculating Pools

Maintaining desired water quality requires the proper use of circulating and filtering equipment. A recirculating swimming pool is similar to a water treatment plant. In a water treatment plant, "new" water is treated; in a swimming pool, the pool is filled in the spring and the water is used (swimming), contaminated, treated, reused, retreated, and so on, all year. The equipment and chemicals used in water treatment plants and swimming pools in most cases are the same — chlorine, alum, filters, pumps, and so on. In fact swimming pools *are* small water treatment plants. Figure 5.1 illustrates the path pool water takes as it is treated.

All pools should be equipped with either gutter drains, surface skimmers, or both (see Figure 5.2). The water pulled through these comes from the surface, where it is most contaminated because the material with specific gravity less than that of water will float. Therefore, this water is skimmed off the top to be filtered. The amount of water skimmed from the top can be controlled by opening or closing the valve to the surface skimmer; usually the gutter drains flow by gravity to the pump. Most of the water to be recirculated is pulled through the main drains. This is helpful in maintaining a chlorine residual throughout the pool. The water from the gutter drains through the make-up tank, which serves to replenish the water lost by splash, evaporation, and the like. There must be an air gap between the fresh water make-up line and the pool water to prevent **backsiphonage** (see Figure 5.3). Water from the make-up tank, surface skimmers, line, and main drains goes through a hair strainer where lint, hair, and other extraneous materials are removed. At this point the water is still on the suction side of recirculating pump.

Next, chlorine is added to the water as a disinfecting agent to kill pathogenic organisms. After chlorination, a filter aid (usually alum) is added to the water. Alum is a general term referring to aluminum compounds of sulfate or potassium, which aid in the flocculation (settling out) of small particles of impurities. The water now goes to the pump, which also serves as a rapid mixer. Once through the pump, the water passes by a manometer, used to measure the rate of flow to the filters.

Six filtration systems are commonly used in swimming pools. All six utilize some type of filter media (sand and gravel or diatomaceous earth). All are acceptable in their ability to remove dirt and impurities. The two basic filter types are classified as perpetual and temporary media. Filters in which the same media can be reused are of the *perpetual media* type and include the following:

- *Pressure sand.* Prior to 1950 this was the standard method of filtration. It employs

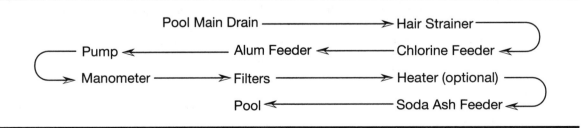

FIGURE 5.1 Path of swimming pool water.

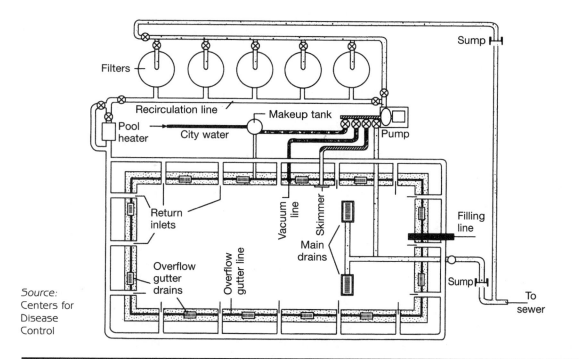

FIGURE 5.2 Swimming pool piping system.

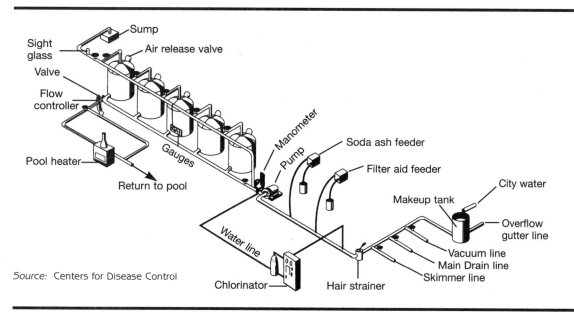

FIGURE 5.3 Swimming pool filtration equipment.

one or more filter tanks filled with layers of sand and gravel. A motorized pump forces water down through the various layers of sand and gravel and back to the pool.

- *Vacuum sand (gravity sand)*. The oldest method of pool filtration, this was the most common until it was replaced by the pressure sand type. Once called the gravity sand method, it has undergone engineering changes and now is known as the vacuum sand method. The filter is a large, open bed consisting of several layers of gravel topped with sand. Water flows through the bed, with a combination of gravity and vacuum forces used to circulate it back into the pool.

- *High-flow sand*. In this more recent type of sand filtration (Figure 5.4), water is forced through sand that is kept in suspension by a rapid flow rate. The system requires half the filter surface area needed with the pressure sand method. Another advantage is that no coagulant (alum) is needed. Some question whether high-flow sand filters can deliver the same quality of water as the regular sand filters.

Filters that require new media after cleaning, the *temporary media* type, include the following:

- *Vacuum diatomaceous earth*. This method of filtration is also commonly referred to as the *open pit* or *open tank* method. Its filter medium consists of fossilized marine plants (diatoms) that form a 1/16 inch thick layer on the elements, which are visible in an open tank. The fossilized diatoms serve as a screen on the surface of filter elements and strain dirt particles from the water. Water flows into the tank via gravity and is drawn through the elements and recirculated back to the pool. The advantage of this method is easier access for maintenance and cleaning.

- *Pressure diatomaceous earth*. D.E. pressure filtration was developed during World War II. The filter elements are housed in pressurized tanks, and water is pushed through the D.E.-coated elements and recirculated back to the pool (Figure 5.5).

- *Regenerative cycle diatomaceous earth*. Regenerative filters are a relatively recent adaptation of pressure D.E. filtration. The elements, several hundred per tank, are small tubes, usually made of spring stainless steel

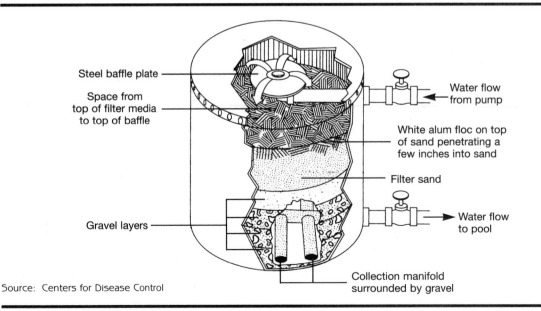

Steel baffle plate

Space from top of filter media to top of baffle

Gravel layers

Water flow from pump

White alum floc on top of sand penetrating a few inches into sand

Filter sand

Water flow to pool

Collection manifold surrounded by gravel

Source: Centers for Disease Control

FIGURE 5.4 High-flow sand filter vessel.

Environmental Health

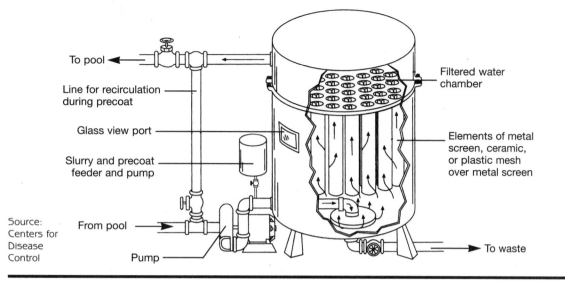

FIGURE 5.5 Pressure diatomaceous earth filter with cylindrical elements.

and covered with an acid- and base-resistant synthetic material. The main difference between the pressure and regenerative types is that the regenerative system automatically removes the previous D.E. coating and re-applies it to the elements, using the same filter media several times a day. This system may require as few as eight 50-pound bags of D.E. per 12-month operating season.

Most of the filtering is done by gelatinous material, usually aluminum hydroxide, that forms on top of the filter media. From the bottom of the filters comes the filtered water that may or may not be heated as it reenters the pool. Soda ash then is added to raise the pH to the desired level. (Recent studies indicate it is best to introduce the soda ash after the filtration process). Urine, body acids, alum, and gaseous chlorine have a tendency to lower the pH level.

Swimming Pool Construction and Maintenance

Pools obviously should be constructed of an impervious material. Concrete pools are common,

and packaged steel panel units are available. The walls and bottom should be smooth and light-colored to facilitate cleaning. Water depth should vary from 3 feet (.9 m) to at least 6 feet (1.8 m) in every 15 feet (4.5 m) at the shallow end. The shallow area — that area less than 5 feet (1.5 m) deep — should comprise from 70% to 80% of the pool area. Areas less than 2 feet (.6 m) deep should be confined to wading pools. Surface area is based on approximately 2 square feet per person at maximum load on the assumption that one-third of the patrons will be outside the pool itself at any given time.

Pool shapes vary from square to bean-shaped and banjo-shaped. Rectangular-shaped pools in which the width is one-third the length probably are most common. Regardless of the shape of the pool, depth markers should be located around the periphery. These markers should be readily visible from the deck, and placed no more than 25 feet (7.5 m) apart, but preferably 10 feet (3.0 m) apart. Their purpose is to prevent nonswimmers from jumping into deep water and divers from diving into shallow water.

Pools should have a runway not less than 4 feet (1.2 m) wide, commencing with the edge of the pool. The deck or runway should slope away from the pool at about ¼ inch per foot to prevent the water from draining back into the pool. A deck drain should be provided for approximately each 100 square feet of deck/runway surface. These drains may connect to a public sewer.

Where submersed lights are used, an electrical inspector should inspect them annually to assure that they are safe. This could prevent electrocution accidents.

The following are various parts of the pool, also shown in Figure 5.6, that must be understood for proper pool operation and maintenance.

Overflow gutter drains: drainage fittings used in the overflow gutter at the uppermost portion of the water.

Vacuum fitting: the place where a hose is connected to the suction piping to allow vacuuming of the pool. No other duty should be assigned to the pump when the pool is being vacuumed.

Return water inlets: located all around the pool and adjusted to control the amount of water entering the various areas of the pool.

Surface skimmer: a device that skims the water after storms, rain, etc. (less important in indoor pools). After each use the strainer basket in the skimmer is removed and cleaned.

Fillspout: located underneath the diving board for safety, its purpose is to fill the pool.

Main drain: outlet fittings at the bottom of a swimming pool through which water passes to the recirculating pump. During recirculation, three-fourths of the pool's total water volume leaves through the main drain and the other one-fourth leaves through overflow gutters or skimmers. The main drain opening should be protected and be at least four times the diameter of the pipe.

Other parts of a pool include:

Filter aid unit: in anthracite and sand filter systems, alum or another coagulant is added here.

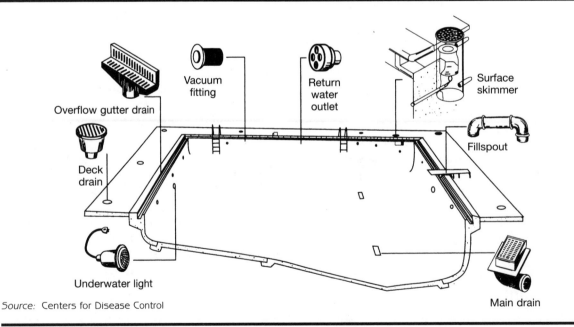

Vacuum fitting

Overflow gutter drain

Return water outlet

Surface skimmer

Fillspout

Deck drain

Underwater light

Main drain

Source: Centers for Disease Control

FIGURE 5.6 Longitudinal section through pool showing fittings.

Environmental Health

Soda ash feeders: may be used to raise pH of pool water.

Pumps: serve three basic functions: to recirculate the pool water, to backwash the filters, and to agitate alum so a large surface area is provided. Centrifugal pumps usually are used in swimming pools.

Manometer: a pressure device that measures volumetric flow to ensure that the desired turnover rate is being met. All pools must be recirculated three or four times daily or must be treated every 6 or 8 hours.

Make-up tank: contains fresh water to fill or refill the pool as a result of water loss. The water level here is the same as the pool's; therefore, it determines the water level in the pool. The make-up tank is connected to the city water supply. The disadvantage of this lies in provision of an air gap.

Gauges: Two gauges that measure the pressure to ascertain when the filters should be backwashed. The difference in the pressure gauges indicates that the filters are dirty.

Sight glass: a device through which one can determine when the filter is clean by observing the water in the backwashing process as it passes through.

Special Pools

Many different types of pools currently are being manufactured. Most are confronted with the same maintenance and public health concerns, though. This discussion will be confined to two specific types, therapeutic and wading pools.

Therapeutic Pools

Therapeutic pools (public spas and hot tubs) are becoming almost as popular as swimming pools. They represent a relatively new development, and many of the new public pools are including a therapeutic pool as a separate system with its own circulating pump and filter. The turbulence and heated water in these pools have enhanced their "spa" effect. Because of the growing demand for therapeutic pools, the following requirements have become important:

- *Circulation.* The contents of a therapy pool should be recirculated quickly. The small volume of water in relation to the number of bathers necessitates rapid turnover to ensure water purity.

- *Surface skimmer and main drain.* Each therapeutic pool should have two main drains and at least one skimmer. The reason for this is to prevent suction and body entrapment accidents and to ensure rapid and complete water turnover.

- *Hydro-therapy system.* To achieve the "spa" or "jetting" effect, a properly sized pump and aid blower should be installed. The temperature of the water should not be higher than 104°F. The therapy pool always should have a thermometer so pool users can make an accurate check.

- *Chlorine/bromine feeding.* Because of the high water temperature in a therapy pool, chlorine/bromine dissipates rapidly. An automatic feeding device, properly sized to the therapy pool, must be installed and operated continuously.

- *Safety requirements.* Skid-proof decking and handrails for steps are necessary. In addition, all steps and seat edges should be delineated so that when the water is agitated, the edges are easily visible. The edges of steps and seats should be marked by installing a solid dark tile in a contrasting color.

Wading Pools

Presenting the worst conditions of any swimming pool, shallow wading pools often are packed with small children who are most susceptible to waterborne diseases. The relative amounts of ammonia and organic nitrogens introduced into a wading pool (mainly by urine) are enormous. The chances of children being immune to diseases spread by pools are less than for older people, and the likelihood of their consuming pool water is greater. To keep a wading pool in good operating condition and as sanitary as possible, the following rules should be adhered to rigorously.

1. The circulation rate should be checked and maintained at the desired levels at least once an hour.

2. Chlorine and pH readings should be taken every hour and adjusted to maintain a minimum of 1.5 ppm of free chlorine and a pH of 7.2–7.6.

3. The pool should be vacuumed and skimmed as often as necessary and *at least once a day.*

A wading pool should not be made a part of another pool. It should be separated by a barrier and should have its own recirculating and chemical feeding systems.

Gas Chlorine Room

When chlorine gas is used as the means of disinfection, special precautions must be taken. There must be a separate room with an outside entrance for the chlorination equipment (see Figure 5.7). The room should have a door with louvers at the top instead of at the bottom, where they normally are located. The chlorine cylinders, both full and empty, must be fastened securely to prevent breaking. A self-contained breathing apparatus (SCBA) should be available in case of a chlorine gas leak. An exhaust fan, which switches on as the door to the chlorine room opens, should be installed and operative. This fan should be at floor level. If the chlorine room is below ground level, the fan duct should terminate above ground level. Chlorine gas is approximately two-and-one-half times as heavy

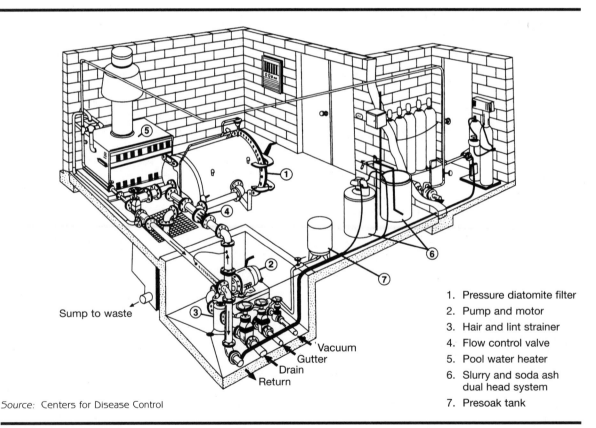

Sump to waste

Vacuum
Gutter
Drain
Return

1. Pressure diatomite filter
2. Pump and motor
3. Hair and lint strainer
4. Flow control valve
5. Pool water heater
6. Slurry and soda ash dual head system
7. Presoak tank

Source: Centers for Disease Control

FIGURE 5.7 Typical pressure diatomite filter system.

as air and therefore will be near the floor. A stationary chlorine sniffer and alarm system are recommended. As a substitute, a can of ammonia should be kept in the chlorine room to check for chlorine leaks after cylinder changes and at other times when needed. Ammonia reacts with chlorine to form ammonium chloride, a white substance with a cloudlike appearance in air.

Chlorine is highly corrosive; therefore, either an inert metal tubing or rubber tubing must be used to transport the chlorine solution to the recirculating line. Another way of ascertaining a chlorine leak before entering the room is to have a glass panel in the door through which one can check periodically to see if a highly polished brass object placed in the chlorine room shows corrosion. Chlorine is highly corrosive to brass, reacting with it in a few minutes.

Because chlorine is so corrosive and hazardous to people, the trend is away from chlorine gas and toward the use of calcium hypochlorite or some other disinfectant.

PLAYGROUNDS

Playgrounds, whether in public locations — such as schools or parks — or in private backyards, are places that allow children to interact socially while they swing, slide, climb, or simply sit and talk. These areas play a vital role in the development of children by providing challenges and testing their skills. The challenges presented should be stimulating and fun within a safe and healthful environment.

Design and Maintenance

When planning a new playground, it is important to consider hazards or obstacles to children traveling to and from the playground. A barrier around the playground site is recommended to prevent children from running into the street or roadway. Even when a barrier is present, however, children never should be left unattended or unsupervised. Playgrounds should be organized

carefully into different areas to prevent possible injuries caused by conflicting games or activities, such as a playing field located too close to a swing set, in which a child runs in front of a swing in motion.

Active, physical activities always should be separated from more passive or quiet activities. Areas for play equipment, open playing fields, and sand boxes should be located in different sections of the playground. In addition, popular, heavy-use pieces of equipment or activities should be dispersed appropriately to avoid crowding in any area of the playground.

The layout of playground equipment and activities should provide for a clear line of sight to every area of the playground, enabling good supervision. All moving equipment on the playground, such as swings, teeter-totters and merry-go-rounds, should be located toward a corner or edge of the playground or play area. Slide exits always should be located in an uncongested area of the playground to prevent possible collisions between children.

Poor or inadequate maintenance of playground equipment can lead to severe injuries on the playground. Because the safety of playground equipment and its stability depend on good inspection and maintenance, the manufacturers' maintenance instructions and recommended inspection schedules should be strictly followed and enforced. A comprehensive maintenance program should be developed for each playground. All equipment should be inspected frequently for any potential hazards, for corrosion or deterioration from rot, insects, or weathering. The playground also should be checked frequently for broken glass and other dangerous debris. Some manufacturers supply, with their maintenance instructions, a checklist for general or detailed inspections. These can be used to ensure that inspections are in compliance with the manufacturer's specifications.

Inspections alone do not constitute a comprehensive maintenance program. All hazards or defects identified during inspections should be repaired as quickly as possible using only replacement parts listed by or obtained from the manufacturer of the equipment. In addition to general maintenance inspections, more detailed inspections should be conducted on a regular basis depending upon the types and amount of equipment on the playground, level of use, local climate, and manufacturer's maintenance instructions.

Playground design and maintenance have improved significantly over the past 15 years, mainly because of the U.S. Consumer Product Safety Commission's (CPSC) publication of a *Handbook on Public Playground Safety*. Thanks to the CPSC guidelines, landscape architects and playground designers no longer are forced to rely solely on intuition and experience when trying to design and maintain a safe play environment. They also can follow specific guidelines for playground equipment established by the American Society of Testing Materials (ASTM) and be confident that new structures from top manufacturers will be unlikely to impale, entrap, cut, pinch, bruise, or otherwise cause serious injury to children. The discouraging side to playground safety is that not all playgrounds are inspected for safety, and few of the inspections that do occur are conducted by well-trained, certified environmental health and safety inspectors.

Equipment-Related Injuries

Approximately 170,000 children are injured on playgrounds throughout the United States each year. Most life-threatening injuries result from falls from equipment, impact with moving equipment, entanglement of clothing, and head entrapment. Many of these injuries can be prevented by the proper design and maintenance of playground facilities. The most common playground equipment-related dangers are as follows.

- *Pinch-crush parts.* Moving or sliding parts on equipment such as seesaws, gliders, and bending coiled springs can cause serious injury to extremities such as fingers and toes. When using these types of equipment, proper clothing (including shoes) should be worn at all times.
- *Rings.* When using this type of equipment, it must be the proper size. The ring should

be bigger than 5 to 10 inches in diameter so a child cannot get his or her head entrapped within the ring. Any ring smaller than the specified minimum size should be discarded immediately.

- *Hooks.* This type of equipment is shaped like a large metal S. Hooks usually are used for attaching chains to swing sets. Large, open-ended S-hooks are the most dangerous, as they can easily grab clothing or contribute to pinching or cutting. With these hooks, the ends of the S always should be squeezed together tightly, which usually can be done with some type of pliers. If this is not possible, the local gym-set dealer should be consulted.
- *Hard, heavy swing seats.* This type of equipment can strike a hard blow to a child's head, inflicting trauma. Features to look for when choosing a swing seat include: light weight, sturdy, round edges, and a grip on the seat. If purchasing a seat made of aluminum or other metal, it should have rolled edges.
- *Inadequate spacing.* When installing a gym set, the set should be a minimum of 6 feet from fences, building walls, walkways, and other play areas such as sand boxes. This allows a safe margin. Adequate spacing of equipment from playground boundaries also is highly advisable for playgrounds near busy streets.
- *Exposed screws and bolts.* Two of the most common injuries to children in the playground are cuts and bruises. An uncapped or unprotected protruding screw is often the offender. Unprotected screws should be covered immediately, either with tape or some type of rubber cap.
- *Hard surfaces.* A gym set never should be installed over a hard surface such as concrete, blacktop, or cinders. Grass, rubber, wood chips, and sand are always better alternatives.
- *Sharp edges.* Some gym sets have sharp edges or points where the parts fit together.

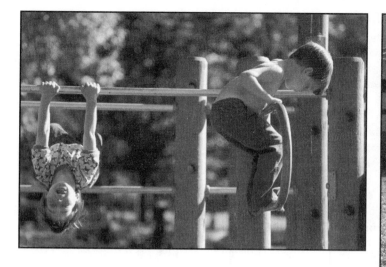

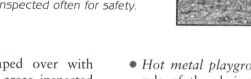

Playground equipment should be inspected often for safety.

These areas should be taped over with heavy tape, and the taped areas inspected regularly for weather damage.

- *Improper anchoring.* Legs of equipment should be set in concrete for stability. All types of anchoring devices should be placed below ground level to avoid a tripping hazard.

- *Strangulation hazard with playground cargo nets.* The U.S. Consumer Product Safety Commission advises parents to check outdoor play equipment featuring cargo nets before allowing children to play on them. Nets having openings with a perimeter length (sum of the length of the four sides) of between 17 and 28 inches could allow head entrapment and possible strangulation. The CPSC cites incidents at fast-food restaurants playgrounds where a child's head was entrapped and an adult had to cut the net to release the child.

- *Strings and strangulation.* Clothing strings, loose clothing, and stringed items placed around the neck can catch on playground equipment and strangle children. When children are playing, they should not be wearing these.

- *Hot metal playground equipment.* A good rule of thumb is to always check for hot surfaces on metal playground equipment before allowing children to play on it. Solid steel decks, slides, and steps in direct sunlight may reach temperatures high enough to cause serious contact-burn injuries in a matter of seconds. Typically affected are the hands, legs, and buttocks.

Playground Surfacing

The CPSC has estimated that approximately 100,000 playground equipment-related injuries resulting from falls to the (ground) surface are treated annually in U.S. hospital emergency rooms. This represents about 60% of all playground equipment-related injuries. Injuries resulting from falls to the ground are potentially fatal, especially when the head is involved. According to the CPSC, about three-fourths of all fall-related deaths involve head injuries.

Until 1981, the preferred playground surfaces were concrete, asphalt, and grass. Schools liked asphalt because it was considered to be softer than concrete and was easily maintained. There was nothing to track into the school building (like sand), and it needed no raking or care. In public parks, grass and hard dirt — the result of grass wearing away — were most commonly seen under playground equipment. Rubber mats soon became popular and were used in some settings; however, they were found to be too expensive for most municipalities and school systems. Sand and pea gravel were fairly inexpensive but required constant maintenance and replacement. Sand could be blown around and was tracked into schools, where it ruined the floors. Sand also attracted animals. Pea gravel could be thrown around and, if dispersed on concrete walks, could cause slip-and-fall accidents.

Not until 1986 did shock-absorbing surfaces with properties sufficient to reduce serious head injuries become the preferred playground surface. Regardless of the material chosen, however, the appropriate depth cannot be expected to prevent or reduce the severity of all injuries from falls. The term used to describe the shock-absorbing performance of a surfacing material is its "critical height."

Two basic groups of materials are acceptable for the surfacing of playgrounds: unitary and loose-fill.

1. *Unitary materials* are generally rubber mats or a combination of rubberlike materials held in place by a binder that may be poured in place at the playground site and cured to form a unitary shock-absorbing surface.

2. *Loose-fill materials* include, but are not confined to, sand, gravel, and shredded-wood products. These materials have acceptable shock-absorbing properties when installed over hard surfaces such as asphalt or concrete. Table 5.2 gives the appropriate depths of loose-fill materials and the critical heights at which the depths will be effective.

All playground supervisors should have a uniform method of reporting and documenting accidents that occur on the playground. Accident forms should include specific information including names and addresses of witnesses, how a particular piece of equipment was being used, and photographs of the accident site, if possible.

Play is critical to the physical and social development of children. Play apparatus alone does not make a playground a functional developmental area. For children to learn through recreation, properly planned programs with supervision — conducted specifically in a safe and healthy environment — are absolutely necessary.

SUMMARY

More Americans now are realizing the importance of recreational activities to good public

Material	Uncompressed Depth		Compressed Depth	
	6 in.	9 in.	12 in.	9 in.
Wood Mulch	7 ft	10 ft	11 ft	10 ft
Double Shredded Bark Mulch	6 ft	10 ft	11 ft	7 ft
Uniform Wood Chips	6 ft	7 ft	12 ft	6ft
Fine Sand	5 ft	5 ft	9 ft	5 ft
Coarse Sand	5 ft	5 ft	6 ft	4 ft
Fine Gravel	6 ft	7 ft	10 ft	6 ft
Medium Gravel	5 ft	5 ft	6 ft	5 ft

TABLE 5.2 Critical Heights (in feet) for Loose-Fill Material Depths (in inches)

Source: Consumer Product Safety Commission

Environmental Health

health. Recreational activities help to renew the mind and body and therefore contribute to mental, physical, and social well-being. Americans make an estimated 7.8 billion one-day visits each year to a variety of recreational areas, participating in numerous activities that involve manmade apparatus and natural environmental resources. Although recreational areas and activities can help to provide a relaxing and rejuvenating environment, they also present major environmental health and safety concerns.

Unintentional injuries and the spread of disease increase as recreational areas become more densely populated. Also, problems associated uniquely with recreational areas — remote locations, seasonal operations, water-oriented activities, vector and animal problems, noxious plants and weeds, age-specific activities, and many others — increase the need for improved environmental health and safety awareness in recreational areas. Many common environmental health and safety problems can be avoided if design, maintenance, and human control measures are strictly enforced. Finally, management of recreational areas must provide adequate staff training and give top priority to the principles and practices of maintaining a safe and healthful recreational environment.

REFERENCES

American Academy of Pediatrics Committee on Accident and Poison Prevention. 1988. Snowmobile statement. *Pediatrics*, vol. 82, pp. 798–799.

Berry, Dennis. 1989. *Pool Managers: Water Quality Handbook*. LaMotte Company, Chestertown, MD.

Carlson, Richard E., Theodore R. Deppe, Janet R. MacLean, and James A. Peterson. 1972. *Recreation and Leisure: The Changing Scene*, 3d ed. Wadsworth Publishing Company, Belmont, CA.

Centers for Disease Control and Prevention, 1995, February 27. Injuries Associated With the Use of Snowmobiles. *Journal of the American Medical Association*, pp. 448–449.

Christiansen, Monty L. 1995. *Playground Safety*. Center for Hospitality, Tourism and Recreation Research, University Park, PA.

Eriskine, A. L. 1970. The Epidemiology of Snowmobile Injuries. *Trauma*, vol. 10, p. 804.

Forgey, William W. 1985. *Death by Exposure*. ICS, Merrillville, IN.

Gabert, Thomas. 1993, December. Recreational Injuries and Deaths in Northern Wisconsin. *Wisconsin Medical Journal*, vol. 92, no. 12, pp. 671–675.

Greenberg, A. 1989, November. How Safe is Skiing? *Skiing*, pp 56–62.

Greenberg, A. 1989, Spring. Is Skiing Overrated? *Skiing*, pp. 12–14.

Hauser, Dan. 1995, Spring. Riding on Thin Ice. *Snowmobile*, p.5.

Johnson, Ralph L. 1994. *YMCA: Pool Operation Manual*, 2d ed. YMCA of the USA, Champaign, IL.

Johnson, Robert J., C. D. Mote Jr., and John Zelcer. 1993. *Skiing Trauma and Safety: Ninth International Symposium*. ASTM Publications, Philadelphia.

Jucker, Karl, Clayne R. Jensen, and Gary Howard. 1983. *Skiing*. Wm C. Brown, Dubuque, IA.

King, Steve, 1996. Prevent Playground Injuries with Professional Inspection. *Parks & Recreation*, vol. 31, n. 4, p. 62.

Koren, Herman, 1996. *Handbook of Environmental Health and Safety: Principles and Practices*, 3d ed. CRC Press, Boca Raton, FL.

Koren, Herman. 1996. *Illustrated Dictionary of Environmental Health and Occupational Safety*. CCR Press, Boca Raton, FL.

Lisella, Frank S. 1994. *VNR Dictionary of Environmental Health and Safety*. Van Nostrand Reinhold, New York.

Miller, Dean F. 1995. *Safety: Principles and Issues*. Brown & Benchmark Publishers, Dubuque, IA.

Moen, Carl. 1970. *Sports Safety*. Division of Safety Education, American Association for Health, Physical Education, and Recreation, Washington, DC.

Morgan, Monroe T. 1993. *Environmental Health*. Brown and Benchmark Publishers, Dubuque, IA.

Patton, Pettis L. 1996. *Urban Playgrounds: An Institution of Learning for Children. Parks & Recreation*, vol. 31, vol. 4, p. 68.

Pope, James R. 1985. *Public Swimming Pool Management: A Manual on Sanitation, Filtration, and Disinfection*. Clemson University, Clemson, SC.

Rea, Phillip S, and Roger Warren. 1986. *Recreation Management of Water Resources*, Publishing Horizons, Columbus, OH.

Salvato, Joseph A. 1992. *Environmental Engineering and Sanitation*, 4th ed. John Wiley and Sons, New York.

Teague, Travis, 1992. Playgrounds: Managing Your Risk. *Parks & Recreation*, vol. 31, no. 4, p. 54.

U. S. Public Health Service. *Environmental Health Practice in Recreational Areas*, PHS Publication No. 1195, Washington, DC.

U. S. Department of Agriculture. 1982. *Snow Avalanche: General Rules for Avoiding and Surviving Snow Avalanches*.

U. S. Department of Agriculture. 1994. *Snow Avalanches: Basic Principles for Avoiding and Surviving Snow Avalanches*.

U. S. Department of Health and Human Services. 1985. *Suggested Health and Safety Guidelines for Public Spas and Hot Tubs*.

U. S. Department of Health and Human Services. 1988. *Swimming Pools: Safety and Disease Control through Proper Design and Operation*.

Wallach, Fran. 1996. An Update on the Playground Safety Movement. *Parks & Recreation*, vol. 31, no. 4, p. 46.

Wilkerson, James A. 1988. *Hypothermia, Frostbite, and Other Cold Injuries*. Mountaineers, Seattle.

Willgoose, Carl E. 1979. *Environmental Health: Commitment for Survival*, W. B. Saunders, Philadelphia.

Wastewater Management

Key Terms

Aeration
Bar screen
Biochemical oxygen demand (BOD)
Box and can
Chemical oxygen demand (COD)
Comminuter
Digester

Dissolved oxygen (DO)
Evapotranspiration
Grinder
Grit chamber
NPDES
Non-point pollution
Pit privy

Primary clarifier
Settling basin
Sewage
Sludge
Storm sewer
Venturi meter
Wastewater stabilization pond

Objectives

🌐 Discuss the need for wastewater disposal.

🌐 Explain non-water-carried systems.

🌐 Define and explain individual water-carried systems.

🌐 Describe municipal wastewater treatment, its purpose, and its function.

🌐 Discuss the principles of water pollution.

The United States is the same size as it was in 1492. Lakes, rivers, and streams are the same size or smaller than when the country was discovered. The population has grown rapidly, however, spawning thermal, noise, air, and water pollution. Today the production of "necessities" and the nation's affluence have generated pollution at the point of production via the use and disposal of the materials generated to satisfy the public's desires.

Water pollution (anything in water that is not water) comes from industry, domestic units, agriculture, and natural sources. Some sources of natural pollution are volcanic ash, dust storms, trees, decomposing vegetation, eroded soil, and excrement.

Industrial plants release waste into the air, onto the land, and into the water. The water used in many industrial processes picks up forms of industrial waste that remain in the water as it is discharged into the environment. This waste can be chemical (organic or inorganic), such as mercury; physical, such as heat; or biological, such as microbes borne by employees working in the plant.

Domestic water pollution constitutes a big portion of the water pollution. Domestic waste consists of kitchen and bathroom waste from homes, schools, hospitals, nursing homes, and other places where people live, work, and travel.

Pesticides, herbicides, and fertilizers are major sources of agricultural waste. Precipitation sometimes washes these compounds into streams, rivers, lakes, and oceans. This is difficult to control because it is **non-point pollution**. Another example of non-point agricultural waste is livestock drinking, urinating, and defecating in ponds, lakes, and streams. In trying to reduce agricultural waste, we can reduce the required food supply if we make mistakes.

Natural sources of pollution include, among others, volcanic ash, dust storms, decomposing vegetation, and eroded soil. Efforts to reduce industrial and domestic water pollution concentrate on minimizing the use of materials that escape to the atmosphere and end up in water. These efforts are exerted mainly through industrial and domestic (city) wastewater treatment plants. In these plants much of the material (waste) that is not water is removed. Much

research is being done throughout the world to improve the technology for wastewater treatment.

The principle of wastewater treatment can be explained by simile. Assume that we run wastewater through a large pipe that has a filter in it, and assume that the filter excludes everything except the water (Figure 6.1). If that were possible, only pure water would flow out of the pipe after being filtered. Purification would be accomplished quickly and painlessly.

Human waste products are harmful to humans. In this chapter we will focus on some techniques of disposing of human urine and feces that are capable of spreading disease. Our concern is mainly the biological causative agents of disease.

Water is a natural resource that too often is taken for granted in human culture. Unlike many other consumer goods, water contaminated by human waste cannot be simply thrown away. Water containing human waste — termed **sewage** or **wastewater** — generally contains more than 99.9% water. The remaining less than 0.1% consists of the waste we remove from the water.

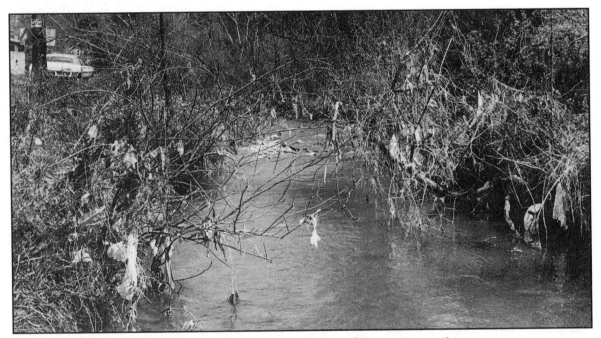

Solid waste adds to water pollution and aesthetic degradation of the environment.

Photo courtesy of East Tennessee State University

Environmental Health

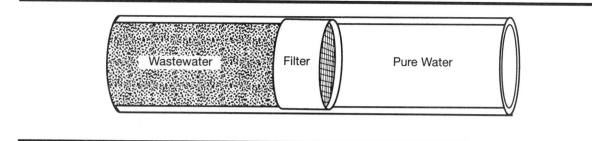

FIGURE 6.1 Hypothetical wastewater treatment system.

Every state in the United States has a law stating that human excrement must be disposed of in a sanitary manner. Reasons for sanitary disposal of wastewaters are to prevent the pollution of surface waters, the pollution of groundwater, and hookworm infestation by refraining from using human excrement as a fertilizer on vegetables and other foods. Further, wastewater should be disposed in a sanitary manner to prevent waste from being accessible to insects capable of transmitting disease, and for many other reasons.

Excreta disposal can be divided into two main types: non-water-carried and water-carried. We also can discuss wastewater disposal according to individual and municipal systems.

NON-WATER-CARRIED SYSTEMS

In many underdeveloped nations and in parts of the United States, dwellings are not equipped with indoor plumbing. If no water is entering the dwelling, no water is available to flush human waste away toward treatment. When these conditions are present, the best solution may be to install a **pit privy**, or pit latrine. An example is pictured.

The objective for pit construction, as it is for all disposal systems, is to construct an underground area where urine and feces can be deposited and retained in a sanitary manner. This means that the pit area is sufficiently above any water table, provides a self-closing door, and screens any openings, such as vents, which would allow access to flies or other vermin

capable of spreading disease. Thereafter, the waste is deposited directly into the pit. If and when the pit becomes full, the building housing it can be relocated to a new pit. The old pit must be covered with at least 18 inches of earth.

Another type of non-water-carried sewage system is the **box and can**. These systems may be found on buses, trains, airplanes, and construction sites, or any areas where people's

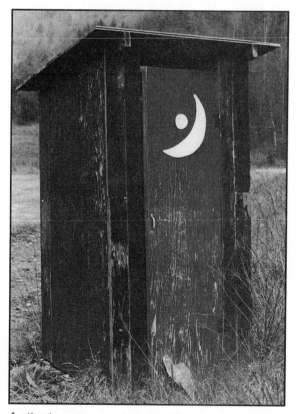

A pit privy.   Photo courtesy of East Tennessee State University

waste must be contained until it can be removed for treatment. The box and can disposal system is found virtually anywhere people gather without a water-carried sewage system. The units, often termed "portable toilets" or "port-a-john," have a self-contained, above-ground chamber to collect urine and feces. A liquid chemical often is added to the chamber to reduce odors, break down the waste, and serve as a disinfectant. The box and can system must be maintained by pumping the contents of the storage chamber as necessary and transporting the waste to an approved wastewater treatment facility.

INDIVIDUAL WATER-CARRIED SYSTEMS

Before purchasing a tract of land, numerous factors must be considered, the most important of which could be the capability of the soil to absorb water. If potable water is available for use within the dwelling, this water must undergo treatment after its use. In this case, no central sewage disposal system is provided; therefore, the property must be evaluated for an on-site, water-carried subsurface sewage disposal system — specifically a septic tank and drainfield system. In subdivisions, the system should be an interim expedient device until a central sewerage system is constructed. In many areas, however, a central sewer, or public sewer, may not be available for decades.

The function of a **septic tank and drainfield system** is to remove as many solids as possible from wastewater and filter this waste through the soil. In many cases, plants draw the wastewater from the soil by transpiration or the soil's capillary action pulls it to the surface in order that evaporation may occur, called **evapotranspiration.**

Soil Evaluation

A critical concern that must be considered prior to construction of any subsurface sewage disposal system is the soil's capacity to absorb the wastewater. Not all soils are capable of absorbing enough water to allow construction of a subsurface system. The health department environmentalist/sanitarian or a soil scientist evaluates the soil for appropriateness by use of (a) a percolation test, (b) soil maps, and/or (c) soil color and texture evaluation.

A percolation test involves digging a hole of a specified diameter to a typical depth of approximately 36 inches (90 cm). The hole is filled with water and allowed to presoak or saturate for a time dependent upon the soil type, generally overnight. After saturation of the soil, the hole is filled with water to a designated level. The depth of the water in the hole is measured at regular time intervals to determine how many minutes are required for 1 inch of water to exit the hole. As a result, a percolation rate, in minutes per inch, is established.

For example, if it took 1 hour for the water to lower an inch, the percolation rate would be 60 minutes/inch (24 min./cm). If the level of water in the hole lowered 1 inch (2.5 cm) in 10 minutes, the percolation rate would be 10 minutes/inch (10 minutes/2.5 cm). The faster the percolation rate — the less time (minutes) required to drop an inch of water in the percolation hole — the better is the percolation rate. Generally speaking, soils with a percolation rate of 60 minutes per inch (2.5 cm) or greater are not acceptable for constructing a conventional drainfield system. The percolation rate also is a factor in determining the size of the drainfield. The smaller the percolation rate, the less drainfield required. Absorption-area requirements for private residences with a disposal and washing machine are given in Table 6.1.

Soil maps also can be helpful when determining percolation rates. Upon knowing the exact location of the tract of land in question, the evaluator may refer to soil maps that tell specific soil types, textures, and applications for the area. These maps provide a general indication of the area considered for a drainfield. A more thorough evaluation may be accomplished by conducting a soil color, structure, and texture evaluation in the exact area of the drainfield.

Environmental Health

TABLE 6.1 Absorption-Area Requirements for Private Residences (Provides for Garbage-Grinder and Automatic-Sequence Washing Machines)

Percolation rate (time required for water to fall 1 inch, in minutes)	Required absorption area, in square feet per bedroom,[1] standard trench,[2] and seepage pits[3]	Percolation rate (time required for water to fall 1 inch, in minutes)	Required absorption area, in square feet per bedroom,[1] standard trench,[2] and seepage pits[3]
1 or less	70	10	165
2	85	15	190
3	100	30[4]	250
4	115	45[4]	300
5	125	60[4,5]	330

1. In every case, sufficient area should be provided for at least two bedrooms.
2. Absorption area for standard trenches is figured as trench-bottom area.
3. Absorption area for seepage pits is figured as effective side-wall area beneath the inlet.
4. Unsuitable for seepage pits if over 30.
5. Unsuitable for leaching systems if over 60.

Source: Manual of Septic Tank Practice. U.S. Public Health Service.

For a soil evaluation, an evaluator bores holes with a soil auger and observes the color, structure, and texture of the soil to a desired depth. Generally speaking, brighter colored soils, as well as soils with greater amounts of sand or loam, tend to be better drained. Through knowledge of soils, an environmentalist/sanitarian or soil scientist can often estimate a percolation rate. Of the three types of evaluations, the percolation test is most accurate.

Before installing a subsurface sewage system, additional factors must be considered. The area must be evaluated to locate any natural drainageways, because it is not desirable to have surface water flowing over the absorption field area. The drainfield area should be located at an adequate distance (generally 100 feet) from bodies of water, water supplies, dwellings, property lines, underground utility lines, and the like. The amount of water used within a day's time must be considered before designing and installing the system. A dwelling with eight people certainly will use more water than a dwelling with two people. Therefore, the dwelling with eight would require a larger drainfield area to absorb the excess water used.

The sanitarian/environmentalist designs the on-site wastewater disposal system according to the specific properties of the evaluation. In most areas the city issues a permit before any construction can begin. The permit specifies the disposal system design. Once installed, the sanitarian/environmentalist inspects the system before the septic tank and absorption trenches are backfilled. The inspection ensures quality control and determines if the installation has been done in accordance with applicable regulations (as specified by the health department).

Septic Tank System

Now let's trace a drop of water from the dwelling through a typical septic tank and drainfield system (Figure 6.2). From a plumbing fixture such as the kitchen sink, water drains through a U-trap. The U-trap's function is to collect water, forming a barrier against gases backing up into the house from the sewer system. From the U-trap the flow continues through a pipe out of the house and into the house sewer line.

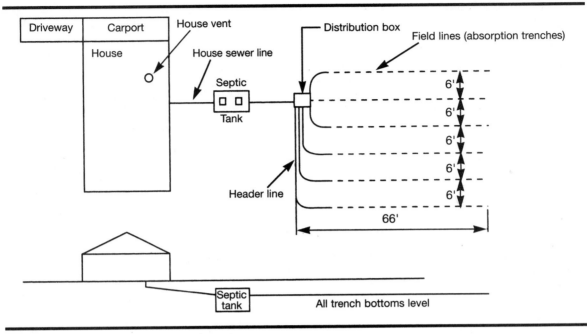

FIGURE 6.2 Layout of septic tank system.

The house sewer line must have sufficient diameter and slope to allow an unrestricted flow of sewage. From this point the flow continues directly into the underground septic tank. As the water enters the septic tank, the influent is diverted downward by an inlet tee. The inlet tee serves two functions: (a) it diverts the solids in the wastewater toward the bottom of the septic tank, and (b) it allows gases to back up into the household sewer line and exit through a vent. The vent, located on the houses's roof, helps the wastewater to flow freely through the plumbing. It also vents into the atmosphere gases produced in the septic tank and avoids loss of water seals by siphoning.

The septic tank itself is a large chamber that is generally rectangular in shape. The tank's length is usually twice the width. The volume of individual septic tanks varies, but the tank itself should be large enough to allow the wastewater a retention time of at least 24 hours.

The septic tank (see Figure 6.3) serves three main functions:

1. It is a settling basin for removal of solids as sludge.

2. It stores the settled sludge and scum until the waste can be removed mechanically.

3. It provides a chamber for biological decomposition.

The biological activity is anaerobic, producing the gases carbon dioxide (CO_2), hydrogen sulfide (H_2S), and methane CH_4), as well as water (H_2O). The gases rise from the septic tank back into the household sewer line and out the vent. The heavier materials — those denser than water — settle to the bottom of the septic tank and produce a sludge. The solid materials — less dense than water — float to the top of the wastewater, producing a scum layer. The objective is to allow water to flow from the septic tank with as many solids removed as possible, and with the scum also removed.

The effluent from the septic tank usually flows through a header line and into the distribution box, if present. The function of a distribution box is to collect the wastewater and distribute it evenly into each of the absorption trenches. Many current designs do not use distribution boxes. If no distribution box is used,

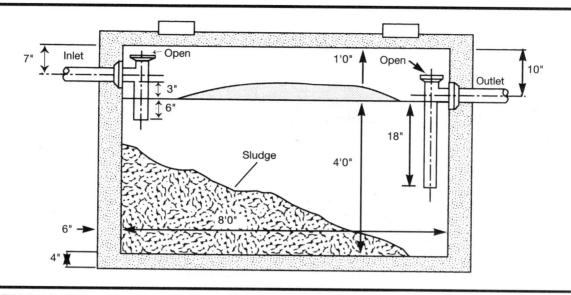

FIGURE 6.3 Septic tank.

the water simply flows directly through header lines into the drainfield or the absorption trench. This is accomplished by the old maxim of water seeking its own level.

If the distribution box is used, the water flows through the sealed lines directly into the absorption trenches. Header lines to the absorption trenches are adjusted to the height of the water in the distribution box, thereby producing an equal flow to each trench (see Figure 6.2). Once the water reaches the trenches, it is evenly distributed by way of drainage tile or percolation pipe (drainfield pipe). In some areas drainfield tile is required. Other areas require a plastic pipe that comes in 10 feet, (3.04 m) or greater lengths, or may even be continuous. This pipe is constructed with holes to allow the wastewater to flow out of the pipe and into the absorption trenches.

Absorption trenches are dug to a predetermined depth, generally about 36 inches, to absorb the wastewater. The tile, or percolation pipe is placed over 6 inches of gravel below, and 2 inches of gravel are placed above (Figure 6.4). Generally, this (including the 5" pipe) should total approximately 13 inches (32.5 cm) of gravel. The gravel should be clean and free of

any fine particles because its void spaces serve as a storage reservoir for excess wastewater until it is absorbed into the ground (see Figure 6.5). Most of the wastewater in a traditional system will be absorbed by the soil in the absorption trenches; the rest evapotranspires.

Let us consider the possible fates of a pathogenic organism as it is transported through such a system. It may settle with the sludge in the septic tank and become food for other microorganisms. If a pathogen is not destroyed by microorganisms or the anaerobic environment in the septic tank, however, it may be passed to the absorption trenches. In the trenches, the soil should have the capability to trap any pathogens as the wastewater percolates through. Subsurface wastewater systems should not be installed in areas of fractured rock. Unlike soil, this rock does not have the capability to filter pathogens from the wastewater, thereby contributing to groundwater contamination.

Some drainfield systems are constructed without distribution boxes. An example is the serial (or hump) system shown in Figures 6.6 and 6.7. In this system all of the wastewater initially flows into the first trench. The water rises

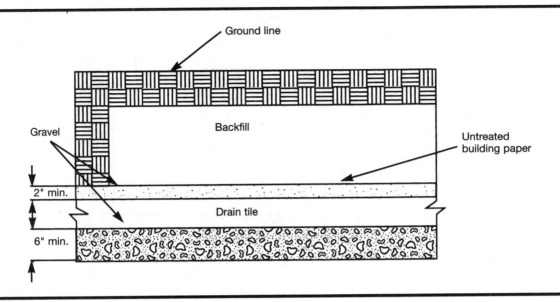

FIGURE 6.4 Lateral view through trench.

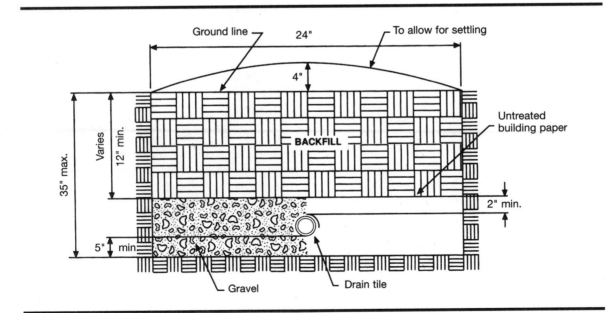

FIGURE 6.5 In-view of a drainfield line.

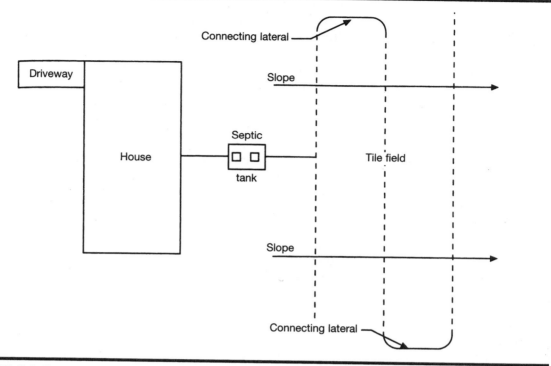

FIGURE 6.6 Field layout for serial system (home system).

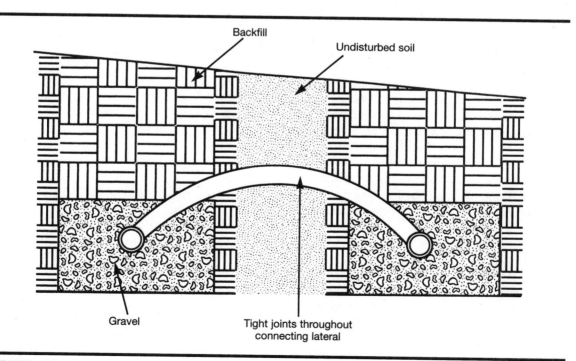

FIGURE 6.7 Serial (hump) system: Section of connecting lateral.

in the trench continually until it reaches the level of a preinstalled "crow over" pipe. This pipe collects the water and carries it to another trench, where the water is absorbed. The backfill in the trenches pulls the water toward the surface by capillary action. As the wastewater gets closer to the ground's surface, plants consume it and the sun evaporates it. Thus, evapotranspiration plays an important role in the serial system.

Seepage pits are used in some areas. They are deep, possibly 10 feet (3.04 m) or more, and are designed to go down until reaching the good soil. A seepage pit typically is 10 feet (3.04 m) wide, 10 feet (3.04 m) long, and 10 feet (3.04 m) deep, with 8 feet (2.40 m) of gravel in it. The void spaces in the gravel hold the wastewater during times of high use for later percolation into the ground. Seepage pits include a septic tank and possibly a distribution box. Various states have several approved types of individual sewage disposal systems.

MUNICIPAL WASTEWATER TREATMENT

Physical, chemical, and biological treatment processes all have been used in wastewater treatment, although modern treatment of municipal wastewater usually involves biological processes. Essentially, the wastewater treatment plant provides a controlled environment that enhances the growth of certain microorganisms that adsorb and metabolize constituents of the waste. General requirements for the growth of microorganisms are described in Chapter 2.

Wastewater treatment processes are either aerobic or anaerobic. The aerobic process is used most frequently. The widely used activated sludge process exemplifies modern aerobic wastewater treatment. Sufficient air has to be forced into liquid in the aeration tank to maintain treatment effectiveness and prevent the unpleasant odors generated by the aerobic processes. Various other conditions — including pH and temperature — must be maintained at levels suitable for microorganisms.

Here we will describe biological filtration, generally in trickling filters or biological towers. Although used less than in the past, biological filtration lends itself well to an introductory discussion of wastewater treatment.

The Process

Wastewater can be collected and treated on a large scale by municipal wastewater treatment facilities. The flow through a conventional wastewater treatment plant looks like this:

Sanitary Sewer → Bar Screen → Grit Basin → Grinder → Primary Clarifier → Activated Sludge or Trickling Filter → Secondary Clarifier → Chlorine Basin → Stream

The wastewater exits a dwelling just as it does with the septic tank system, through the house sewer line. From the house sewer, the wastewater flows into a domestic or sanitary sewer. The sanitary sewer system consists of a series of pipes that collect the wastewater. This collection system transports the waste to a wastewater treatment plant.

Another type of sewer, the storm sewer, can be found in many areas. Unlike the sanitary sewer, the storm sewer collects surface runoff only from rainwater; it does not collect domestic waste. The storm sewer water should not flow into a wastewater treatment plant, nor should it be connected to the sanitary sewer at any point.

As the wastewater enters the treatment plant via the sanitary sewer, it flows through a **bar screen**, which strains out large materials that may damage the treatment plant. The individual bars are located about 2 inches (5.1 cm) apart to remove floating sticks and other large objects. The bar screen can be cleaned and waste taken to a landfill.

From the bar screen the flow continues into a grit basin or chamber. Until now water has flowed rapidly through the pipe. As the wastewater enters the **grit chamber**, however, the rate of flow slows as the water is spread over a large area. The purpose of the grit chamber is to slow down the water just enough to allow time for heavy particles, such as grit, sand, and other dense materials, to settle out. The settled materials are removed and taken to a landfill. The lighter materials in the wastewater, unable to settle in the grit chamber, travel through a comminuter or grinder. This unit grinds up the large solids to prepare them for digestion by microorganisms in the treatment plant.

The flow may proceed through a **venturi meter**, a device for measuring the rate of flow through the treatment plant, and then the **primary clarifier**. This clarifier, also called a settling basin, allows materials to settle out. In a circular tank, the water enters through the center of the clarifier and moves outward slowly, exiting by overflowing around the rim of the unit.

The water moves slowly enough through the clarifier to allow a large amount of suspended solids to accumulate on the bottom, producing **sludge**. Machines scrape this sludge from the bottom of the clarifier and pump it away. A scum layer forms on top of the clarifier. As with sludge, a machine scrapes the scum off, feeds it into a hopper, and pumps it to a sludge treatment processor.

One type of processor is a digester. The effluent from the primary clarifier enters activated sludge tanks or a trickling filter. Trickling filters are large and have a medium of rocks about the size of a fist, or a synthetic material, with a depth of about 7 feet (2.1 m). The water enters the trickling filter through large arms that spray and distribute the wastewater evenly over the surface of the filter. Numerous biological organisms grow on these rocks. As the wastewater flows down through the rocks, the organisms on the rocks metabolize many of the suspended solids that were not settled in the primary clarifier. This process is much more effective if the rocks are kept wet at all times. Hence, the water is recycled in periods of low wastewater flow to create a high-rate trickling filter.

Materials continue to build up on these rocks and eventually slough off. The trickling filter is not actually a physical filter but, rather, an area of biological decomposition. The activated sludge tank serves the same purpose as the trickling filter — to remove waste from the wastewater.

Aeration tank digestion is also called the **activated sludge process**. Effluent from primary treatment is pumped into the tank and mixed with a bacteria-rich slurry. Air of pure oxygen pumped through the mixture encourages bacterial growth and decomposition of the organic material. Water is siphoned off the top of the tank, and sludge is removed from the bottom.

The water collected at the bottom of the trickling filter flows into a secondary clarifier, moving just as it does through the primary clarifier. The secondary clarifier settles any remaining suspended solids. These solids are collected and pumped into the digester.

The effluent from the secondary clarifier should be clear by this point. Before being discharged into a stream, this effluent is chlorinated and often aerated. As the water enters the stream, it is free of most causative agents of disease.

The Digester

Recall that all of the sludge and scum collected in the clarifiers and trickling filter is pumped into a digester. The **digester** is a large sealed unit where anaerobic decomposition takes place. The sludge and scum provide food for the decomposition. Metabolization of these organic materials produces methane (CH_4), hydrogen sulfide (H_2S), and carbon dioxide (CO_2). Water (H_2O) is also a product of this metabolism.

The gases are collected and processed to produce a gas that can be readily burned. The gas, mainly methane, then can be used to heat the digesters, as well as buildings at the wastewater treatment plant and even homes and businesses. During periods of the year when heating is not required, the gas can be bottled and stored for later usage.

The sludge is stored in the digester and subjected to anaerobic decomposition for a specified time. After sufficient decomposition, the sludge is pumped out of the digester and into sludge-drying beds. The drying beds, composed of sand, are flooded with approximately 6 inches (15 cm) of wet sludge. The sludge is mainly liquid at this point. The sun evaporates the water, leaving behind a quantity of material that dries, cracks, and rolls up. You may have seen dried mud after a flash flood, where it cracks and rolls up. The sludge appears similar to that. The sludge generally takes two or three weeks to dry. Once dried, it is collected and transported to fill in eroded fields and pastures or composted.

Quality Control

Recall that 70% to 80% of all pathogens are aerobic. This sludge has just spent approximately 60 days in the anaerobic environment of the digester. Pathogenic aerobes cannot survive such stressful conditions, and they die off. As a result, the sludge is improved in sanitary quality but it still is not fully safe. It should not be applied to areas where the public gathers, such as playgrounds, football fields, and the like, or to soil growing vegetables that will be eaten raw.

Many other wastewater treatment processes — activated sludge, rotating biological contactors, contact aeration — are used in municipal and package treatment plants. Activated sludge has become more common than trickling filters in new construction. No matter what the complexity of the chemistry or physics, the objective is the same: to remove the less than 0.1% of waste dissolved in the more than 99.9% aqueous medium.

Now the question may arise: Is the effluent leaving the wastewater treatment plant and entering a river or stream free of pathogens? Some pathogens may settle out in the grit basin or in the primary clarifier, either by settling to the bottom as sludge or by floating to the surface as scum. In these cases the pathogens are transported to the digester and subjected to an anaerobic environment. Other pathogens may be passed over in the primary clarifier and trapped in the trickling filter, where they become food for other microorganisms. If some pathogens manage to escape the trickling filter, they may settle out in the secondary clarifier, where they will be subjected to the fate of the anaerobic digester. If pathogens manage to survive all of these processes, they will be passed on to the chlorine basin. In this basin, chlorine destroys the hazardous microorganisms. At this point the treated effluent from the wastewater plant is microbiologically safe to discharge into a river or stream.

Wastewater treatment plants have a quality control laboratory, in which tests are run on the affluent and the effluent. Some tests run on wastewater are the dissolved oxygen (DO), biological oxygen demand (BOD), settlable solids, and chemical oxygen demand COD).

A permit system under NPDES (National Pollutant Discharge Eliminations Systems), was established to control wastewater discharges. Publicly owned utilities and industries both are required to obtain permits to discharge pollutants to surface waters. The purpose is to ensure that existing treatment plants comply with effluent limitations and performance standards, and that new plants have the best available technology and operating methods. The program also includes requirements for monitoring and reporting discharges and requires adequate funding and staffing with qualified personnel.

Effluent quality rules and regulations of the Environmental Protection Agency describe the minimum level of effluent quality that secondary treatment must attain under the NPDES. Acceptable secondary effluent is commonly defined in terms of BOD, suspended solids, fecal coliform bacteria, and pH. For BOD, the arithmetic mean of the values for effluent samples collected in a period of thirty consecutive days must not exceed 30 milligrams per liter, and the arithmetic mean of values in any period of seven consecutive days must not exceed 45 milligrams per liter.

Dissolved Oxygen (DO)

In liquid wastes, dissolved oxygen (DO) is the factor that determines whether the biological changes are brought about by aerobic or by anaerobic organisms. Aerobic action is associated with desirable conditions and anaerobic action as being undesirable because of the foul odors it produces, such as hydrogen sulfide. Both types of organisms are everywhere in nature, so conditions favorable to the aerobic action (aerobic conditions) must be maintained; otherwise the anaerobic organisms will take over and nuisance conditions will develop. Thus, dissolved-oxygen measurements are important for maintaining aerobic conditions in natural waters that receive potentially polluting materials and in aerobic treatment processes intended to purify domestic and industrial wastewaters.

One of the most important single tests, dissolved-oxygen determination, is used for a wide variety of purposes. For example, dissolved oxygen is necessary to support normal populations of fish and other aquatic organisms. This requires the presence of dissolved-oxygen levels that support the desired aquatic life in healthy condition at all times.

Determinations of dissolved oxygen serve as the basis of the BOD test. Thus, they are the foundation of the most important determination used to evaluate the pollutional strength of domestic and industrial waste. The rate of biochemical oxidation is measured by determining residual dissolved-oxygen in a stream at various time intervals.

Biochemical Oxygen Demand (BOD)

Biochemical oxygen demand (BOD) usually is defined as the amount of oxygen microorganisms require while stabilizing decomposable organic matter under aerobic conditions. The term "decomposable" means that the organic matter serves as food for bacteria, and energy is derived from the oxidation process. The test is one of the most important in stream pollution control activities. The BOD test is essentially a bioassay procedure that measures oxygen consumed by living organisms (mainly bacteria) while utilizing the organic matter present in a waste, under conditions as similar as possible to those that occur in nature. Care must be taken in running the BOD test because, for example, if additional air is introduced, the results will not

be correct. If the temperature is not 20° C — which is, more or less, a medium value as far as natural bodies of water are concerned — the test will not be correct. The organisms used to break down organic matter and the organisms in this test utilizing the oxygen are native to the soil. Generally, a 5-day BOD test is used in environmental monitoring.

Chemical Oxygen Demand (COD)

The **chemical oxygen demand (COD)** test is used widely as a means of measuring the pollutional strength of domestic and industrial waste. This test allows measurement of waste in terms of the total quantity of oxygen required for oxidation to carbon dioxide and water. It is based upon the fact that all organic compounds, with a few exceptions, can be oxidized by the acts of a strong oxidizing agent under acid conditions. During the determination of the COD, organic matter is converted to carbon dioxide and water regardless of the biological assimilability of the substances.

COD values are greater than BOD values — and may be much greater when significant amounts of biologically resistant organic matter is present. Hence, when running the BOD and COD on a sample, COD results are expected to be higher. The COD test is limited in that it is unable to differentiate biologically oxidizable and biologically inert organic matter. In addition, it does not provide any evidence of the rate at which the biologically active materials would be stabilized under conditions that exist in nature. The results of the dissolved oxygen test, BOD test, and COD test are all reported in milligrams per liter.

Wastewater Stabilization Ponds

Many small communities simply cannot afford the initial construction, continuous maintenance, and operation of a conventional wastewater treatment plant. In these areas the wastewater may be produced primarily in homes and small businesses and thereby are void of any significant industrial waste. Circumstances such as this usually are ideal for the installation of a wastewater stabilization pond.

A **wastewater stabilization pond** is engineered to utilize biological decomposition as a means of wastewater disposal. A wastewater stabilization pond looks similar to a large pond or a small lake. The wastewater stabilization pond is generally rectangular or oval in shape, the banks dropping sharply into the water. The size of the ponds varies. Those designed to treat large volumes of water are generally larger than those designed to treat smaller volumes. The depth of the pond often is around 4 feet and should be constant over the entire area.

Once the pond is filled and in operation, microbiological decomposition of the waste occurs. The wastewater is simply piped into the pond at a location and depth where water movement through the pond causes breakup of floating solids. This condition creates an extended detention time of the wastewater, allowing many solids to settle to the bottom of the pond. These organic solids serve as food for microorganisms. There is often a large volume of these solids on the bottom, which results in an accelerated rate of microbial decomposition. As the microbes feed rapidly on this matter, they reproduce continuously, eventually depleting the oxygen supply at the bottom of the pond. This creates an anaerobic environment. This anaerobic environment is limited to only the bottom half of the pond. At the top half an aerobic environment still exists.

Because the majority of the solids have settled to the bottom of the pond, there is not as much organic matter available for decomposition in the upper half. Therefore, the microbes in the upper half do not have to work as hard metabolizing the waste and do not require as much oxygen — although abundant oxygen is introduced from the atmosphere by diffusion, and from small plants and algae by photosynthesis. On the bottom, waste products from the anaerobic microbes will be released. These include carbon dioxide (CO_2), hydrogen sulfide (H_2S), and methane (CH_4). As these gases rise from the bottom toward the surface, the aerobic organisms use them in the upper half of the pond.

OIL SPILLS

With the increased need for energy, particularly oil, accidents that spill oil into the environment are becoming more frequent. Although oil spill clean-up technology is increasing, oil companies and transporters of oil should be required to research and implement improved, safer means of transporting oil.

The waste entering a stabilization pond should be limited to only those materials that can be degraded — those that provide food for microorganisms. Toxic materials with the capacity to kill the microorganisms should not be discharged to this type of sewage treatment facility.

The wastewater in the pond is subjected to evaporation as well as percolation (usually minimal) into the soil beneath. The remaining water exits the pond via an effluent pipe that controls the maximum water level. The maximum volume of the pond is set, and introducing new wastewater may cause the pond to overflow into the effluent pipe. Though it has a high chlorine demand, this effluent may be chlorinated, then discharged into a moving surface water supply.

Wastewater stabilization ponds should be maintained continuously by controlling excessive plant and algae growth. This keeps the areas around the banks well groomed and monitors the effluent to assure adequate disinfection.

SUMMARY

To protect the health of the public, every state requires that human waste (urine and feces) be disposed of in an approved sanitary manner. Water pollution from excreta is of particular concern because it provides a favorable environment for disease-causing organisms. Knowing the point of origin is helpful. More difficult is non-point pollution, such as that introduced by pesticides, herbicides, and fertilizers from agricultural waste.

Human waste disposal systems can be classified as non water-carried and water-carried. The former are exemplified by the pit privy and the box and can. Individual water-carried systems generally consist of a septic tank and drainfield.

The location of a subsurface sewage disposal system must be predicated on a soil evaluation, a percolation test, soil maps, and evaluation of soil color and texture. Modern municipal wastewater treatment plants usually use biological processes, which encourage the growth of microorganisms that render waste constituents harmless. Wastewater treatment is either aerobic or anaerobic, of which the former is used most often, particularly an activated sludge process and biological filtration.

REFERENCES

Hammer, Mark. 1986. *Water and Wastewater Technology*. 2d ed. John Wiley and Sons, New York.

Issac-Renton, Judith. "Longitudinal Studies of Giardia Contamination in Two Community Drinking Water Supplies: Cyst Levels, Parasite Viability, and Health Impact." *Applied and Environmental Microbiology*. Jan 1996. v. 62 n. 1. pp. 47.

National Environmental Health Association. 1979. *On-Site Wastewater Management*. Denver.

Rhyner, Charles R., et al. 1995. *Waste Management and Resource Recovery*. CRC, Boca Raton, FL.

Saluate, Joseph A., Jr. 1972. *Environmental Engineering and Sanitation*. 2d ed. John Wiley and Sons, New York.

Sawyer, Clair N., and Perry L. McCarty. 1994. *Chemistry for Environmental Engineering*. 3d ed. McGraw-Hill Book Company, New York.

Silverstein, Kenneth. "Everything in the Kitchen Sink (nonpoint pollution threatens city water supplies)." *American City & County*. March 1994. v. 109 n. 3. pp. 26.

U. S. Public Health Service. 1967. *Manual of Septic Tank Practice*. U. S. Government Printing Office. Washington, DC.

Vesilind, Arne. 1996. *Environmental Engineering*. PWS Publishing, Boston.

Solid and Hazardous Waste Management

Key Terms

Ashes
Autoclaving
CERCLA
Composting
Corrosive
Deep wells

Energy recovery
Garbage
Ignitable
Incineration
Reactive
Refuse

Rubbish
Secure landfill
Sanitary landfill
Superfund
Toxic
Waste to energy (WTE)

Objectives

- Identify the classifications of solid waste.
- Explain the storage of waste.
- Describe the collection of solid waste.
- Discuss the history of solid waste management and evaluate the various methods.
- Discuss the need for recycling.
- Explain the transportation of hazardous waste.
- Identify and explain hazardous waste disposal.

Ecosystems are sustainable because they dispose of waste and replenish nutrients by recycling all elements. Cavemen and early civilizations did not have a problem with waste because it consisted mainly of organic waste and the decomposers converted it into useful materials. Also, there were few people, and they generated little waste. The problem became large with more people generating more and a variety of waste — chemical, liquid, solid, nuclear, and hazardous. Little of this waste is food for the decomposers. Thus, a variety of methods must be used to manage the waste.

Until relatively recently, solid waste was dumped, buried, or burned, and some of the garbage was fed to animals. The public was not aware of the links of refuse to rats, flies, roaches, mosquitoes, fleas, land pollution, and water pollution. People did not know that the solid waste in open dumps and backyard incinerators supported vectors of diseases including typhoid fever, endemic typhus fever, yellow fever, dengue fever, malaria, cholera, and others. Thus, the cheapest, quickest, and most convenient means of disposing of the waste were used. Rural areas and small towns utilized the open dump or backyard incinerator. Larger towns and cities used municipal incinerators. Later, landfilling became the method of choice for disposing of solid waste.

As people became more affluent and demanded greater convenience, the "single service-era" began. With it came a drastic increase in the amount of waste generated. The increase in waste per person, plus more and more people — with these same people needing the land for homes, shopping centers, roads, parking lots, and so on, — led to a shortage of land suitable for landfills. New York City sent a large load of "garbage" on a "cruise." New York sent a boxcar of garbage to Kansas City and, later, Wisconsin, where these areas refused to dispose of it at any price.

In the 1950s, solid waste could be buried in a sanitary landfill for 75¢ per ton. Now costs start at $25 per ton in small towns and $100 per ton in densely populated areas such as New Jersey. With more people and more waste, the problem has reached a critical point in many areas of the United States.

We would not be in this mess if in the past solid waste had been viewed as a resource rather than something of no value. Future generations may look at the old landfills as "resource centers." Now, as we approach the 21st century, we realize our past mistakes and are taking a new look at "garbage." Contrary to the practices of open dumping, burning, or burying waste, solid waste "disposal" methods must change.

CLASSIFICATION OF SOLID WASTE

The United States is a "throw away society." We use many materials for a short time and then dispose of them. Think about the last time you visited a fast-food restaurant. Your hamburger was wrapped in paper or boxed in a container. After the meal, you likely threw away these wrappings along with your paper cup and napkins. The car you drove home from the restaurant will wear out eventually and it will be thrown away also. These are typical examples of the increasing amount of solid waste that humans generate. Americans now generate more than 190 million tons of solid waste a year (see Figure 7.1). That's more than 1,000 pounds of trash per person per year, and it is projected to increase by 20% per year by the year 2000.

The solid waste products generated by humans can be divided into two general categories: **refuse** and larger items (such as old cars, trains, and refrigerators) that are not disposed of easily. Refuse is composed of garbage, rubbish, and ashes. **Garbage** is the organic putrescible matter from scraps of food, not only from

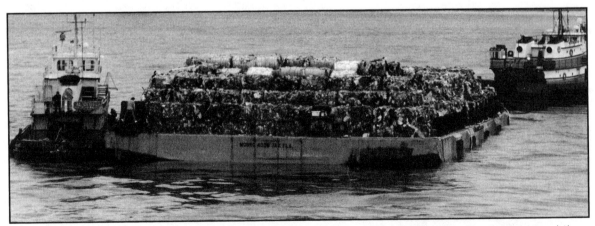

The garbage barge Mobro traveled on a 6-month odyssey of more than 6,000 miles, to six states and three other countries, before it found a home in New York, where it came from!

Environmental Health

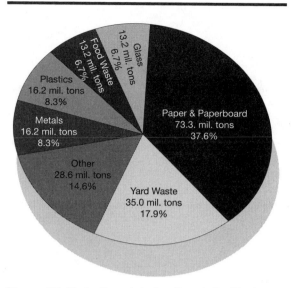

Source: EPA Waste Characterization Report, Franklin Assoc., 1992

FIGURE 7.1 Total waste generation in United States, 1990 (195.7 million tons before recycling).

the table but also during the growth and harvest of food on the farm and its transportation and storage.

When you buy sealed and packaged food from the grocery store and remove the food from its packages and prepare it, you produce two types of refuse. One is garbage, or food scraps, and the other is rubbish from the container. **Rubbish** is the combustible and noncombustible solid waste generated from people's activities. It includes waste such as paper, plastic bags, beverage cans, yardwork trimmings, and many other materials. Most of the solid waste generated in the United States is in the form of rubbish.

Ashes, another form of refuse, are combusted materials that someone has burned to total breakdown. A person often can dump these relatively inert ashes onto the surface of the ground with few problems. Other forms of refuse may not be handled and disposed of as conveniently. Solid waste that is handled improperly can provide a breeding ground for

insects and rodents. These pests can become annoying, frightening, and, most important, may spread disease to humans.

A comprehensive solid waste management program encompasses the storage, collection, and disposal of solid waste. Proper management in these three areas helps greatly in controlling insects and rodents.

STORAGE OF SOLID WASTE

A home may contain several types of solid waste receptacles. People put small wastepaper baskets in bathrooms and bedrooms. They put larger, covered containers in the kitchen to collect the garbage and rubbish from food preparation. Some people equip their homes with mechanical devices that compact waste into a storage receptacle. Others use still larger solid waste receptacles outside the dwelling to serve as a central storage point. Most homes use 20- or 30-gallon garbage cans that must be fly-tight and noncorrosive and are of sufficient number to store all of the solid waste generated until it is collected. Where recycling is practiced, receptacles are changed to accommodate recycling.

Larger facilities such as multi-dwelling units, businesses and industries may use large-volume, non-compacting, bulk receptacles, commonly termed "dumpsters." Many rural areas use these centrally located, large-volume receptacles as a temporary means of storage. The residents in these areas simply bring their waste to the large receptacles, the contents of which are later transported to a disposal area.

COLLECTION OF SOLID WASTE

Solid waste should be collected a minimum of once per week, and preferably twice per week. The collection frequency is based on the life cycle of the house fly. Under ideal conditions, a house fly develops from an egg into an adult in 8 days. These flies breed in refuse. Collecting and disposing of the solid waste within 8 days, interrupts the flies' life cycle. By collecting

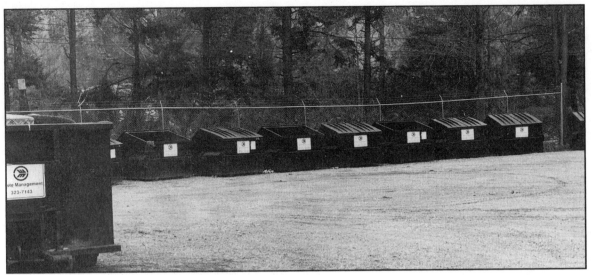

A rural community refuse collection center may look like this.

refuse in a timely manner, people can control fly populations to a large extent. Waste also provides food and harborage for other insects, as well as rodents capable of transmitting diseases to humans. Combustible materials, too, may build up and increase the chances of fire.

Home collection of solid waste generally is done by a private collector or a local government-owned and financed operation. Private collectors usually charge a fee to each individual homeowner, or a government contract will pay the fees. The government contract enables solid waste collection in a uniform, sanitary manner. Without such a contract, some individuals may be reluctant to pay the collector for the service and the refuse may go uncollected.

Many cities and towns require homeowners to use certain types of receptacles. Collectors usually pick up at the curb in front of the dwelling. In some neighborhoods the collectors pick up the receptacles in the backyard, as the people who live there consider receptacles too bulky to handle and unsightly in front of dwelling.

The solid waste collection vehicle should be covered and able to compact the refuse collected. It may load from the rear, side, or top. The storage areas in these vehicles should be kept relatively clean and water-tight.

Some hog-feeding operations collect only garbage. The collectors often heat garbage to 212°F for 30 minutes to kill any infectious microorganisms before farmers feed it to their livestock. If farmers feed uncooked garbage to their hogs, trichinosis is one disease that may result.

SOLID WASTE MANAGEMENT

In the past, common practice in the United States was to designate an area for solid waste disposal and simply dump this waste on top of the ground. In such an operation, old cans, tires, and other objects retained water, producing a breeding ground for mosquitoes. Further, rats, roaches, flies, and other vectors used this readily accessible garbage as food. In short, these open dumps provided an area for a variety of pests to live and breed.

People often visited these dumps in search of valuable items that others may have discarded. This created a danger from broken glass, old medicine that children may ingest, dangerous chemical compounds, and many other hazards. Open dumps also caused surrounding property to depreciate and produced noxious odors. In addition to polluting groundwater, surface water runoff from the areas often carried waste into adjacent lakes and streams, increasing water pollution. The combustible materials in these areas often caused fires. Open dumps are undesirable, and these facilities now are illegal in the United States.

Some coastal areas formerly disposed of their solid waste at sea. Workers loaded the waste into barges and transported it away from the city. Today, this practice is illegal because it produces water pollution. Another means of disposal that is now illegal is "back yard" **incineration**. Incinerators burned refuse collected in the home and produced excessive amounts of air pollution. Still used today in some areas are large municipal incinerators; however, many are converting waste-to-energy plants. The required pollution control equipment ensures that the emissions do not exceed pollution standards. The open dump, disposal at sea, and backyard incineration still are used in many countries of the world.

The EPA has recommended that solid waste management be emphasized in the following order of preference:

1. Source reduction
2. Recycle – Reuse
3. Waste heat recovery — waste to energy (WTE)
4. Burying (landfill)

SOURCE REDUCTION

Years ago, children looked forward to opening new jars of peanut butter and jelly. After the contents were eaten, the jars became new drinking glasses. Bakers in the family bought new sacks of flour. The flour was eaten, and the flour sacks were transformed into clothing. Many of the food containers were reusable. Milk was picked up at the store or delivered to the doorstep in returnable bottles.

Later we entered the disposable era. Soft drink bottles and milk bottles were "nonreturnable." Salt, sugar, pepper, and catsup containers were replaced by individually wrapped packages

that came to be known as "single-service" items. In restaurants, cafes, and fast-food places the dishwasher was replaced by paper, plastic, and styrofoam plates. Thus, the amount of refuse generated per person to satisfy our desire for convenience grew in alarming proportions.

The practice of single service, together with more people, 70% of whom were living in towns and large cities, led to a solid waste crisis. The problem was caused by more people creating more waste in congested areas with limited disposal sites. It was complicated by little regard for the environment or means of managing effluent from an affluent society. Now managing effluent has become big business as some have realized "there are dollars in that waste."

Although solid waste management has become big business, we still should emphasize source reduction. Probably the best way to illustrate source reduction is by the example of the old kerosene oil can. From the 1920s to the 1940s, oil was used to illuminate homes by oil lamp, and oil was used to start fires in the fireplace. Families had their own galvanized metal oil can, which they took with them to the store, where the can was filled with oil and returned to the home. These cans were not found in fields, on creek banks, or in rivers. They were reusable. A single oil can usually lasted a family a lifetime.

I have seen plastic gallon milk jugs in creeks, rivers, fields, and lots. Could we not develop a multi-use milk container that could last a family a lifetime? This certainly would keep much waste out of landfills. Further, we could develop containers for soft drinks, beer, cooking oil, and so forth, that would reduce waste at the source with many far-reaching advantages. This could be done while meeting environmental and public health standards.

Some other ways to reduce sources of waste are as follows:

- Use fewer materials. American Indians, for example, generated little waste.
- Package things such as toothpaste in tubes instead of pump-type dispensers.
- Use cloth napkins instead of paper napkins.

- Use cloth grocery bags that go to and from the store with you again and again.
- Legislate the use of only returnable bottles.
- Use bulk sugar dispensers instead of individually wrapped packages.
- Use stainless steel instead of plastic when possible.
- Use cloth diapers instead of disposable diapers.

These measures can be reality if the public will demand them through its purchasing power.

RECYCLE-REUSE

The requirement of placing deposits on bottles has done a lot to save space in landfills and resources. Led by the Coors Brewery, the first company to produce aluminum cans, aluminum recycling has gained great acceptance and has done a lot to alleviate the solid waste dilemma. Paper, plastic, metal, and glass recycling is being practiced more in recent years.

Antique stores can be considered a form of reusing materials, as are flea markets. Also, some places take adult clothing and make it into children's clothing. Oil, rubber, asphalt, and appliances are being "recycled" more and more. Small businesses repair furniture, old stoves, refrigerators, and other appliances, and sell them.

Recycling is one solution to the solid waste problem. Vanishing natural resources, limited amounts of land suitable and available for landfills, and economic reward are reasons that recycling is fast becoming a feasible and popular method of waste disposal.

In lesser developed countries, solid waste is not a problem because people use almost all of it. For example, they burn the wood, paper, and plastic products and reuse many of the glass and metal containers for food storage and even as drinking cups. In the United States, in contrast, there is a need to recycle and in some areas recycling plants are highly successful. Home recycling and resource recovery plants should replace landfills as the major means of disposing of solid waste. Recycling of materials will alleviate future shortage of resources, greatly reduce pollution, and cut energy demands. Rather than burying them, wastes should be returned to factories, melted down, and reshaped for reuse.

In the United States, we recycle approximately 90% of our beverage cans (Figure 7.2). Like recycling aluminum and steel, we could recycle much of our other waste.

Even though recycling is good for the environment and is a good way to save resources, it is not utilized as much as it should be. Some reasons are:

- People have become accustomed to convenience, and separating waste is an inconvenience.
- People are used to throwing things away.

COMPLETE RECYCLABLE AUTO GOAL

In this present day of conservation, the automotive industry is giving the recycling of cars serious consideration. Approximately 75% to 80% of an automobile is recycled today. The goal of the Vehicle Recycling Partnership, a 5-year old consortium of General Motors, Ford Motors, and Chrysler, is to eliminate the last 20% to 25% from eventually being deposited in a landfill.

One innovative new technology is *pyrolysis* — which is basically the decomposition of a substance in the presence of heat alone. Superheating the car's remains to a scorching 1,400°F changes the once invaluable material into a substance that can be used as filler in concrete, shingles, and asphalt coatings.

The USCAR (U. S. Council for Automotive Research) has combined forces with the "big three" automakers and established a jointly operated Vehicle Recycling Development Center, where they study how to best recycle all parts of a car. Some examples are: a quick and efficient way to eliminate the fluids from a car in under 20 minutes, oil-eating bacteria that can effectively remove the lubrication and oil originating from the car's parts, and carpet, seat, and foam materials that can be recycled and used as padding or insulation in other products.

Source: Johnson City Press, Oct. 8, 1996

- The market for waste is not sufficient. Locating a recycling store beside the grocery store would help.

- Stronger laws are needed to require recycling.

- Recycling programs lack sufficient funding for research and start-up demonstrations.

- Some people just do not care.

Scientists have done research to find ways to recycle various materials, thereby reducing the cost of solid waste management and overloads on landfill space. We still need to find ways to recycle more plastics, cloth, asphalt, glass, leather, wood, and other materials. Industry also is encouraged to recycle its solid and liquid waste. In addition, laws should be passed to require reduction in the generation of solid waste.

WASTE TO ENERGY AND INCINERATION

The municipal incinerator (Figure 7.3) is a means of solid waste treatment. These incinerators can be centrally located close to the sources of the solid waste prior to processing. The temperatures within the incinerator must be very high (1800°F) to prevent air pollution. These incinerators often are expensive to construct and they must include a site location to dispose of the ashes. Burning refuse to generate electricity is another possibility, and selling the electricity or steam helps offset the cost of the incinerators. This technology commonly is called **energy recovery** or **waste-to-energy (WTE)** because the heat derived from incinerating refuse is a useful resource. Burning refuse can produce steam used directly for heating buildings or generating electricity. Internationally, well over 1,000 waste-to-energy plants are operating in Brazil, Japan, Russia, and Europe. In the United States, more than 110 waste incinerators burn over 45,000 tons of refuse daily. Some are simple incinerators, and others produce energy. Figure 7.4 portrays the waste-to-energy incinerator.

SANITARY LANDFILL

One of the most widely used means of solid waste disposal is the **sanitary landfill**. Briefly, in a sanitary landfill, the solid waste is buried in

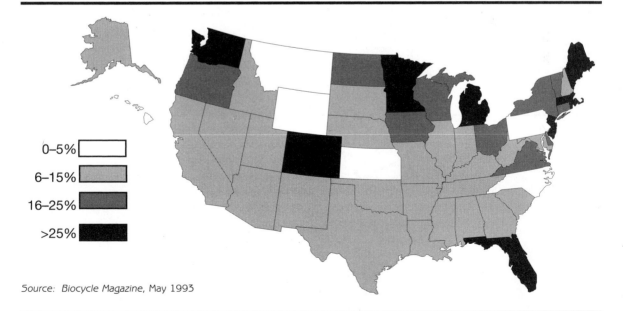

0–5%
6–15%
16–25%
>25%

Source: Biocycle Magazine, May 1993

FIGURE 7.2 State recycling rates.

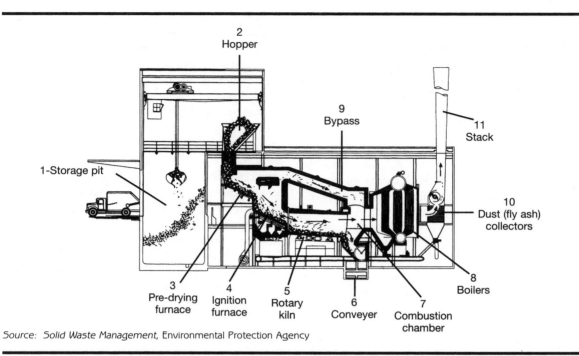

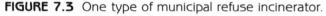

Source: Solid Waste Management, Environmental Protection Agency

FIGURE 7.3 One type of municipal refuse incinerator.

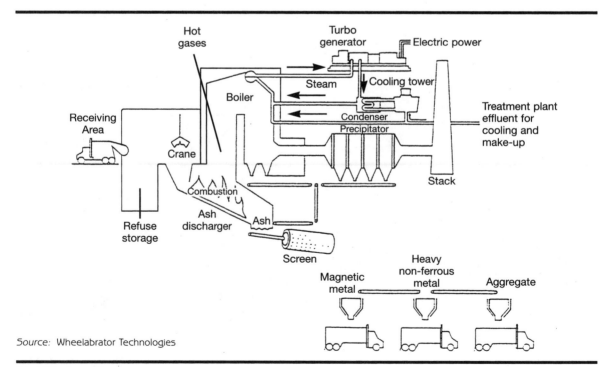

Source: Wheelabrator Technologies

FIGURE 7.4 Waste-to-energy incinerator.

Environmental Health

sections and covered with soil. If the landfill is operated properly, it can be located near populated areas. A landfill should not be located in areas with high groundwater tables, and preferably where the soil is a sandy loam. Roads leading into the landfill should be constructed to handle traffic from heavy collection vehicles.

A properly operated sanitary landfill eliminates insects, rodents, safety hazards, fire hazards, and other problems that exist in open dumping. Figure 7.5 gives an example of regulations for sanitary landfills. This one closely resembles federal guidelines.

Buffer zone standards for siting new landfills apply to Class I disposal facilities. A Class I disposal facility is a sanitary landfill that serves a municipal, institutional, or rural population to be used for disposal of domestic, commercial, institutional, municipal, demolition/construction, farming wastes, discarded automotive tires, and dead animals. According to the standards, Class I facilities must be located, designed, constructed, operated, and maintained such that the fill areas are a minimum of:

— 100 feet from all property lines

— 500 feet from all residences

— 500 feet from all wells determined to be downgradient and used as a source of drinking water by humans or livestock

— 200 feet from normal boundaries of springs, lakes, and other bodies of water.

Landfills also must operate under leachate migration control standards. The facility must have a liner designed to last the estimated life of the site as well as the post-closure care period. The facility also should be designed, constructed, and installed to prevent any leaching of waste or waste constituent from the facility into adjacent subsurface soil, groundwater, or surface water. This waste migration must not occur at any time during the use of the facility or during the post-closure period.

The facility's liner must be constructed of materials that have the appropriate chemical properties and sufficient strength and thickness to prevent failure. Failure of the liner may result

from pressure gradients, physical contact with the waste or leachate to which it is exposed, climactic conditions, stress of installation, and stress of daily operation.

The liner must be placed on a foundation or base capable of providing support. The foundation also must provide resistance to pressure gradients both above and below the liner. This prevents failure of the liner from settlement, compression, or uplift.

Any surrounding earth likely to be in contact with the waste leachate must be covered by the liner. The liner also must be designed to meet a minimum performance standard of 3 feet of recompacted soil; this achieves a maximum hydraulic conductivity of 1×10^{-7} cm/sec.

A geologic buffer must be located directly beneath the liner. It shall measure not less than 5 feet from the bottom of the liner to the seasonal high water table of the uppermost unconfined aquifer or the top of the formation of a confined aquifer.

If compacted earth liners are used, the minimum allowable thickness shall be 3 feet unless otherwise approved. If geomembrane liners are used, they must be used in conjunction with a compacted earth liner that must be at least 3 feet thick. Together the two liners also must achieve a maximum hydraulic conductivity of 3 feet or 1×10^{-6} soil. The compacted earth liner used with the geomembrane liner also shall be free of sharp objects, and compatible with supporting soils and with leachate expected to be generated. The geomembrane liner also shall have sufficient strength and durability to function for the life of the facility plus the post closure care period.

A leachate collection and removal system is required immediately above the liner. It is designed, constructed, maintained, and operated to collect and remove leachate from the facility. This system must be constructed of materials that are chemically resistant to the waste managed in the facility and the leachates expected to be generated. The materials also must be of sufficient strength and thickness to prevent collapse under the pressures exerted by overlying wastes, waste cover materials, and

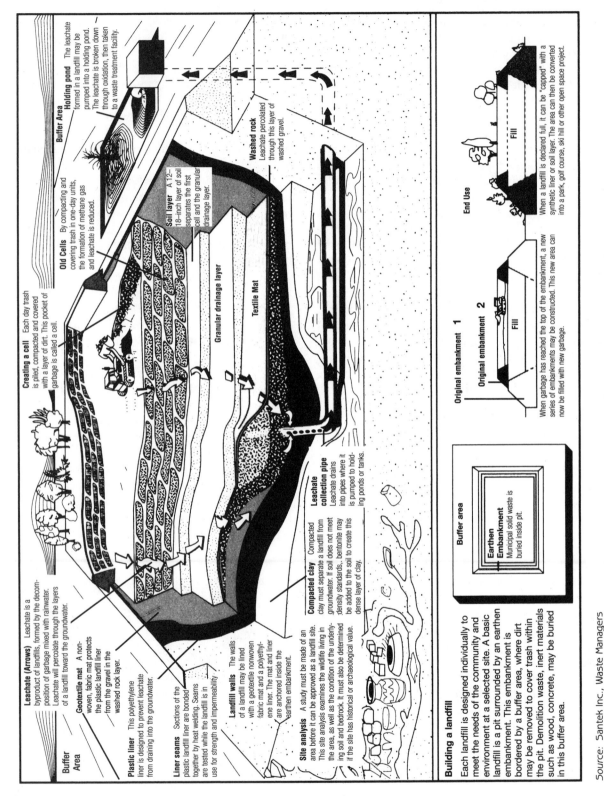

Buffer Area

Leachate (Arrows) Leachate is a byproduct of landfills, formed by the decomposition of garbage mixed with rainwater. Leachate will percolate through the layers of a landfill toward the groundwater.

Plastic liner This polyethylene liner is designed to prevent leachate from draining into the groundwater.

Geotextile mat A nonwoven, fabric mat protects the plastic landfill liner from the gravel in the washed rock layer.

Liner seams Sections of the plastic landfill liner are bonded together by heat welding. Seams are tested while the landfill is in use for strength and impermeability.

Landfill walls The walls of a landfill may be lined with a geotextile nonwoven fabric mat and a polyethylene liner. The mat and liner are anchored inside the earthen embankment.

Site analysis A study must be made of an area before it can be approved as a landfill site. This site analysis examines the wildlife living in the area, as well as the condition of the underlying soil and bedrock. It must also be determined if the site has historical or archaeological value.

Compacted clay Compacted clay must separate a landfill from groundwater. If soil does not meet density standards, bentonite may be added to the soil to create this dense layer of clay.

Leachate collection pipe Leachate drains into pipes where it is pumped to holding ponds or tanks.

Textile Mat

Granular drainage layer

Soil layer A 12–18-inch layer of soil separates the first soil and the granular drainage layer.

Creating a cell Each day trash is piled, compacted and covered with a layer of dirt. This pocket of garbage is called a cell.

Old Cells By compacting and covering trash in one-day units, the formation of methane gas and leachate is reduced.

Buffer Area

Holding pond The leachate formed in a landfill may be pumped into a holding pond. The leachate is broken down through oxidation, then taken to a waste treatment facility.

Washed rock Leachate percolated through this layer of washed gravel.

Building a landfill

Each landfill is designed individually to meet the needs of the community and environment at a selected site. A basic landfill is a pit surrounded by an earthen embankment. This embankment is bordered by a buffer area, where dirt may be removed to cover trash within the pit. Demolition waste, inert materials such as wood, concrete, may be buried in this buffer area.

Buffer area

Earthen Embankment Municipal solid waste is buried inside pit.

Original embankment 1

Original embankment 2

Fill

When garbage has reached the top of the embankment, a new series of embankments may be constructed. This new area can now be filled with new garbage.

End Use

Fill

When a landfill is declared full, it can be "capped" with a synthetic liner or soil layer. The area can then be converted into a park, golf course, ski hill or other open space project.

Source: Santek Inc., Waste Managers

FIGURE 7.5 Operational standards for sanitary landfill.

any equipment used at the facility. Other equivalent or superior protection may be substituted for this buffer. The leachate collection and removal system must be protected, by design or operational features, or both, from equipment mishandling that might reasonably be expected during operation.

These landfill facilities must be designed, constructed, operated, and maintained such that the final cover includes a cap that will: provide long-term minimization of migration of liquids through the closed facility, function with minimum maintenance, promote drainage, accommodate settling and subsidence so the cap's integrity is maintained, and meet specific closure requirements.

Further, the leachate collection reservoirs shall be constructed (e.g., lined) such that collected leachate is contained. The reservoir also must have sufficient capacity to store the volume of leachate expected to be generated in 30 days. The facility must have a reliable and convenient means of detecting the level of collected leachate in the reservoir and sampling the leachate.

During construction or installation, liners and cover systems (e.g., membranes, sheets, or coatings) must be inspected for uniformity, damage, and imperfections (e.g., holes, cracks, thin spots, foreign materials) immediately after construction or installation. For example, geomembrane liners and covers must be inspected to ensure tight seams and joints and the absence of tears, punctures, or blisters. Further, soil-based and admixed liners and covers must be inspected for imperfections including lenses, cracks, channels, root holes, and other structural nonuniformities that may cause an increase in the permeability of the liner or cover.

COMPOSTING

Composting is an effective method of solid waste disposal. In **composting**, biodegradable materials break down through natural processes and produce humus. The metabolism of microorganisms is what breaks down the waste aerobically or anaerobically.

Materials that are nonbiodegradable must be separated from the degradable materials and disposed of in some other manner. Some common nonbiodegradable materials are glass, plastics, rubber products, and metals. Once nonbiodegradable materials have been removed and a totally biodegradable waste has been established, it is brought to a grinder. Grinding increases the surface area of the waste and enhances biological degradation.

Aerobic composting involves decomposition in the presence of air (free oxygen). Anaerobic implies decomposition in the absence of the atmospheric oxygen. Most modern compost systems are aerobic rather than anaerobic for several reasons.

1. Aerobic processes are not accompanied by the foul stench present at an unsealed anaerobic composting operation.
2. In crop production industries, composting is safer because temperatures do not reach pasteurization temperatures that exceed the thermal death point of most plants, animals, and parasites.
3. Aerobic composting is more rapid than anaerobic composting.

An aerobic compost operation ideally is an optimal environment for the growth of aerobic organisms. The material to be composted is the food. Therefore the "food" should have a C/N* ratio favorable for decomposition. The microbes desire a C/N of 25:1 to 30:1. If the C/N is too low (l20:1), the ammonium compounds will volatilize into the air, causing an unpleasant odor. Various groups of organisms have different optimum temperatures (some prefer 25°C, some 37°C, and others 55°C), though the optimal temperature for a process as a whole integrates the optimums of the various microbes. The pH of aerobic composting varies depending on the organisms' need for oxygen. Aeration is important and is provided by turning the compost mechanically to expose it to oxygen to speed decomposition. Microbes must have moisture, and such is the case in composting. The amount

---

*CN = carbon nitrogen ratio

of moisture needed varies, as does the composition of the material being composted. The moisture content should be approximately 45% to 50%. If the moisture is too low, microbial activity slows, and biological activity ceases at a moisture content of about 12%. If the moisture content is too high, it reduces the amount of free oxygen present and slows the process so that it may become anaerobic. Many times sludge is added to waste for composting to provide microbial food and trace elements.

The three main types of composting are: windrow, static pile, and in-vessel.

1. *Windrow.* A sludge/refuse mixture configured in long rows (windrows) that are aerated by convection air movement and diffusion or by turning periodically through mechanical means to expose the organic matter to ambient oxygen.

2. *Static pile.* A stationary mixture is aerated by a forced aeration system installed under the pile.

3. *In-vessel composting.* Composting takes place in enclosed containers in which environmental conditions can be controlled. The waste decomposes into a harmless organic material that can be used as a soil conditioner and enhancer for agricultural applications.

MEDICAL WASTE DISPOSAL: METHODS AND PROBLEMS

Because of great concern about the spread of infectious diseases through contact with blood-borne pathogens, one of the major challenges facing the healthcare industry is the safe handling and disposal of medical waste. According to the American Hospital Association (AHA), the average hospital generates about 25 pounds of waste per day per patient bed. Infectious waste accounts for about 20% of that total. Hospitals and other generators of medical waste are at financial as well as legal risk for the safe and timely disposal of infectious waste.

The Environmental Protection Agency (EPA) and Centers for Disease Control and Prevention (CDC) recognize as medical infectious waste, contaminated sharps (needles, etc.), objects, blood and blood products, pathological wastes (anatomical waste and tissue samples), and laboratory waste capable of producing disease. Thus, consideration of several factors is necessary, including the presence of a pathogen of sufficient virulence, dose, portal of entry and resistance of host. For a medical waste to be infectious, it has to contain pathogens with sufficient virulence and of sufficient quantity so that exposure to the waste by a susceptible host would result in an infectious disease. In 1987 the CDC indicated that, though any items that have had contact with blood, exudes, or secretions are potentially infective, to treat all waste as infective is not usually practical or necessary. Differentiating infectious and medical waste is difficult, as the terms often are interchanged.

Health Concerns

From a safety standpoint, a twofold problem exists when handling medical waste.

1. Healthcare workers, waste haulers, and the public must be protected from the risks that medical waste poses to their health.

2. Government and industry must minimize the amount of medically related waste released into the environment.

The health problems are primarily occupational, as the greatest concerns are the health and well-being of healthcare workers and waste haulers. Cases of public exposure to wastes generated by health facilities are rare and isolated. Far more common are occupational illnesses, resulting from exposure to infectious materials. Therefore, efforts should be focused on educating and training workers, managing waste on- and off-site, and diminishing the demand for disposable medical materials.

The American Hospital Association (AHA) established perhaps the most meaningful interpretation of medical waste by offering the following classes of waste materials:

1. Cultures and stacks

2. Pathological waste
3. Human blood and blood products
4. Used sharps
5. Animal waste
6. Waste from patients with highly virulent diseases
7. Unused sharps.

Methods of Disposal

Several treatment technologies are available to dispose of medical waste. The most commonly encountered methods are steam sterilization, shredding/chlorinating, microwave disinfection, incineration, and other combustion technology.

Steam Sterilization

The advantages of steam sterilization, or **autoclaving**, are low capital investment and operating costs, relatively small space requirements, and simplicity of operation. Disadvantages include limited capacity, the requirement of special waste packaging and handling, and odor and drainage problems. Autoclaving is not recommended for pathological wastes, waste with high liquid content, and waste contaminated with volatile chemicals. After autoclaving, the appearance of waste remains unchanged. Although needles, syringes, blood bags, and the like, are sterile, they also are recognizable. This has the effect of making much of this waste unacceptable for disposal in a landfill or other disposal setting. Also, compacting autoclaved waste tends to break open waste bags and other containers, exposing and spilling their contents. Consequently, waste haulers and landfill operators may not be willing to accept autoclaved waste in spite of its sterile condition.

Shredding/Chlorinating Technology

In the past few years, a technology has been promoted featuring a combination of shredding and chemical sterilization. Currently two models are available. One size treats small, limited quantities of laboratory wastes and sharps. The other model is a relatively large-capacity system that treats almost all infectious waste a hospital generates. With the large-capacity system, waste is loaded manually onto an inclined conveyor belt, which feeds into a high-torque, low-speed shredder. Waste is discharged from the bottom of this shredder into a high-speed hammermill that granulates the waste. During both shredding stages, waste is sprayed continually with a sodium hypochlorite solution. An inclined, perforated conveyor at the hammermill's discharge separates the granular waste from the excess liquid (slurry). The slurry is collected in a basin and piped to a sewer drain. The solids are discharged into a cart, where they are retained for off-site disposal. The shredding rate is adjusted so the sodium hypochlorite contact time is sufficient for complete sterilization.

The principal advantages of shredding/chlorination systems are simplicity, substantial reduction in volume, alteration of appearance, and wide range of use. Disadvantages are their relatively high costs, limited throughput capacities, and potential slurry contamination. Noise levels and chlorine concentrations also are high. The slurry discharged to the sewer may have concentrations of heavy metals, organics, and other contaminates requiring a discharge permit. In addition, special precautions may be needed to ensure compliance with workplace standards.

Microwave Disinfection

Microwave technology represents an innovative alternative to common waste disposal systems in that it offers waste treatment and volume reduction without introducing undesirable treatment byproducts into the environment (air, ground, or water). Briefly, the medical waste is transported mechanically to a closed chamber, where it is injected with steam under pressure and then shredded. The waste then is conveyed through chambers where a series of 12 microwave units maintain a constant high temperature (greater that 200° F) for 45 to 60 minutes depending on load density. Final shredding at the discharge point further reduces the volume and renders the waste completely unrecognizable. This process can accommodate large quantities of waste, making it acceptable for large, multi-system operations and commercial establishments. Disadvantages are the high initial cost and the need to provide alternative means for disposing of certain medical wastes, primarily chemotherapy waste.

Incinerator Technology

Incineration uses controlled, high-temperature combustion to destroy organics in waste materials. Modern incineration systems are well-engineered, high-technology processes designed to maximize combustion efficiency and completeness with a minimum of emissions. Three basic hospital/institutional technologies currently in use are multiple-chamber, rotary kiln, and controlled air incinerators.

1. *Multiple-chamber incinerators*. Also referred to as Incinerator Institute of America (IIA) technology, the multiple-chamber incinerator was developed in the mid-1950s and was virtually the only system installed in hospitals through the mid-1960s. Multiple-chamber incinerator processes are designed for pumping air in excess levels, and they use settling chambers to control combustion and limit emissions. Despite this emission-limiting function, most of these devices require emission control systems to comply with standard emission regulations. Further, they cannot meet the current performance and operating requirements of many states without substantial upgrading and the addition of state-of-the-art combustion control equipment.

2. *Rotary kiln incineration*. Rotary kiln incineration features a cylindrical, refractory, lined, combustion chamber. The chamber rotates on a slightly inclined horizontal axis. Waste is loaded at the elevated end of the kiln. The rotary action moves the waste through the system. The kiln rotation promotes good burnout and superior ash quality. These systems require secondary combustion chambers and air pollution control equipment to ensure compliance with emission regulations.

3. *Controlled air incinerators*. Also called modular combustion and starved-air incineration, controlled air incineration is basically a two-stage combustion process. In the first-stage chamber, solid waste is burned in a starved air (reducing) environment. In the second-stage chamber, combustion products and volatile gases are burned under excess air conditions. The first controlled air incinerators were installed in the United States around 1962. This technology was popular initially because of its relatively low cost. Its popularity grew quickly because most of these systems could comply with air pollution control regulations readily without having to add costly air pollution control equipment. More than 95% of all hospital/infectious waste incinerators installed during the past 20 years have been of this type. Soon, however, this type of incineration will not be in compliance with stringent emission control regulations being legislated in many states. Installation of pollution control equipment will be required on a great many of these systems.

Thermal Plasma Technology

Thermal plasma treatment represents an innovative departure from the more conventional incineration technology. Invented by Vance IDS of Florida and known commercially as Incandescently Heated Bio-Hazardous Waste Disposal, this process exposes medical waste to intense incandescent heat, electrically generated in an inert (argon gas) plasma ion cloud and controlled atmosphere. Chamber temperatures reach approximately 20,000°F, which literally vaporize materials introduced into the chamber to their basic molecular components. Because of near complete ionization, temperatures outside the chamber do not exceed 90°F.

This process yields pure carbon black, which is a marketable byproduct and can be used in road construction. The process has a greater than 99% waste reduction factor. Argon gas is reclaimed and returned to the system, and the balance of the residue, a non-leaching aggregate cinder, is pulverized and can be released safely into the sewer system or accumulated indefinitely on-site, available for sale to concrete manufacturers as a hardener. The cleaned byproduct gases, consisting of oxygen and carbon monoxide, are vented out through the sewer trap and pipe vent. Temperature, time, pressures, waste weight, and generation location are recorded and saved so a complete report can be generated.

While exceedingly promising, this technology is largely unproved and is expensive. Its greatest potential at this time exists where large regional waste processing and disposal facilities are feasible. Many states currently mandate that infectious waste be treated on-site. They also restrict off-site transport of the waste or prohibit it from being landfilled, or both. Many additional states are planning similar restrictive legislative measures. At present, incineration is the only method the EPA recommends for disposing of virtually all types of infectious wastes. Offset disposal difficulties and limitations probably are the greatest incentives for hospitals and other institutions to select a type of on-site treatment. Many hospitals that are unable to utilize on-site treatment may be required to ship their waste across the country to the disposal facilities. These services typically are costly, and at times prohibitively expensive.

This method has several advantages, however, as off-site disposal is simple and requires relatively short implementation time. It avoids problems with locating and permitting on-site treatment systems. Also, building space and associated support systems are not required. These benefits usually are not enough, however, to make an off-site facility the most attractive alternative. The Medical Waste Tracking System of 1988 and comparable state legislation have imposed additional difficulties with this treatment option. Packaging, manifesting, and tracking requirements, with their accompanying severe penalties, for noncompliance, provide the most recent major deterrent to off-site waste disposal.

Healthcare providers face several sets of new and complex requirements. Federal and state laws have extended a facility's liability for waste handling beyond the walls of the hospital itself. The insurance industry labels this increasing exposure to liability as "environmental impairment risks." If current trends continue, legal regulations faced by generators and disposers of medical waste will only get tougher and more complicated. Commercial insurers currently are limiting liability coverage for the transportation and disposal of medical waste. These factors have increased the need for hospitals to protect themselves from a dangerous liability situation. The plethora of new regulations coming from different directions warrants care in determining which regulations take precedent.

As we approach the 21st century, the disposal of medical waste will become more complex and problematic. It is a serious problem now, and all indications point to a future full of legal and insurance fights, dangerous and deliberate violations, and vast room for improvement. For these reasons, healthcare providers not only must become more responsive to changing regulations but also more proactive and responsible in dealing with the overall medical waste issue.

HAZARDOUS WASTE

As the nation becomes increasingly industrialized and more technologically advanced, more wastes are generated. Some of the waste is hazardous. In the code of Federal Regulations, the U.S. Environmental Protection Agency identifies more than 400 hazardous wastes. The EPA defines the four characteristics of hazardous waste as: toxicity, ignitability, corrosivity, and reactivity.

1. *Toxicity.* **Toxic** means potentially poisonous to humans. Toxicity is determined by a toxicity characteristics leeching procedure (TCLP). Technicians expose a waste to laboratory-created landfill conditions and allow it to equilibrate. After 24 hours, water samples are tested for levels of substances high enough to be hazardous.

2. *Ignitability.* **Ignitable** compounds are liquids with a flashpoint below 60° C or non-liquids liable to cause fire via friction, moisture absorption, or spontaneous chemical change. Organic solvents, oils, plastics, and paints are ignitable compounds.

3. *Corrosivity.* **Corrosive** wastes, those with a pH below 2 or above 12.5, can eat away living tissues or corrode materials through chemical reaction. These corrosive materials, such as acids, alkaline substances, cleaning agents, and battery residues present a threat to people who come into bodily contact with leaky containers.

4. *Reactivity.* **Reactive** wastes include obsolete munitions and certain chemical wastes that react vigorously with air or water. They may explode and generate toxic gases. An example is the waste from the firecracker industry.

An example of a hazardous waste problem (though not regulated under hazardous waste law) is the former use of polychlorinated biphenyls (PCBs). These are organochloride chemicals structurally similar to the pesticide DDT. Because PCBs have excellent insulating properties, they were used widely in transformers and other electrical components. They also had a wide range of use in soap, paint, glue, waxes, brake lining, caulking compounds, and epoxy resins. In 1968 in Japan, cooking oil was contaminated accidentally with PCBs, and several thousand people suffered subsequently from enlarged liver, disorders of the intestinal tract and lymphatic systems, and loss of hair. In the early 1970s, PCBs were found in cow's milk, inland and deep-sea fish, meats, and humans. Tests have indicated that PCBs interfere with reproduction in fish, rodents, and many species of birds and monkeys. PCBs are suspected of being carcinogenic. Moreover, PCBs are not easily biodegradable — which raises concern where even small quantities have been spilled in the environment. Compounding the problem is that when PCBs decompose, their products are even more poisonous than the original material. Production of PCBs stopped in the United States in

1977. Decades more will have to go by for the compounds to be removed from the environment.

Sometimes workers must dispose of a batch of chemicals because of overheating or some other problem. Many of these wastes are toxic, and some are deadly. Thus, they should not be mixed with domestic waste or pumped into streams, lakes, or oceans. In the past, the easiest way to dispose of the wastes was to pack them in 55-gallon steel drums (the "garbage cans" of the chemical industry) and store them elsewhere. As the drums accumulated, often in the thousands, they created new toxic waste sites.

Some examples of hazardous waste incidents are as follows.

- At a rural site 25 miles south of Louisville, Kentucky, 6,000 drums full of toxic chemicals and 11,000 more partly full were found. The corroding drums oozed hazardous chemicals into the soil. An investigation found that the deceased owner of the land had pocketed money that was supposed to be used for proper disposal of the waste.

- Iberville Parish, Louisiana, was the site of a truck driver's death. The driver had dumped a load of hazardous chemicals into a waste pit. The dumped chemicals reacted with chemicals already in the pit, producing a cloud of hydrogen sulfide gas that paralyzed the driver's respiration. Investigators noticed later that the disposal site was operating without proper permits.

- Montaque, Michigan, was a site of water contamination. Illegal dumping of carbon tetrachloride and chloroform, as well as tetrachloride othylene, poisoned well water in the area. This accident was uncovered in 1977, when a former employee of Hooker Chemical complained to Michigan authorities about the hazardous wastes. Investigators also discovered a secret dump site and many drums that had been allowed to drain onto the property. Hooker subsequently had to pay to provide local residents with a proper waterline or take water to them. As a result of the legal action, Hooker was forced to construct a huge clay-lined vault to contain its wastes and begin efforts to decontaminate the groundwater.

- Residents of Seymour, Indiana, were evacuated from their homes in March 1980 when hydrogen gas reacted with solvents from more than 60,000 containers of hazardous

In the early 1940s, Hooker Chemical Company of Niagara Falls, New York, dumped approximately 19,000 tons of waste into a canal site. In 1953, the company covered the dump site with dirt and sold the land to the Board of Education of Niagara for $1. The deed of the sale indicated that the site contained "waste products resulting from the manufacturing of chemicals." The deed further stated that Hooker would not be responsible for the condition of the land. The site later was used for an elementary school and playground, with housing also in the area.

The steel drums eventually rusted, corroded, and leaked. The contents seeped into the soil and groundwater and eventually entered the lakes, rivers, and streams. Heavy rain during the spring of 1977 raised the level of the groundwater and turned the area into a muddy swamp. Many of the school children and people living in the neighborhood suffered serious illnesses. The citizens reported skin sores, epilepsy, rectal bleeding, liver malfunctioning, miscarriages, severe headaches, and birth defects.

An environmental survey revealed that the drums were leaking and that several other dumps contaminated with hazardous waste were scattered around the city. Almost overnight, a new and serious environmental concern was brought to the attention of the public. The dump site was evacuated, families were relocated at a cost of $37 million to the State of New York, and cleanup began (and may never really end). The hazardous waste era had arrived.

An estimated 1000 kg of wastes containing dioxin had been buried in that area. Dioxin is a highly toxic substance — one of the deadliest known. Through this unfortunate incident, it was found that dioxin could enter drinking water supplies and cause severe problems.

wastes that a company had dumped improperly in the nearby area. The EPA declared a water emergency at Seymour. The cost of complete removal of the waste was estimated at $12 million.

Federal officials believe there may be as many as 50,000 dangerous chemical dumps in the United States.

Transportation of Hazardous Waste

Railroads, trucks, and barges transport hazardous waste in the United States. The transportation of hazardous wastes can pose a threat to the public. To promote safety and protect the public's health, companies follow four basic control measures for the movement of hazardous waste from a generator to disposal.

1. *Hazardous waste manifest.* The concept of a cradle-to-grave tracking system is considered a key to proper management of hazardous waste. Manifest copies accompany each barrel of waste that leaves the site where it is generated and are signed and mailed to the receiving sites to indicate the transfer of waste from one location to another.

2. *Labeling and placarding.* Each container is labeled and marked. The transporting vehicle is placarded before a waste is transported from the generating site. Companies post warning labels such as: explosive, strong oxidizer, compressed gas, flammable liquid, corrosive material, and poisonous/toxic substances.

3. *Haulers.* Because of the dangers involved, haulers of hazardous waste are subject to operator training, insurance coverage, and special registration of vehicles transporting hazardous waste. Handling precautions include restrictive use of the transport trucks and the use of gloves, face masks, and coveralls for the workers' protection.

4. *Incident and accident reporting.* Accidents involving hazardous waste must be reported immediately to the state regulatory agency,

as well as local health departments. Necessary information that will help responders contain the material should be made available.

Hazardous Waste Disposal

When choosing a hazardous waste disposal site, evaluators must consider many factors. These include hydrology, geology, climatology, ecology, and public and environmental health. Some disposal options include the so-called secure landfill; chemical, physical, and biological treatment processes; incineration; and deep-well injection.

Secure Landfill

In the past, the **secure landfill** was one of the more frequently used methods of disposing of hazardous waste. Regulations now drastically limit their use. A secure landfill consists of ground excavation and some sort of insulation to prevent waste from escaping into air, water, and land. This is accomplished by locating the landfill away from aquifers that are used for drinking water supplies. The operated area is lined with concrete or some approved impermeable liner. Compacted earth (preferably clay) is placed over the liner, then another liner is poured. The barrels, many times specially lined, coated with concrete, and so on, are placed in the area and covered with earth. Secure landfills now are covered by the "land ban," which specifies treatment methods for wastes before they can be placed into or on the ground. Treatment methods are designed to ensure that contaminants do not migrate from the disposal area.

Builders design each level of the landfill so workers can monitor leachate. Preferably, surface waters are diverted away to reduce the chance of water entering, covering the barrels, and causing rust.

Chemical, Physical, and Biological Treatments

The goal for **chemically, physically,** and **biologically** oriented treatment processes is to reduce the volume of waste and the hazardous characteristics of the waste. Chemical methods include neutralization, precipitation, solidification, and oxidation reduction. Physical processes include evaporation and compaction of some material. Biological techniques depend largely upon microorganisms to decompose toxic organic compounds. These treatment methods greatly reduce the volume of waste to be landfilled or incinerated and avoid migration of hazardous components from the disposal area.

Incineration

Incineration, burning at high temperatures, is a significant means of handling hazardous waste. Combustion is intended to convert waste to a less bulky, less toxic, and less noxious material. The products of combustion are mainly carbon dioxide, water, and ash. Some products of incomplete combustion (PICs) are harmful. If the water or gaseous products of combustion contain undesirable compounds, further treatment is necessary. This treatment usually consists of scrubbing for the gaseous material and wastewater treatment for the water. The residue is disposed of in secure landfills.

Incineration reduces the volume of landfilled hazardous waste, thus saving landfill space. Incinerators are expensive, however, and the waste, ash, gases, and water must be controlled to prevent damage to the environment and the public' s health.

Remediation

Deep-Well Injection

In hazardous waste management, as with radiological health, emphasis should be placed on reducing the amount at the source of generation. Sometimes this can be accomplished by reusing and recycling the waste and by modifying the industrial process to eliminate or reduce the waste generated. Presently, waste minimization is the preferred method of hazardous waste management. All facility permits issued effective September 1, 1985, and thereafter specify that a waste minimization program must be in place. Further, all generators, upon completing a manifest, must specify that they have such a program.

In 1980, the U. S. Congress passed **CERCLA**, the Comprehensive Environmental Response, Compensation and Liability Act, known as the Superfund program, to clean up contaminated waste sites. In 1984, Congress added amendments to the 1976 Resource Conservation and Recovery Act, to better manage hazardous waste. The Superfund Amendments and Reauthorization Act was passed in 1986. These acts are summarized in Chapter 14.

SUMMARY

Solid waste management begins by reducing the generation of waste and by recycling. Waste that remains may be treated, for example, by incineration or disposed of in a sanitary landfill. Requirements for landfills have been strengthened and now include liners, leachate collection and treatment, management of gases produced by decomposition, and more. Composting has been revived in the United States, with plants in many communities. Techniques have developed to manage infectious waste, though this remains a challenge.

Hazardous waste programs have developed over the last 20 years. The manifest system provides a mechanism to track transfers of hazardous waste. Reduction in generation of hazardous waste is important, and recycling is growing. Simple disposal of solid waste on land has been replaced largely by burial of treated waste. Remediation of contaminated sites is increasing, as necessary specialized technology is developed.

REFERENCES

American Public Works Association. 1970. *Municipal Refuse Disposal*. Public Administration Service, Chicago.

Blackman, William C., Jr. 1995. *Basic Hazardous Waste Management*. 2d ed. Lewis Publishers.

Doucet, Lawrence G. 1990. Infectious Waste Treatment and Disposal Alternatives. Peekskill, NY: *Professional Development Series #057005*.

Griffin, Roger D. 1989. *Principles of Hazardous Materials Management*. 2d ed. Lewis Publishers.

LaGrega, Michael D., P. L. Buckingham, J. C. Evans, and Environmental Resources Management Group. 1994. *Hazardous Waste Management*. McGraw-Hill, New York.

Miller, Tyler. 1988. *Living In the Environment*. 5th ed. Wadsworth Publishing, Belmont, CA.

Martin, William F., John F. Martin, and Timothy G. Prothero. 1987. *Hazardous Waste Handbook for Health and Safety*. Butterworth-Heinemann. Boston.

Pfeffer, John T. 1992. *Solid Waste Management Engineering*. Prentice Hall, Englewood Cliffs, NJ.

Public Health Service. 1982. *Sanitation in the Control of Insects and Rodents of Public Health Importance*. U. S. Government Printing Office, Washington, DC.

Rhyner, Charles R., Leander J. Schwartz, Robert Wenger, and Maty Kohrell. 1995. *Waste Management and Resource Recovery*. CRC, Boca Raton, FL.

Slavik, Nelson S. 1988. OSHA/EPA Handling and Disposal of Hazardous Materials. *Technical Document Series #055970*.

Vesiland, Anne. 1996. *Environmental Engineering*. PWS Publishing Company, Boston.

Vesiland, P. A. 1983. *Environmental Pollution and Control*. 2d ed. Ann Arbor Science, Michigan.

Vectors and Their Control

By Darryl Barnett, Dr. P.H.
East Kentucky University

Key Terms

Arachnids
Arthropods
Cyclo-propagative
Dermatitis
Maggot
Metamorphosis

Myiasis
Ootheca
Pediculosis
Proboscis
Proventriculus
Scabies

Synanthropic
Transovarian transmission
Transstadial transmission
Tumbler
Vector
Wriggler

Objectives

- Identify the rodent that is of greatest public health interest.
- Identify the arthropods of greatest public health interest.
- Name the most prominent disease agents.
- Describe the transmission route from the vector.
- Discuss the habitat of public health-related rodents and arthropods.
- Discuss the most important control methods for the vectors.

A **vector** is any organism that transmits a pathogen, or disease-causing agent. Among vector-borne diseases are murine typhus, bubonic plague, leptospirosis, salmonellosis, rat bite fever, ricettsialpox, trichinosis, lymphocytic choriomeningitis, toxoplasmosis, and listeriosis. Two types of vectors that are most problematic are discussed in this chapter: rodents (mainly rats) and insects of the arthropod class. Money spent on managing solid wastes to control these vectors pays off because it reduces the need for spending on vector control programs and vector-borne diseases.

RODENTS

Rodents are undesirable for several reasons. They destroy property, frighten people, spread disease, and compete with humans for food. Improperly managed solid waste creates an ideal habitat for insects and rodents.

Rats plague many store owners and farmers. Rodents are undesirable in feed and seed stores because they destroy the seed, corn, and other supplies. Rats also are undesirable in poultry houses and bird farms. They destroy and contaminate structures, as well as harm young birds and chicks. In some areas of the world, rats destroy as much as one-third of the entire harvest.

Because rats gnaw and burrow, they can cause structural damage to buildings. They have been known to gnaw insulation off wiring, which has started fires in buildings. Norway rats prefer to burrow and live below the ground. Therefore, they have been known to burrow and weaken the foundation bulkhead of dams and thus create the condition for flooding and other forms of destruction.

We wish to control rodents to protect our property and enhance our health. If we are going to control them, we must know something about their biological characteristics and habits.

Biological Characteristics

Domestic rodents include Norway rats, roof rats, and house mice. They are members of the order *Rodentia*, family *muridae*. Rats are "commensal," which means they live at people's expense. They eat their food, live in their houses, and share with them their diseases — without contributing anything beneficial to the relationship.

Rodents are characterized by a single pair of incisor teeth on each jaw and by the absence of canine teeth. They usually have a tail with fine scales and few hairs, although many American rodents, such as field mice, wood rats, squirrels, and chipmunks, have hair and a bushy tail.

The *Norway rat (Rattus norvegicus)* (see Figure 8.1) is predominantly a burrowing rodent. The most common and largest of the domestic rats, it is found throughout the temperate regions of the world including the United States. Some common names of this species are: brown rat, house rat, barn rat, sewer rat, and wharf rat. The Norway rat has a heavy, stocky body and averages 7 to 18 ounces in weight and between 7 to 10 inches in length. A distinguishing characteristic of the Norway rat is that the combined head and body are longer than the

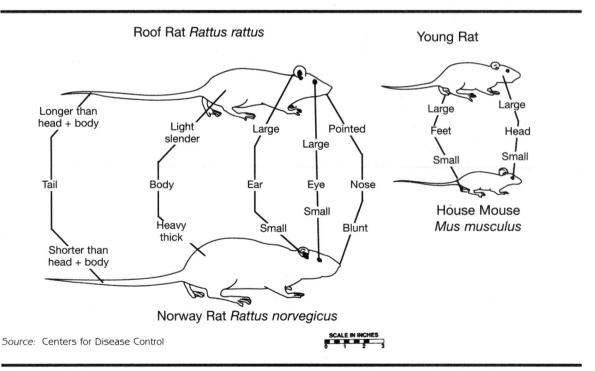

FIGURE 8.1 Field identification of three domestic rodents.

tail. The total length of Norway rats (tail plus body and head) is between 13 and 18 inches. The Norway rat has coarse fur, usually brownish or reddish gray, a blunt nose, and small, close-set ears that appear to be half buried in fur. The eyes are small compared with those of other rats. The gestation period for Norway rat averages 22 days; and the rats reach sexual maturity in 3 to 5 months after birth. Norway rats have from four to seven litters per year, with the average female weaning 20 rats per year. The rats' life expectancy is about 1 year. Preferable food is garbage, meat, fish, vegetables, fruits, and cereal. The Norway rat needs only ½ to 1 ounce of water per day.

The *roof rat (Rattus rattus)* is somewhat smaller than the Norway rat (see Figure 8.1) and is a more agile climber. In the United States, the roof rat is found mainly in the South, across the entire nation to the Pacific coast. It is found in Hawaii as well as colder regions of the world. The roof rat's body is slender and graceful. It weighs 4 to 12 ounces and is 6 to 8 inches long. A distinguishing factor of the roof rat is that the tail is longer than the combined body and head. Tail length is from 7 to 10 inches, and total length of the roof rat is from 14 to 18 inches. The roof rat has a pointed nose, large ears, and large eyes. The average gestation period of the female roof rat is 22 days; the young reach sexual maturity in 3 to 5 months. Females average four to six litters per year, with an average of six to eight offspring per litter. The roof rat prefers to live above ground, indoors, in attics, between floors, in walls, in enclosed spaces, or outdoors in trees and dense vine growth. The roof rat's preferred foods are vegetables, fruits, and cereal grains. It also competes with people for other foods.

The *house mouse (Mus musculus)* is abundant throughout the United States, as well as the rest of the world. It has a long, slender, graceful body (see Figure 8.1), with an average weight of ½ to ¾ ounce. Its tail is 3 to 4 inches long, which is little longer than the head plus the body. It has a pointed nose, large ears, and large eyes. The house mouse reaches sexual maturity in 1½ to two months after birth. The

gestation period is 19 days, and the mother has an average of eight litters per year. The offspring range from five to six per litter. Longevity for a house mouse is usually less than 1 year. These mice prefer convenient indoor spaces between walls and cabinets, in furniture, or in stored goods. Outdoors they live in weeds, rubbish, and grasslands. The preferred food is cereal grains, but they will eat most types of the other edible food that people consume.

Rodents are sensitive to touch. They have guard hairs (vibrissae) all over their bodies, which serve as feelers or sensitive whiskers. Hence, rats and mice prefer to run along walls and between objects where they can keep their sensitive whiskers in contact with vertical or side surfaces. This compensates for their poor vision; and they also are believed to be color-blind. Having an extremely keen sense of smell, rodents can readily detect the odors of most foods that humans consume. Rodents also have well-developed tastebuds and will eat most foods that humans eat, preferring fresh food to spoiled food. Rats tend to associate sickness caused by poison bait with the bait and will not take the poison again, thus becoming bait-shy.

The Norway rat prefers to burrow and live below the ground. The roof rat prefers to live above the ground. As its name suggests, the house mouse prefers living in human quarters. The rodents' burrows seldom are far from a source of food and water.

Rodents must gnaw to wear off the average growth of 4 to 6 inches per year on their incisors. If they do not gnaw, the incisors will grow around and seal their mouths. Therefore, rats gnaw to gain entrance and to obtain food. In so doing, they are destructive to human belongings.

Some signs that indicate the presence of rodents are seeing live or dead rats, hearing rats, and seeing rodent droppings, runways, burrows, nests, and signs of gnawing. Further evidence is seeing feeding stations, or spots where rats have pulled food scraps and left them after eating what they wanted. Additional signs are urine, rat hair, and rat body odors.

Four Rodent Control Measures

Rodent control management is divided into four distinct areas:

1. Eliminating sources of food.
2. Eliminating breeding and nesting places.
3. Rat-proofing buildings and other structures.
4. Killing them.

A good job of solid waste management goes a long way toward creating an unfavorable environment for rodents. Storing, collecting, and disposing of refuse in a sanitary manner does much to deprive the rodents of their requirement for survival: food.

Rats prefer to consume people's food while it is in the pantry, grocery store, or on shelves. If they cannot get to this food supply before people do, however, they will survive easily on people's garbage. Therefore, garbage storage, collection, and disposal are vital to eliminating rodents. Another situation in which rats obtain food is the feeding of pets. Sometimes owners overfeed cats or dogs and after dark the rodents come in and eat the food. Interestingly, rats can live for a long time by eating apples. Hence, apple trees in a community can serve as a food supply for rodents if other basic requirements for survival, such as harborage, are provided. Because rats prefer to live close to people's food supply, people must be careful to make the food unavailable for them. This includes food in the home, restaurants, grocery stores, schools, and other places where humans live, work, travel, and recreate.

Elimination of breeding and nesting places is another way to control rodents. The rubbish in an open dump provides a home, or harborage, for the rodents, and their food source is readily available. Some communities require that all lumber, fire wood, and the like be stored at least 6 inches above the ground. At this height, the materials do not provide a home for rats, which prefer dark, moist places in which to burrow. For this reason, wood should not be piled directly on the ground, and trash and other rubbish should be removed from the premises periodically to prevent nesting. Old appliances such as washing machines, televisions sets, and refrigerators, as well as cars, trucks, and other solid waste also provide a living place for rats. A common mistake made while building a house is to pour the patio and steps before the ground (fill dirt) has settled adequately. When the dirt finally settles, it leaves a space under the patio and other areas that is suitable for rat harborage.

If the rats cannot be starved to death and, for some reason, their breeding and nesting places cannot be removed, we must concentrate on building them out (see Figure 8.2). Most modern homes are rat-proofed. The crawl space under the house usually has ventilators, each having a grid with a screen behind it to prevent rodents from entering. Likewise, attics typically have ventilators with screens on them. Because the Norway rat prefers to burrow, the footings on houses are poured in an L-shape with the boot (the toe of the L), on the outside. The rats will burrow down, encounter the concrete, and not burrow further. This prevents them from entering buildings where food is stored. Other means of rat-proofing are to put metal strips on doors where rats may tend to gnaw to gain entrance and putting hardware cloth (rat wire) over windows. All potential entrances to buildings — such as openings around pipes, cracks in walls, and other places where a rat could gain entrance — should be sealed with concrete. In sum, one has to do everything possible to build out dwelling places and businesses so rodents cannot gain entrance.

The final measure to control rodents is to kill them. If we need a killing program, we have failed in the first three endeavors: starving them to death, denying them a home, and building them out. Extermination then becomes necessary. The preferred method is by natural means. Traditionally, this meant the household cat. No chemicals are added to the environment and the cat becomes part of the family. Cats are not recommended for restaurants, grocery stores, and other food establishments, however.

Also, many rodenticides are available on the market, many of which are toxic to humans. When selecting rodenticides and making them available to rats, people must be extremely careful. Two rodenticides recommended for use by laypersons are red squill and warfarin.

Red squill generally comes wrapped in paper similar to candy or gum. Red squill is a one-time rodenticide. A sufficient amount of red squill must be made available to the rats to kill them the first time, because they tend to become bait-shy. If rats eat enough of the red squill, they will be killed by paralysis of the heart muscles. Because red squill is an emetic, any human who eats red squill accidentally would regurgitate the poison immediately. Rats cannot regurgitate, so, once ingested, the red squill will kill them.

The second recommended rodenticide is a group called *anticoagulants*, of which the most common is warfarin. Warfarin generally is put in corn meal. The rats come back continuously during the night and eat the poisoned corn meal, not realizing that it thins their blood. Eventually they begin hemorrhaging. The blood seeps through the blood vessels, weakening the rats until they eventually die. Warfarin is considered safe around children (unless they live in a famine area) because they do not often eat dry corn meal. If a child ingests warfarin, Vitamin K is given to thicken the blood. Foods high in Vitamin K include leafy vegetables. Warfarin

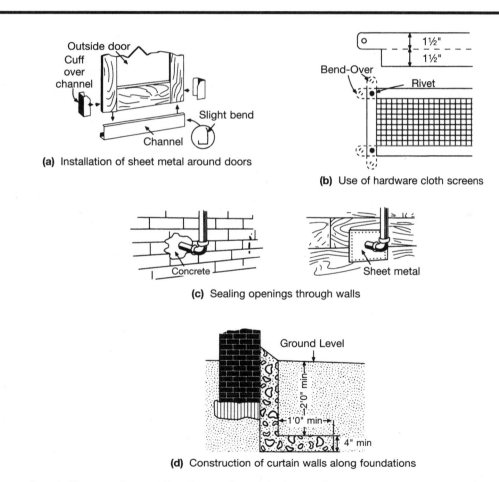

(a) Installation of sheet metal around doors

(b) Use of hardware cloth screens

(c) Sealing openings through walls

(d) Construction of curtain walls along foundations

Source: Control of Domestic Rats and Mice, National Centers for Disease Control

FIGURE 8.2 Common measures to build out rats.

should be made available to rats in adequate quantities until the rat population is completely killed. This is a good choice as rats do not tend to become bait-shy to warfarin as they do with red squill and some other rodenticides.

A patch test may be used to determine if a poisoning program is effective in killing all the rats. This consists of spreading flour on the floor and around the walls. If the next morning five- and four-toed footprints and tail marks are seen in the flour, the rats have not been killed and the program must continue.

Another common way to kill rats is by traps. Mousetraps have been used for many years. They are placed along walls, near runways, burrows, and the like so the rats will encounter them. The traps have attractive bait such as peanut butter or cheese, with the hope that rats will be attracted to the traps, trigger them, and be caught. Rats do tend to become trap-shy. If the rat is caught squealing and suffering in the trap, other rats tend to associate this and stay clear of this strange object in their environment.

The most desirable, most economical, ways to control rats are to try to starve them to death and to deny them a place to live. These measures also create a clean environment for humans.

ARTHROPODS

Arthropods are animals belonging to the phylum *Arthropoda*, meaning "jointed foot." Insects, the largest class of arthropods, typically have three pairs of legs, a segmented body with a head, thorax and abdomen, plus mouthparts consisting of a palpi and a proboscis. The proboscis is utilized by mosquitoes, fleas, lice, cockroaches, and flies to pierce the skin and suck the blood. In the case of some flies, a sponging mouthpart can be used to spread disease organisms. Insects generally are acknowledged as the arthropods of greatest public health significance.

The second most prominent class of arthropods of public health significance are the arachnids, which include ticks and mites. Arachnids typically have the head, thorax and abdomen unified into one body region. As adults, they have four pairs of legs and no antennae. Mouthparts consist of a cutting organ called the *chelicerae*, which enables insertion of the hypostome. This anchors the arachnid and allows blood feeding from the host. The tick is among the most efficient of the arthropod vectors.

Insects

Mosquitoes

Mosquitoes, a member of class *Insecta*, are a formidable public health problem, as they are responsible for spreading disease organisms to millions of people each year. These pathogens include arboviruses, which cause yellow fever; various encephalitides; dengue and its hemorrhagic fever; the protozoans, which cause the various forms of malaria; and the nematodes, which cause filariasis.

Mosquitoes have a complete **metamorphosis**, a four-stage life cycle, as shown in Figure 8.3. The first three stages occur in water. The *Anopheles* and *Culex* genuses lay their eggs on water, and the eggs of the *Aedes* genus mosquito, of public health interest, are found on the sides of containers or in tree holes just above water level. This knowledge is valuable when determining the proper strategy for eliminating egg-laying areas for specific mosquitoes. The next two stages, larva and pupa, known in the mosquito as the **wriggler** and the **tumbler,** must have access to air. This necessity enables a means of killing them by spraying larvacides on the surface of water. The adult mosquito, both male and female, is an active flyer, varying in both range and preference for meal sources. Mosquitoes typically are active at evening and night and during the day rest in shaded areas. Most prefer temperatures in the 80° to 90°F range. The male feeds on plant juices, and the female feeds upon the blood of warm-blooded or cold-blooded animals.

Thus, the female is responsible for transmitting disease organisms. Most, but not all, female mosquitoes require a blood meal before they are able to lay each batch of fertile eggs. Only one

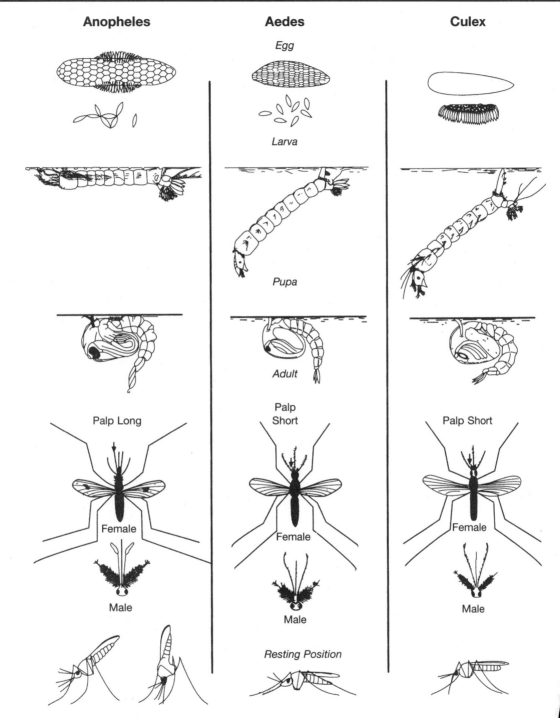

Anopheles   **Aedes**   **Culex**

Egg

Larva

Pupa

Adult

Palp Long   Palp Short   Palp Short

Female

Male

Resting Position

Source: U. S. Public Health Service

FIGURE 8.3 Stages in life cycle of mosquitoes.

Chapter 8   Vectors and Their Control

mating is required, however, to fertilize egg production for a lifetime.

The mosquito transmits the disease agent primarily with its salivary glands and **proboscis** or biting part; the proboscis is designed for piercing the skin and sucking blood. While the mosquito is taking blood, salivary secretions from the gland are injected as an anticoagulant. The disease-causing agent, which normally has migrated from the intestinal system, is injected with the salivary secretion. In this manner mosquitoes spread the disease organisms.

Mosquito control is founded in an integrated approach, including the use of

— chemicals such as insecticides and larvacides.
— biological control such as the *Gambusia affinis*, a predatory fish, and parasites such as the nematode *Romanomermis culicivorax*
— sanitation efforts.

The latter includes good solid waste control, eliminating artificial containers favored by *Aedes aegypti* and vehicle tires, favored breeding spots for *Aedes albopictus*. Sanitation also includes other types of habitat elimination such 's eliminating transient water pools (ditches, nals, etc.), which are ideal habitats for *Culex salis*. Proper storage, collection, and disposal solid waste results in the elimination of ding areas and ultimately can save money me in the control of arthropods.

e mosquitoes, belong to the class nd have a complete metamorphosis. and pupa stage are seen rarely. We r with the adult stage. The larval nown as a **maggot**, is viewed with n the eggs are laid in the flesh of resulting larvae invade the sur- tissue, resulting in a condition is. Medical researchers however, und that the larval stage of the amily that includes common bluebottles — can be used

beneficially to devour dead tissue around infected wounds. Be that as it may, people historically have viewed flies as carriers of disease-causing agents and as destroyers of food. From a public health viewpoint, flies can be classified as *biting flies* (sandflies, horseflies, deerflies) or *nonbiting flies* (houseflies, bottleflies, screwwormflies). The latter also are called **synanthropic** flies, referring to their close association with humans. (see Figure 8.4) Today, the presence of flies often is viewed as a gauge or sentinel that sanitation efforts are not being carried out properly. Flies are sources of annoyance, painful bites and disease transmission. Thus, they currently are considered one of the greatest public health hazards facing humans.

In the southern United States, the most abundant synanthropic fly is the housefly (*Musca domestica*). In the northern part of the country, the most common is the blowfly. The former is considered to be the greater threat to human health. The housefly and the blowfly do not bite but, rather, have "spongelike" mouthparts. This fly can devour only liquids. It tests for food sources constantly by excreting saliva which dissolves the food. This is evidenced by the light brown spots left on areas in which large numbers of flies have visited.

Domestic flies spread the causative agents of disease in the following ways:

1. On their mouth parts
2. Through their vomitus
3. On their body and leg hairs
4. On the sticky pads of their feet
5. Through the intestinal tract by means of fly feces.

These are the mechanical transmission methods that spread the causative agent of the diseases and conditions including typhoid fever, paratyphoid, dysentery, and diarrhea.

In addition to being annoying, the biting flies also contribute to the spread of disease. The stablefly (*Stomoxys calcitrans*), blackfly (*Simulium venustrum*), and tsetse (*Glossinia palpalis*) are examples of vicious biters. Enormous numbers of blackflies have been known to

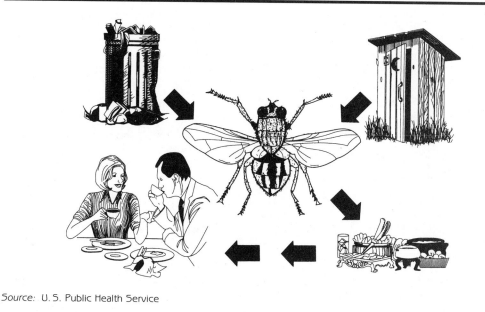

Source: U. S. Public Health Service

FIGURE 8.4 Mechanical transmission of disease-causing organisms by flies.

attack cattle and kill them. Deerflies, horseflies, sandflies and other biting flies attack humans, causing great discomfort. These flies require a blood meal to produce eggs and they typically transmit the disease agent from the salivary gland while feeding. Diseases spread by these flies are categorized as biologically transmitted diseases of the **cyclo-propagative** type. This means that the causative agent undergoes a change in its form and additionally proliferates within the fly. Diseases transmitted in this manner include African sleeping sickness, onchocerciasis, loiasis, and many others, causing suffering and death to millions of people the world over. Thus, control of these flies is essential to the control of many serious and widespread diseases.

Controlling the fly is based upon a of the fly's life cycle and other biological factors. Eliminating breeding media, such as horse manure, cow manure, privies, and garbage, is necessary for effective fly control. Thus, good solid waste management is basic to denying breeding areas and as food sources for adult flies.

Cockroaches

The cockroach, a member of the class *Insecta*, has a three-stage life cycle consisting of the egg, nymph, and adult. The three-stage rather than four-stage life cycle is known as incomplete metamorphosis. Cockroaches have become well-adjusted to living with and near humans. The hardiness of the cockroach is well known. It has been found to withstand radiation doses 50 times that which can kill a human. In addition, immunologists have found that cockroaches have an immune system comparable to that of mammals. Cockroaches also are purported to be the source of allergens to many people living in inner-city crowded conditions. They harbor in cracks and crevices in and around human habitats. Like many other household pests, they travel between sources of disease pathogens (privies, sewers, garbage) and food intended for human consumption. Little evidence supports the outbreak of specific diseases as a result of cockroaches. Because their activity is well known, however, and they have been shown to carry *Salmonella typhimurium, Entamoeba histolytica,* and the virus for poliomyelitis, they are assumed to be a threat to human health. They carry the organisms on their feet, body hairs, and mouthparts, and in their intestines.

Cockroaches eat almost anything from fingernails to steak. They are fond of starchy items such as cereals, bakery products, and book bindings. These roaches also will feed upon beer, cheese, leather, wallpaper, and dead animals. They discharge a nauseating liquid from the mouth and thoracic glands, which imparts an unsavory odor and taste into infested food. They regurgitate partly digested food from their mouths and defecate while feeding, both of which are loaded with microorganisms.

Roaches do not fly; rather, they move by a gliding motion. Most cockroaches are nocturnal, appearing during daylight only if disturbed or very hungry. They prefer to live in warm, moist areas such as cracks and crevices near stoves, refrigerators, hot water heaters, coffee urns, and warm water pipes.

Of the several species of cockroaches, the three most common are discussed here.

1. The American cockroach, *Periplaneta americana*, is believed to have originated in Central Africa but now is found worldwide. The nymphs are white but soon turn a grayish brown and eventually become dark brown in color. This roach has a particular appetite for beer and sweets and often is called the "water bug."

2. The German cockroach, *Blattella germanica*, is native to Europe. It is the pest found most commonly in restaurants and homes. It can enter homes from infested establishments (grocery stores) by means of bottled drinks, packaging, potatoes, onions, other foods, and used furniture. This roach is a pale, yellowish brown and is easily identified by two, dark brown stripes on the pronotum (head). German cockroaches are prolific reproducers. The female carries the eggs in an egg pouch or **ootheca**, protruding from the abdomen until one day before they hatch. These roaches also are known as "Croton bugs."

3. The Oriental cockroach, *Blatta orientalis*, is a dark brown or black species that probably is the third most common cockroach in the United States. It is somewhat less domesticated than most species. The habitat includes sewers, damp basements, outbuildings, and the like. This roach has a strong, repulsive odor. It has the longest life cycle of the three discussed here, and it tends to favor colder climates.

Fleas

Fleas have complete metamorphosis and are members of class *Insecta*. Their effect on people varies from a red spot at the site of the bite to an intense generalized rash. Flea bite sensitization also may occur. The most severe effect is the transmission of disease organisms to people. Although fleas tend to have a preferred host, they will freely utilize another in the absence of their normal host.

Normal flea hosts range from avians to rats to people. The flea normally lays its eggs in the host's hair or feathers. The eggs fall from the host, with the larval stage feeding on organic debris and the pupal stage being spent in a cocoon. Within 24 hours of emergence from the cocoon, adult fleas, both male and female, are ready to feed. Similar to the mosquito, the flea needs the blood meal in order to lay eggs. Fleas are characterized as capillary feeders, using stylets to penetrate the skin and to form a tube to transmit the blood. This enables them to transmit disease pathogens through regurgitation or salivary contamination. They also may transmit disease through fecal contamination. The most noted flea-related diseases are typhus fever and plague. The most notable flea in these diseases is probably the *Xenopsylla cheopis*. This flea is especially vulnerable to blockage of the **proventriculus** by the plague organism *Yersinia pestis*, which causes the flea to regurgitate into a bite wound, thus transmitting the organism to the host.

The control of fleas centers on repressing the flea, either on the host or on a premise area such as pet bedding. Treatment with pesticides to eliminate the flea in yards and lawns is central to their control. In addition, control of the hosts, such as rats, is paramount in eliminating disease outbreaks.

Lice

The final member of the class *Insecta* of public health importance is the louse. Liceborne conditions and diseases historically have been associated with people living in crowded or wartime conditions when bathing and clothes-washing facilities have not been available. Louse hosts are as diverse as that of fleas and, similar to fleas, they are not exclusively selective to that host. The three lice of public health interest are the similar appearing body louse (*Pediculus humanus humanus*) and head louse (*Pediculus humanus capitis*), plus the infamous crab louse (*Pthiris pubis*). These species are known as sucking lice because they take blood meals, and they are found only on mammals.

They undergo incomplete metamorphosis, beginning as an egg (nit) either attached to a hair (head and pubic louse) or attached to clothing (body louse). Heat from the head or body incubates and hatches the eggs into the nymph. The adult is similar to the nymph, but larger. The adult is equipped with mouthparts similar to that of the flea for puncturing and pumping blood, as the louse depends upon blood for sustenance. All three types are responsible for **pediculosis,** heavy infestations of lice characterized by hardened, scarred, pigmented skin and secondary infections, usually a result of intense scratching.

Only the body louse is associated with diseases of public health interest such as louseborne-typhus (*Rickettsia prowazeki*), trench fever (*Rickettsia quintana*), and relapsing fever (*Borrelia recurrentis*). Although these lice are blood feeders, transmission of the causative organism in these diseases typically does not occur from the bite of the louse. It normally occurs through contamination of the bite site from scratching. Fecal material enters these wounds directly or from the louse being crushed and spilling intestinal contents into the wound.

Control of lice focuses on treatment of the host and the host's clothing. Common laundering of clothing with hot water or dry cleaning is satisfactory. Approved insecticides may be used for dusting the host or for treating non-clothing items. Emulsifiable concentrates in the form of a head and body shampoo also are available for elimination of all three types of lice. Prevention is the best tool for eliminating louse outbreaks. Proper hygienic habits — especially teaching children not to share clothing, hats, combs, and brushes with peers — is the most effective means of eradicating pediculosis.

Arachnids

Ticks and mites are of high public health concern. They are of the order *Acarina,* specified by its members' nonsegmented bodies. They belong to the class *Arachnida,* along with mites, spiders, and scorpions.

Ticks

The effects of ticks on humans vary from tick bite paralysis, caused by neurotoxic salivary secretions, to the transmission of disease organisms including protozoa, rickettsiae, viruses, and bacteria. Some species of tick can transmit pathogenic organisms from the adult to the egg, called **transovarian transmission,** and from one developmental stage to another, call **transstadial transmission.**

Ticks are divided into two main groups:

1. Hard ticks (*Ixodidae*)
2. Soft ticks (*Argasidae*)

These are easily defined by the location of the head (capitulum), presence of the scutum, and body shape. Ticks have a four-stage life cycle. Adults mate on the host and the female lays eggs when she drops to the ground. The larvae, also called "seed ticks," develop and attach to a vertebrate host, which leads to the nymph stage. The nymph then finds another host for feeding, and molts to the adult. Depending on the species, the life cycle varies by the number of hosts necessary for development to an adult; these ticks are known as "one host," "two-host," "three-host," or "plural-host."

The method of transmitting disease pathogens varies with the pathogen and with the tick. Some pathogens, such as *Rickettsia rickettsii* (Rocky Mountain spotted fever) and *Borrelia burgdorferi* (Lyme disease), are transmitted by tick bite and by contamination of an open wound by crushed tick tissue or feces. These are related to the hard ticks *Dermacentor andersoni*, *D. variablis* and *Amblyomma americanum*. The soft tick genus *Ornithodoros* transmits the pathogen for tickborne relapsing fever (*Borrelia sp*) by salivary secretions and also by infectious fluids from the coxal glands on the body.

Because the tick is such a significant public health vector of disease, prevention and control is of great importance in disease reduction. Strategies for individuals include tucking trouser legs into sock tops, keeping clothing buttoned, inspecting the body during and after possible exposure to the tick, and using tick repellents such as DEET (N, N-diethyl-meta-toluamide) prior to potential exposure. Additional efforts in residential areas include keeping lawns and yards closely cut. This helps control both the tick and the small rodent hosts. Larger vegetated areas can be sprayed with the appropriate insecticide. Control efforts, too, must focus on hosts such as domestic animals, including the use of tick/flea collars, plus the dipping, spraying, and dusting of animals. Buildings, kennels, homes, and bedding areas must be treated simultaneously with the host to ensure proper control and elimination.

Mites

The final group of arthropods of public health importance is the mite. Like ticks, mites belong to order *Acarina* and have four life stages. Mites may be found in vegetation, on various hosts such as mice, rats, and birds, on organic material such as straw and wood, and living on people. They are responsible for transmitting to humans dermatitis, scabies, allergies, and, most importantly, disease pathogens. These diseases include scrub typhus (*Rickettsia akamushi*) and rickettsialpox (*Rickettsia akari*).

The life cycle of the mite is important in its effects on people.

Scabies, a mite infestation of people causing itching and irritation, often leads to secondary infections induced by scratching. Scabies is caused by the female (*Sarcoptes scabiei var. hominis*) burrowing, after mating, into the epidermal stratum corneum, where she feeds on lymph. There she lays the eggs and leaves scybala (fecal material).

The larva of the chigger (redbug) cause the intense itching of **dermatitis**. It also feeds on lymph and the lysis of tissue. The reaction to the saliva contributes to the itching and general reaction.

The scrub typhus agent is passed by a chigger mite (*Leptrotrombidium akamusi*) transstadially to its larva stage, which feeds on a person, thus passing the disease agent to a new host. The adult does not feed on vertebrate hosts. The agent for rickettsialpox is passed similarly, by the bite of the house mouse mite (*Liponyssoides sanguineus*), which carries the agent in its saliva.

Management of mites depends upon the type of mite. Those that are host-related can be reduced by controlling the host (birds, rats, house mice) by modifying buildings, trapping, and poisoning. Those that live on vegetation are best approached by keeping lawns cut short, eliminating tall weeds, and removing vegetation from near buildings. Pesticides also are used for outdoor residual treatment, fumigation, and by personal treatment after exposure. Preexposure repellents also are recommended. Personal hygiene is paramount, as scabies is passed from person to person in many ways. Hot water and soap are recommended after exposure.

SUMMARY

Throughout history insects and rodents have plagued humans. These pests have destroyed human food supplies and spread disease-causing agents to humans. Thus, vector-borne diseases — one of the four classifications of disease —

have caused much suffering and death. An example occurred during the 1340s when one-fourth of the world's population died of bubonic plague, a disease spread by rats and fleas. Vectors still are prominent in spreading some vector-borne diseases, particularly in developing countries. Thus, efforts to prevent these diseases are aimed at preventing and controlling the vectors.

Control measures, in order of desirability, first should utilize natural measures — remove the food or breeding places. The second most preferred method is biological control, such as having a cat around to hunt mice or fish to eat the larvae of mosquitoes.

Third, and least desirable, is to kill the adults, such as poisoning or spraying chemicals to kill mosquitoes.

REFERENCES

James, M. T., and Robert F. Howard. 1969. *Herms's Medical Entomology.* 6th ed. Macmillan, New York.

U.S. Public Health Service. 1986. *Control of Domestic Rats and Mice.* Government Printing Office, Washington, DC.

———.1982. *Sanitation in the Control of Insects and Rodents of Public Health Importance.* Centers for Disease Control, Atlanta.

———.1988. *Fleas of Public Health Importance and Their Control.* Centers for Disease Control, Atlanta.

———.1988. *Flies of Public Health Importance and Their Control.* Centers for Disease Control, Atlanta.

———.1988. *Household and Stored-Food Insects of Public Health Importance and Their Control.* Centers for Disease Control, Atlanta.

———.1988. *Lice of Public Health Importance and Their Control.* Centers for Disease Control, Atlanta.

———.1988. *Mites of Public Health Importance and Their Control.* Centers for Disease Control. Atlanta.

———.1988. *Mosquitoes of Public Health Importance and Their Control.* Centers for Disease Control. Atlanta.

———.1989. *Ticks of Public Health Importance and Their Control.* Centers for Disease Control, Atlanta.

Ware, George W. 1989. *The Pesticide Book.* Thomson Publications, Fresno, CA.

Principles of Toxicology

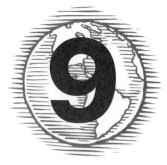

By Larry Curtis, Ph.D.
East Tennessee State University

Key Terms

Acute toxicity

Chemical sensitivities

Chronic toxicity

DNA

Dose-response relationship

Ecological system

Mode of action

Pharmacology

Tolerance

Toxicology

Objectives

🌍 Define toxicology.

🌍 Identify ways in which chemicals damage the body.

🌍 Recognize that humans and other animals are not equally sensitive to the toxicity of specific chemicals.

🌍 Explain why understanding the fundamentals of toxicology is important in environmental health.

🌍 Identify ways in which humans and other animals are exposed to potentially toxic chemicals in the environment.

The study of poisons is called **toxicology**. A chemical acts as a poison when it produces injury, illness, or death. When we hear the word "poison," many of us think of a bottle with a skull and crossbones on it. Although dangerous chemicals indeed can be labeled as poisons, concern over chemical toxicity is broader than this. Any chemical can be toxic if the amount that enters the body — the dose — is great enough. Taking one or two tablets of aspirin can effectively reduce minor aches and pains in an adult; 12 or 15 tablets taken at once can cause nausea and vomiting; consuming 40–50 tablets at once can be life-threatening as a result of severe vomiting, disturbance of blood acid/base balance, and convulsions. The dose determines whether aspirin is a medicine or a poison.

TOXIC DOSES

One responsibility of environmental health practitioners is to assure that exposures to environmental chemicals does not result in a toxic dose. Any chemical can be toxic. The primary role of toxicology in environmental health is to determine the likelihood that environmental exposure to a chemical will result in toxicity. One must consider two types of questions in addressing this issue:

1. What dose of the chemical in question will produce toxicity? Generally, the percentage of individuals who exhibit a certain response to a chemical increases with the dose given. This is called the **dose-response relationship.**

2. What dose do we expect to result from an environmental exposure to a given chemical?

In the examples given for aspirin, the doses are readily apparent. They are simply the number of tablets consumed. In most scientific work the amount taken is adjusted for the individual's body weight. The metric system is used, so doses frequently are given in milligrams of chemical per kilogram of body weight. For most environmental exposures, the situation is not so simple. Chemical exposure may be through the air we inhale, through chemical contact with our skin, or in the food we eat or the water we drink. In cases of exposure from inhalation, chemical concentration in the air and the volume of air we breathe jointly determine the dose. Estimation of dose in this case is not simple because neither of these factors is easy to measure and neither is constant over time.

The time that elapses between exposure and observable response varies for different chemicals. **Acute toxicity** occurs with minutes, hours, or days of exposure. Environmental exposure to some highly toxic chemicals can lead to death almost immediately. Carbon monoxide is an odorless gas produced by incomplete combustion. Headache and confusion, followed by unconsciousness, are signs and symptoms of carbon monoxide poisoning. Exposure to a low concentration of carbon monoxide might produce a single response, a headache. At a significantly higher concentration, a person may lose consciousness and collapse before becoming aware of the problem. Breathing air containing about 1% carbon monoxide leads to death in a few hours. This is why burning any material in an area without good air flow is extremely dangerous.

Chronic toxicity occurs after years of chemical exposure. Benzo[a]pyrene, for example, is produced during incomplete combustion and is present in cigarette smoke. It is not an immediate threat to life, but repeated exposure to it over years can produce lung cancer in cigarette smokers. Deciding whether chronic responses are likely to occur after environmental chemical exposures is the most difficult and demanding problem that toxicologists face.

MODES OF CHEMICAL TOXICITY

The human body contains about 75 trillion cells. Among this number are hundreds of functionally distinct types of cells. These different cell types are organized into the tissues and organs of the body. The interaction between a chemical and a living organism that results in a response is the **mode of action** for that chemical. This way of thinking originated among scientists working in **pharmacology,** the study of drugs and their actions. Most of the work in modern toxicology involves explaining modes of chemical action at the level of injury to individual cells. We are learning a great deal about how specialization in structures of different cell types allows them to serve the functions of various tissues and organs. Mode of action typically involves an interaction between a given chemical and a specific cell structure.

Some cell types contain components unique to them. For example, red blood cells contain hemoglobin, the protein that carries oxygen in the blood. This protein is not found in other cell types. Carbon monoxide binds to hemoglobin tightly and prevents it from carrying oxygen. Therefore, carbon monoxide binding to a certain structure in a specific cell type lessens the ability of blood to carry oxygen to the other tissues of the body. If the dose of carbon monoxide is high enough, the blood cannot deliver sufficient oxygen to the body, and death by suffocation results.

Chemical injury can result in outright cell death if the mode of action inactivates or destroys structures essential to life. In many cases, however, cells are damaged and then recover. Even if a cell repairs the damage inflicted by a toxic chemical and survives, a potential for adverse effects remains. For example, repair of damage to **DNA** may be imperfect. Imperfections in DNA repair result in mutations (you might think of them as genetic scars) and play a role in the development of cancer. Mutations in genes that code for proteins that control cell growth are especially likely to contribute to the development of cancer. Benzo[a]pyrene in cigarette smoke, for example, damages the DNA of lung cells, and imperfect repair of this damage results in mutations that occur in about 60% of human lung cancers.

DIFFERENCES IN SENSITIVITY TO TOXICANTS

One important factor in determining the potential toxicity of a chemical is the amount of it necessary to produce an adverse effect. A chemical is a potent toxicant if a small amount produces an adverse effect. A chemical is of low potency if only large amounts produce an adverse effect. For example, a dose of 10,000 milligrams of ethyl alcohol per kilogram body weight will kill about 50% of the mice receiving it. When a dose of 2 milligrams of strychnine per kilogram body weight is given to mice, 50% of them will die. Clearly, strychnine is a much

Hydrogen sulfide is a gas that bacteria produce as they digest organic matter in oxygen-depleted environments. It is highly toxic and acts by deactivating mitochondria, the subcellular structures that supply chemical energy to cells. Cells cannot operate for long without energy, and hydrogen sulfide poisoning can kill quickly. These poisonings occur mostly in enclosed spaces where the gas can accumulate over time.

more potent toxicant than ethyl alcohol — 5000 times more potent.

The dose of a chemical that produces a response often differs between species and within individuals of the same species. For example, molds that grow on peanuts and corn produce aflatoxin, a chemical that causes liver cancer in experimental animals and humans. The percentage of rats that develop liver cancer after eating a diet contaminated with 15 milligrams of aflatoxin per kilogram of diet increases. Mice can consume a diet containing hundreds of times more aflatoxin without increasing their chance of developing liver cancer. Rats are much more sensitive than mice to aflatoxin-induced liver cancer.

The opposite of sensitivity is **tolerance** — the power of resisting the action of toxins. Mice are much more tolerant than rats to aflatoxin. There are many examples of differences in **chemical sensitivities** — the quality of being sensitive to chemicals — between species. This is a major consideration when we use chemical toxicity information from experimental animals to estimate human responses to the same chemical.

APPLICATIONS OF TOXICOLOGY IN ENVIRONMENTAL HEALTH

Toxicology provides important information for environmental health practitioners. The potential for chemical exposure exists virtually everywhere in our environment: within the home, outdoors, and in the workplace.

Chemical Threats to Humans

Products intended for home use are tested carefully to reduce potential problems, and labeling of hazardous materials is required. Unfortunately, household chemical poisoning still presents a significant public health problem. Poison control centers, usually operated by state governments, provide information to assist the public in cases of such poisonings.

The health concern over chemical contamination of air, water, and food is a longstanding issue. Use of pesticides, releases of chemical manufacturing wastes, and consumption of fossil fuels are most often associated with these pollution problems. Examples of adverse human health effects of chemicals are found in outdoor air, drinking water, and food.

During 1952, air pollution in London is estimated to have caused 4,000 premature deaths. Preexisting poor health is certainly the major factor in the high death toll, but poor air quality over many years probably contributed to this. Examples of pollution producing such obvious responses in human populations are now rare in developed countries like the United States. This does not eliminate the public demand for protection against pollution impacts, though. There is widespread concern over pollution contributing to chronic diseases, especially cancer. People often object strongly to the presence of environmental contaminants even when the potential for toxicity is unclear. This may be largely because of their lack of personal control over exposure. Assessing the likelihood that chemical exposures through outdoor air, drinking water, and food will produce responses in humans is a major challenge in environmental health.

People frequently encounter chemicals in the workplace. Occupational exposures often are in much higher doses than those that occur in the general environment and therefore are of special interest to environmental health practitioners. Working directly with chemicals creates opportunities for exposure that are many times higher than those from air, water, or food contamination. Further, occupational exposure can occur regularly, even daily, over many years.

Environmental health practitioners help develop and enforce government regulations that limit chemical exposures in the workplace. The two major categories of occupations with substantial potential for chemical exposures are industrial and agricultural. *Industrial* activities involve processing or producing virtually every known chemical. Pesticides are of special concern for *agricultural* workers. Limiting occupational exposures through safe handling procedures and protective clothing is essential to environmental health.

Threats to Ecological System

Environmental health practitioners also are responsible for preventing damage to the **ecological system** by chemical releases. Chemicals can be directly toxic to plants or animals and

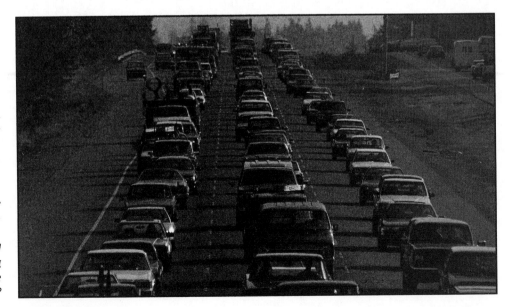

No wonder carbon monoxide levels are high in some cities. As we see only one person in each car, should carpooling become mandatory?

Environmental Health

reduce their likelihood to survive or ability to reproduce. Past declines in numbers of eagles, pelicans and other birds of prey are attributed to extensive use of the insecticide DDT in the 1950s and 1960s. DDT residues are highly persistent and accumulate in animals, including the prey of eagles and pelicans. When feeding on contaminated prey, these birds can accumulate concentrations of DDT residues that poison the gland that deposits minerals in their egg shells. Thin egg shells and a high incidence of egg breakage during incubation explain these reductions in the population. Banning the use of DDT in many industrialized countries is certainly an important factor in the recovery of many bird-of-prey populations over the past 20 to 25 years.

Direct toxic responses of some members of an ecological system can result in indirect responses in other members of the same system. Suppose an animal depends on a certain plant for food. If a chemical is released into the ecosystem that is toxic to this plant but not the animal, only the plant suffers direct toxicity. If the toxicity is severe enough to kill large numbers of plants, the animals will suffer an indirect effect from the loss of an important food resource. Relationships between members of ecological systems often are more complex than this example describes. To accurately predict indirect responses of chemical releases into ecosystems is extremely difficult, if not impossible.

In deciding whether a situation presents a hazard, the environmental health practitioner considers characteristics of the potentially toxic chemical and likely exposure conditions. Accepting the professional judgment of the practitioner is one approach to justifying a decision as to whether a chemical use or release presents a toxic hazard. Risk assessment is a more formal method for making these decisions. Risk assessments characterize the potential for an increase in incidence of adverse health effects from environmental exposure to chemicals. Dose-response information from chemical toxicity studies and assessment of chemical exposure are considered together to estimate the extent of a health problem that a use or release will produce. Risk assessment provides a numerical estimate of hazard and measures uncertainty associated with the estimate. These features make this approach popular with people responsible for setting environmental regulations that might require justification in a court of law.

SUMMARY

Widespread environmental releases of household, industrial, and agricultural chemicals create public concern over the potential for adverse impacts on the health of humans and ecosystems. The study of these poisons is called toxicology, and a chemical is toxic if it harms health. The percentage of individuals who exhibit a certain response to a chemical increases with the dosage, called the dose-response relationship.

Acute toxicity occurs rapidly, whereas chronic toxicity is more difficult to identify as the effects of a chemical may not become apparent until being exposed over several years. The potential for chemical exposure can be present in the home (drinking water and food, for example), outdoors (automobile exhaust and other air pollutants), and in the workplace; the two major occupational categories with potential for chemical exposure are industrial and agricultural.

Also, chemicals can be directly toxic to plants or animals. For example, use of the insecticide DDT, now banned, accumulated in animals, impairing their ability to survive and reproduce.

REFERENCES

Denissenko, M. F., A. Pao. M.-S. Tang, and G. P. Pfeifer. 1996. "Preferential Formation of Benzo[a]pyrene Adducts at Lung Cancer Mutational Hotspots in P53." *Science* 274: 430–432.

Guyton, A. C. 1981. *Textbook of Medical Physiology,* 6th ed. W. B. Saunders, Philadelphia.

Hayes, W. A. 1989. *Principles and Methods of Toxicology,* 2d ed. Raven Press, New York.

Klaassen, C. D. 1996. *Casarett & Doull's Toxicology: The Basic Science of Poisons,* 5th ed. McGraw-Hill, New York.

Radiological Health

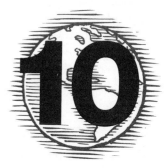

By Albert F. Iglar, Ph.D.
East Tennessee State University

Key Terms

Dosimeter
Geiger counter
Half-life
Ionization chamber instruments

Ionizing radiation
Proportional counter
RAD
REM

Radioactivity
Radon
Scintillation detector
Stochastic effects

Objectives

- List the major sources of radiation.

- Identify major forms of radioactive decay and major types of ionizing radiation.

- Describe units of measure important in radiological health.

- Identify the types of radiation-monitoring instruments and their applications.

- Discuss how to control radiation from internal and external sources.

- Describe the nuclear power cycle as a potential source of exposure to ionizing radiation.

Radiological health, sometimes termed health physics, refers to the protection of humanity from hazards to health, balanced against the benefits of radiation. This means that programs of protection against radiation do not aim at reducing exposure to radiation to zero, because benefits of radiation (such as the use of X-rays to diagnose disease) should be maintained, and because an exposure of zero is not possible (if only because of background radiation from cosmic radiation, terrestrial sources, and body burden).

Radiological health also is limited to **ionizing radiation**, that which interacts with matter to form charged particles. This is defined to include certain electromagnetic radiation (x-radiation and gamma rays) and particle radiation (alpha, beta, neutron, and other radiation). Other radiation that is ionizing under limited circumstances, such as ultraviolet, visible light, and others, is not considered in radiological health.

A distinction often is made between directly ionizing radiation, which includes only radiation composed of charged particles, and indirectly ionizing radiation, which includes neutral particles and electromagnetic radiation. Directly ionizing radiation produces relatively large numbers of ions, mainly by magnetic interaction with the orbital electrons of atoms from a distance. By contrast, indirectly ionizing radiation produces relatively small numbers of charged particles, and these produce additional ions.

SOURCES OF RADIATION

In the United States, diagnostic use of X-rays is a particularly significant source of nonoccupational exposure to ionizing radiation. Thus, state regulatory agencies typically attempt to minimize exposure by assuring that safe X-ray equipment is provided and that it is properly installed, maintained, and operated.

In recent years, radon (or, to be specific, certain of its decay products) has come to be viewed as an important source of nonoccupational exposure to radiation. **Radon** is found naturally in soils, although to widely varying degrees. Various factors in the construction of buildings (such as openings that can admit gases) can increase the entry of radon. Testing of the air in homes for radon is recommended, and sampling can be done easily, by exposure of an activated carbon collector or by other methods. If excess levels are found, various construction measures are available to relieve the problem. The guideline for radon is 4 picocuries per liter.

Other sources of exposure to radiation also can be significant. Use of radionuclides (especially technetium-99m) in medicine, as well as in industry and research, represents multiple sources of exposure. The nuclear fuel cycle (nuclear power) generally presents little nonoccupational exposure to ionizing radiation, but there is concern for catastrophic releases and for an increased number of sources in the future. Consumer products such as smoke detectors provide limited exposure to ionizing radiation. Nuclear weapons present a concern, both from the viewpoint of testing in the atmosphere (now lessened) and from the possibility of use in war.

RADIOACTIVITY

Atomic structure is closely related to emission of radiation. Figure 10.1 shows the general structure of selected isotopes of hydrogen and uranium. Numerous nuclides (a nuclide has a particular atomic number and mass number), including both natural and manmade ones, undergo spontaneous disintegration to more simple forms. This process, which involves emission of radiation, is termed **radioactivity**. This disintegration of given nuclides occurs in such a way that the nuclide approaches stability. An important criterion of the stability of a nuclide is its neutron-to-proton ratio. For atoms with low atomic weight, a neutron-to-proton ratio of approximately 1 is required for stability. Higher ratios are required for stability in atoms with higher atomic weight.

Forms of decay of radioactive nuclides include:

1. *Alpha emission.* Alpha particles have a relative charge of +2 and a mass number of 4, and are identical in structure to helium nuclei. They are emitted by nuclides of relatively high atomic weight, and the loss in mass forms a product that tends toward stability. All comparable alpha particles from a given nuclide have the same energy, although a given nuclide may emit multiple alpha particles of different energy. Thus, all comparable alpha particles from a given nuclide travel the same distance in a homogeneous material. Alpha particles produce high ionization, per unit length of path, although they travel relatively short distances because of their charge. Alpha emitters are of particular concern if they enter the body and become internal sources. Thus, radiation protection means taking measures to prevent alpha emitters from entering the body. One important approach is to keep levels of radionuclides low in the workplace atmosphere.

2. *Beta emission.* Beta particles have a relative charge of −1 and a mass number of zero

Environmental Health

(although they have a small mass). While identical to high-speed electrons, beta particles are emitted by the nucleus. Beta emitters have neutron-to-proton ratios that are too high for stability, and the emission of a beta particle causes a neutron to be replaced by a proton, thus decreasing the neutron-to-proton ratio. Beta particles from a given nuclide have a range of energies but characteristic mean and maximum energies. Beta particles penetrate farther than alpha particles in general, which corresponds to the lesser degree of ionization produced in matter. Beta radiation is of potential concern as an internal source, so measures such as avoiding contamination of air or skin are required. Beta emission also may be significant as an external source, though shielding can be relatively simple (such as with plastic).

3. *Positron emission.* Positron particles have the same mass as beta particles, but the opposite relative charge, +1. They are emitted by the nuclei of atoms with neutron-to-proton ratios too low for stability, and they produce a product with a higher ratio. Positron emission is a form of decay of some radionuclides, but positrons are not a radiation hazard because virtually all positrons are annihilated when they combine with orbiting electrons, the result being production of energy.

4. *X-ray and gamma ray emissions.* These are forms of electromagnetic radiation, consisting of photons traveling in waves at the speed of light. Gamma rays, however, are emitted by nuclei, typically following particle emission, whereas X-rays originate in the orbiting electron structure. An example of the emission of an X-ray photon is found in orbital electron capture, also termed k-capture, in which the nucleus captures an orbiting electron, usually from the k-shell.

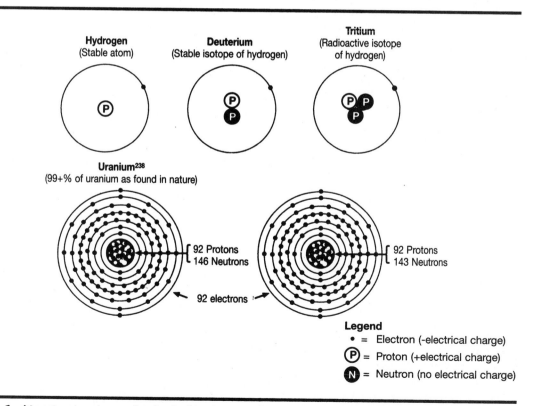

FIGURE 10.1 Atomic structure of selected isotopes of hydrogen and uranium.

An electron with a higher energy level fills the vacant position, with its excess energy given off as an X-ray photon. Orbital electron capture tends to occur in nuclides that have neutron-to-proton ratios too low for stability, and this form of decay causes an increase in the ratio. X-rays and gamma rays have characteristic energies for particular nuclides. X-rays and gamma rays are highly significant if from external sources, and nuclides that emit X-rays and gamma rays also are hazardous as internal sources.

5. *Neutron emission.* Neutrons have mass numbers of 1 (though the mass is somewhat greater than that of a proton) and no net charge. They are highly penetrating in part because they lack a great tendency to produce ionization. Neutron radiation can be significant from both internal and external sources and is associated especially with nuclear fission.

6. *Other forms of decay.* Various other sorts of decay include internal conversion (a gamma photon from a nucleus transfers sufficient energy to an orbiting electron to eject it from the atom) and isometric transition (a higher energy nuclide emits a gamma photon and reaches a lower energy ground state). All atoms of a given radionuclide decay in a defined manner. Although many nuclides have multiple modes of decay, each occurs in a definite proportion of the instances. The result of radioactive decay is, in some cases, transmutation into a new radionuclide. Three radioactive series are found in nature, one nuclide decaying to form another, until a stable nuclide is reached. These are the uranium, thorium, and neptunium series. A fourth series, the actinium series, can be generated artificially.

Radiation from a specific nuclide exhibits a given energy pattern, with energies being expressed in units of mega electron volts (MeV). Further, the decay occurs with regularity for a given radioactive species. That is, a constant fraction of the total number of atoms present decays per unit time. This fraction is unchangeable, except for fissionable nuclides.

Related to this is the concept of **half-life**. The half-life is a constant length of time for any radionuclide, and refers to the time required for half of the atoms of a particular radionuclide to decay. As an illustration, Figure 10.2 shows the decay of a hypothetical substance with a half-life of 24 hours.

UNITS OF MEASURE IN RADIOLOGICAL HEALTH

Activity refers to the quantity of a radionuclide with regard to its rate of undergoing radioactive disintegration. The customary unit of activity in the United States is the Curie (Ci), essentially defined as that quantity of any radionuclide that produces $3.7 \times 10^{1°}$ disintegrations per second. This is a huge quantity of activity, so smaller units are used, including millicuries (1 mCi = 10×10^{-3} Ci), microcuries (1 µCi = 10^{-6}Ci), and picocuries (1 pCi = 10^{-12} Ci). The recommended unit of activity for many purposes is an SI unit, selected as an international standard; the Becquerel (Bq), defined as the quantity of any radionuclide that produces 1 disintegration per second (1 Ci = 3.7×10^{10} Bq).

Radiation monitoring instruments — at least the ones used most commonly — measure exposure based on gas ionization, and related to a unit termed the roentgen. One roentgen is defined as the amount of X-rays or gamma radiation, that together with the associated particle radiation, produces, per standard cubic centimeter of air under standard conditions, in air, one electrostatic unit of positive ions plus one electrostatic unit of negative ions.

Other units of radiation that are especially important in estimating dose of radiation for comparison with standards are:

1. *Units of absorbed dose.* The unit customarily used in the United States has been the **RAD.** One RAD is defined as the dose of any form of ionizing radiation that produces energy absorption of 1×10^{-5} joules/gram

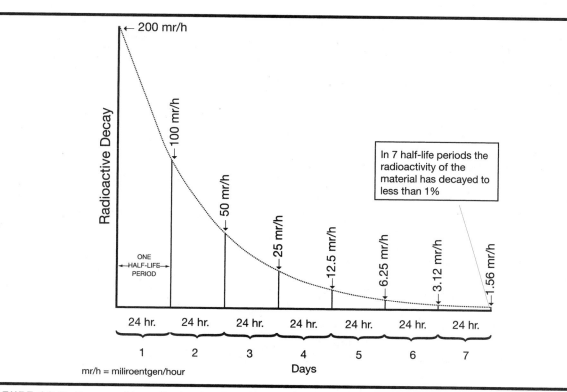

FIGURE 10.2 Decay of hypothetical substance with half-life of 24 hours.

in any specified material. For the SI system, the unit of absorbed dose is the Gray (Gy), defined such that one Gray refers to absorption of 1×10^{-3} joules/gram (1 Gy = 100 RAD).

2. *Units of dose equivalency.* The basis for the approach is that the same absorbed dose can yield very different effects depending on the type of ionizing radiation involved. The common U.S. unit of dose equivalency, the **REM**, is calculated as follows:

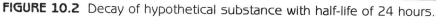

Dose Equivalency = Absorbed Dose × Quality Factor
(in REMs)   (in RADs)

The quality factor (QF) indicates the approximate relative tendency of each type of radiation to produce a biological effect. The quality factors of x, gamma, and beta radiation are taken as 1. The quality factor for neutrons, however, depends on their energy but usually ranges from about 2 to 11, and for alpha the QF is listed as 20.

Basic standards for radiation exposure may be expressed in REMs, such as maximum annual whole body exposure of 5 REMs (occupational). For the SI system of units, dose equivalency is expressed in Sieverts, defined by a similar equation.

INSTRUMENTS FOR MEASURING RADIATION

The most familiar instruments for measuring radiation operate on the principle of gas ionization. The Geiger-Muller counter (sometimes termed **Geiger counter** or GM counter), the best known of these, is a portable survey monitor. In this application, it provides a sensitive means of locating environmental contamination by detecting radiation at an approximate measure of radiation exposure level. The **proportional counter**, also a gas ionization instrument, is used particularly for differentiating radiation in field surveys. **Ionization chamber instruments**, which also utilize the gas ionization principle, are less sensitive but highly accurate. In their most common application, they are used as portable instruments to measure somewhat higher levels of radiation.

The **scintillation detector** is primarily a laboratory-based instrument, often in a system that includes a dedicated microcomputer. Liquid scintillation counters are used especially for measuring and identifying nuclides that emit beta radiation. They find application in the life sciences, most notably for detection of carbon-14 and hydrogen-3. Solid scintillation detectors are used for evaluation of gamma emitters. The semiconductor detectors used in some instruments, however, bring greater sensitivity and improved resolution.

The **dosimeter** indicates cumulative exposure to radiation over time. The most familiar is the nuclear emulsion monitor, more often known as the film badge. Although it provides a permanent record, like other dosimeters it is under the control of the person being monitored. Other devices that serve a similar purpose are thermoluminescent dosimeters (TLD detectors) and pocket chamber dosimeters.

CONTROL OF EXPOSURE TO RADIATION

Radiation can have effects ranging up to loss of life in acute exposure (see Figure 10.3). At present, concern centers on the effects of *chronic* exposure to radiation. In this case, the most notable effects are cancer and hereditary defects. These are called **stochastic effects**, meaning that the dose of radiation determines the probability that the effect will occur. In addition, the stochastic concept includes the non-threshold basis, that no dose of radiation is so low as to avoid these effects totally. Under the stochastic principle, certain control of radiation exposure is required based on the ALARA (as low as reasonably achievable) principle. Radiation

protection includes control of occupational exposure, which involves minimizing exposure to X-rays, controlling exposure by food, air and water, and other measures. One important distinction concerns control of exposure from external sources versus control of exposure from internal sources.

Control of External Sources

External sources refer to those outside the body, such as diagnostic X-ray equipment, a fission reactor, and other sources. The three major methods of control for radiation from external sources are time, distance, and shielding.

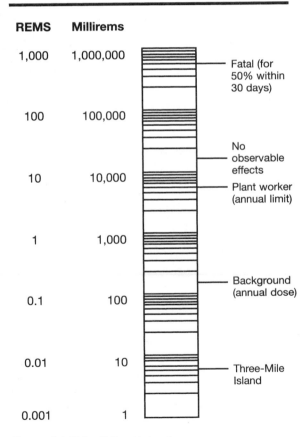

Source: Oak Ridge National Laboratory

FIGURE 10.3 Effects on humans expected at various doses of radiation.

Time

The basis for limiting time is that dose of radiation is the product of dose rate multiplied by time. For example, consider an occupational situation where radiation exposure is 5 mREM per hour, and it is desired to limit total exposure of any worker to 20 mREM per week. The desired limit would be met if each worker were exposed for only 4 hours per week (20 mREM/week divided by 5 mREM/hour = 4 hours/week). This administrative control is relatively simple and inexpensive to implement, although it requires effective supervision (as well as the availability of alternative jobs for workers) and probably is most applicable to low to moderate levels of exposure to occupational radiation.

Distance

Distance as a means of control is predicated on an important characteristic of non-laser electromagnetic radiation: that intensity of the radiation is inversely proportional to the square of the distance from the source. Thus, for example, if the distance from a point source of gamma radiation were doubled, the intensity would be only one-fourth as great. Similarly, if the distance from the source were tripled, the intensity would be only one-ninth as great. Because the range of alpha and beta radiation is relatively limited, this concept usually is limited to X-rays and gamma radiation. The concept also is more difficult to apply to multiple sources and to sources that are too large to be approximated as points. Depending on distance for occupational radiation protection requires effective supervision.

Shielding

Shielding often is the preferred means of protection against external sources of radiation because it creates an environment that is inherently safe. That is, there may be no direct dependence on administrative limitation of exposure time of workers or distance from the source. An important principle of shielding is that a constant fraction of incident radiation is lost in successive equal increments of thickness of the material. In the case of gamma rays and X-rays, the loss in energy occurs by three mechanisms: the photoelectric effect, the Compton effect, and pair production. The same effect of shielding also may be described in terms of the half-value layer, which is the thickness of a particular shielding material that will reduce the intensity of X-rays or gamma radiation of a particular energy by one-half. Although various examples of shielding could be cited, the most familiar probably is the shielding in a room where diagnostic X-rays are performed. Shielding commonly can be found in walls, doors, and floors, depending on the situation. Figure 10.4 illustrates the concept of half-value layer in shielding.

Control of Internal Sources

In the occupational context, control of exposure from internal sources requires preventing contamination of the person, the workplace air, and the workplace itself. A first measure is to enclose the processes that might spread radionuclides in the air or other parts of the workplace environment. A glove box is a simple example of an enclosure that seals radionuclides from the environment of the workplace, yet allows manipulation. With some processes, a combination of at least partial enclosure, supplemented by exhaust ventilation, can be effective in preventing the spread of contaminants into the workplace. Generally this also means that the exhausted air must be treated. For radionuclides in particulate form, this usually involves a roughing filter followed by a HEPA (high efficiency) filter.

For some industrial work, at least minimal potential or actual contamination of the workplace apparently is likely. Standard practice is that access to these areas be limited to employees whose jobs require that they be present and who have received appropriate training. They may wear protective clothing over the entire body. In some situations, workers use respirators to avoid inhaling radionuclides. Before leaving the regulated area, the usual procedure is for workers to remove clothing in a contaminated area, shower, cross carefully into a designated clean area, dress in uncontaminated clothing, and be checked for contamination by use of a radiation monitor.

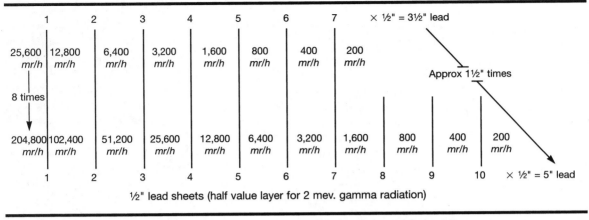

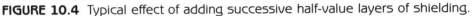

½" lead sheets (half value layer for 2 mev. gamma radiation)

FIGURE 10.4 Typical effect of adding successive half-value layers of shielding.

NUCLEAR POWER

Nuclear power, or more precisely nuclear fission for generation of electricity, is a particular focus of public concern. Potential sources of exposure to radiation encompass the total nuclear fuel cycle (see Figure 10.5), including mining, refining enrichment, generation of power, reprocessing of spent fuel elements, management of waste, and others. The discussion here emphasizes generation of electricity.

In most nuclear power plants, uranium-235 is used as a source of energy. Nuclei of the element tend to disintegrate naturally, with the emission of neutrons and heat. In a nuclear reactor, the neutrons cause the disintegration of more atoms of uranium-235 in a controlled chain reaction. The heat generated is used to produce steam, which turns a turbine and then a generator to provide electricity.

The intention is to design safety into the plant at a fundamental level. The fuel is limited to a maximum of approximately 4% uranium-235, depending on design, and the geometry of fuel materials is such that a compact mass cannot be assembled easily. These measures make it impossible for a nuclear power plant to explode as a fission bomb. Further, the uranium fuel is in a form (often uranium dioxide) that is resistant to solution in water and is sealed inside corrosion-resistant metal tubes.

Redundancy is an important principle in the design of nuclear power plants. This means that plant features critical to safety, such as cooling systems, are represented by replicate units to assure safety under various equipment failure scenarios. In practice in the United States, reactors are enclosed in massive concrete and steel containment structures, designed to preclude disastrous release of radioactive material in the maximum credible accident. Control rods made of neutron-absorbing materials are available for insertion in the reactor.

Despite these precautions, fear of radiation and safety issues are present. Certain discharges of radioactive material are permitted to air and water, although the amounts have been judged to be safe. Further, considering the large release of radioactive material in 1986 from the nuclear power plant at Chernobyl in the Ukraine, renewed attention to safety is surely appropriate. In the United States, future reactors are expected to be designed to be inherently safe by emphasizing negative reactivity. This means that if the fission should start to go out of control, it would have the effect of suppressing the reaction. Figure 10.6 shows the proposed design of a modern reactor.

Breeder reactors represent a way to increase the supply of fissionable fuel for reactors. The basis for the most frequently discussed breeder reactors is the high concentration of uranium-238 found in natural uranium. The fissionable

Environmental Health

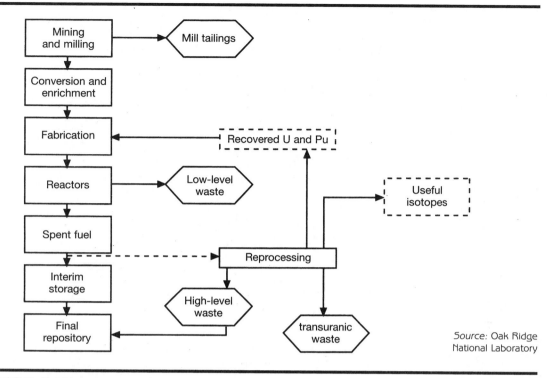

FIGURE 10.5 Nuclear power cycle.

isotope, uranium-235 typically is only 0.71% of the total, and nearly all of the remainder is uranium-238. In fission reactors, uranium-238 can react to form plutonium-239, which is also fissionable. A breeder reactor is designed to enhance this formation, with the result that it produces considerably more fissionable material than is destroyed. In the United States, the Clinch River Breeder Reactor plant was canceled as a result of concern about safety. (One major concern was over the safety of liquid sodium as a coolant.) There is reason to believe, however, that breeder reactors could be important to energy supplies in the future.

Problems with the management of radioactive waste are noteworthy. Low-level radioactive waste usually has been disposed of by near-surface burial in the United States, although this brings concern for contamination of groundwater and other problems. High-level radioactive waste can be sealed deep in the ground in a mined geologic repository. Poor public acceptance (sometimes termed the NIMBY or "not in my backyard" reaction), however, has presented barriers to the development of these disposal facilities.

SUMMARY

Radiological health requires the control of ionizing radiation, that which interacts with matter to produce charged particles. The major types of ionizing radiation are alpha, beta, gamma, X-ray, and neutron, Major sources of exposure include radon, medical use of X-rays, occupational sources, and others.

Exposure may be external (controlled by time, distance, and shielding) and internal (controlled by preventing radionuclides from entering the body). Exposure from the nuclear power cycle and from waste management is presently low but still is a subject of concern.

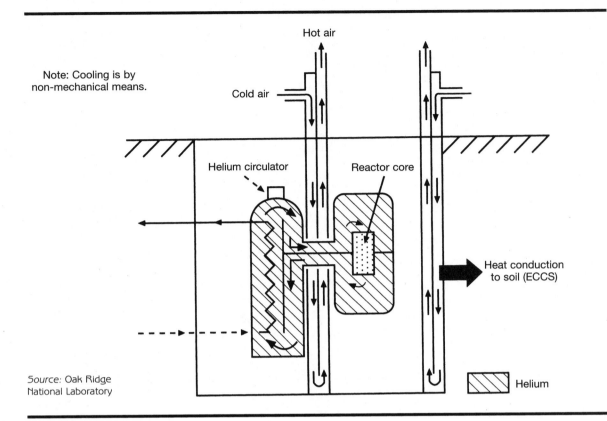

Note: Cooling is by non-mechanical means.

Hot air

Cold air

Helium circulator

Reactor core

Heat conduction to soil (ECCS)

Source: Oak Ridge National Laboratory

Helium

FIGURE 10.6 High-temperature, gas-cooled reactor.

REFERENCES

Eisenbud, Merril. 1987. *Environmental Radioactivity*. 3d ed. Academic Press, Orlando, FL.

Gershey, Edward L., Robert. C. Klein, Esmerelda Party, and Amy Wilkerson. 1990. *Low-level Radioactive Waste*. Von Nostrand Reinhold, New York.

International Physicians for the Prevention of Nuclear War and the Institute for Energy and Environmental Research. 1992. *Plutonium: Deadly Gold of the Nuclear Age*. International Physicians Press, Cambridge, MA.

Martin, Alan, and Samuel A. Harbison. 1986. *An Introduction to Radiation Protection*. 3d ed. Chapman and Hall, New York.

Murray, Raymond L., and Judith A. Powell (editors). 1994. *Understanding Radioactive Waste*. 4th ed. Battelle Press, Columbus, OH.

National Research Council. 1995. T*echnical Bases for Yucca Mountain Standards*. National Academy Press, Washington.

Mettler, Fred A. Jr., and Arthur C. Uptoin. 1995. *Medical Effects of Ionizing Radiation*. 2d ed. Saunders, Philadelphia.

Stannard, J. Newell. 1988. *Radioactivity and Health: A History* (Prepared for U. S. Department of Energy under contract DE-AC06-76RL0 1830). Office of Scientific and Technical Information, Washington, DC.

Wagner, Henry N. 1989. *Living with Radiation: The Risk, the Promise*. Johns Hopkins University Press, Baltimore.

Food Quality Control

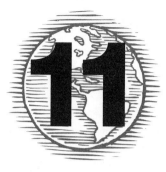

Key Terms

Canning
Desiccation
Drying
Fermentation

Food additives
Osmosis
Osmotic balance disturbance
Pasteurization

Pickling
Plasmolysis
Psychrophilic

Objectives

- Discuss the various aspects of preservation of food.

- Explain the history, significance, and function of food additives.

- Describe food quality management.

- Define and explain foodborne diseases.

- Enumerate the general principles of prevention of foodborne diseases.

- Identify and discuss the importance of milk sanitation principles.

Centuries before microorganisms were first observed under a microscope, their effects on foods were evident to primitive people. Humans learned by experience that fresh foods changed in taste, odor, and appearance with the passage of time. They acquired a liking for certain changes, particularly the alcoholic and lactic acid fermentations, and developed empirical methods of inducing them to add variety to their diet and to preserve seasonal foods for later use. They recognized other changes as spoilage and avoided the spoiled foods as unpalatable or associated with sickness. The ill effects often were attributed to evil spirits, to gods such as Bacchus, or to the influence of the moon and stars.

During the last century scientists recognized the ubiquity and variety of microorganisms and their immense power to decompose food, cause disease, and create new products. On the basis of the pioneering work by Louis Pasteur, Robert Koch, Joseph Lister, Nicholas Appert, and their colleagues, evidence was accumulated to show that microorganisms occur in nature almost everywhere in greater abundance and variety than any other form of life. Not only did scientists show that specific bacteria, yeast, and molds cause particular kinds of fermentation, proteolysis, and fat decomposition, but they also identified the resulting acids, gases, toxins, and other end-products and determined the conditions that would prevent or promote various types of microbial action. These scientists helped to establish the basic principles of food preservation and sanitation on which the U.S. food processing and service industries depend for the preparation of safe, wholesome products.

Bacteria, yeast, and molds play leading roles in the food industry, both in the production of foods such as bread, sauerkraut, cheese, and wine, and in the destruction of foods as a result of rotting and spoilage.

As foods appear in nature, they are essentially free of microorganisms. Microorganisms and other contaminants may be found on the food's surface, but only under unnatural conditions are microorganisms found below the skin or protective outer layer. Some experts think that without the outer skin, microorganisms would invade human bodies so rapidly that within weeks no one would be left on earth. Meats, fruits, and vegetables are similar to humans in that their skin is a protector. If the skin or peeling is cut or removed, microorganisms invade and cause them to rot or deteriorate.

Adding to the above complexities, food no longer is grown where it is consumed, nor is it consumed the day it is harvested. Little of the food served in New York City is grown in New York City or even in that state. The food is shipped many miles from where it is grown to where it is served. Shipping requires time. The food may lie in supermarkets for days before it is sold. Then it may remain in people's dwellings for several days. The longer the food is stored, the greater is the risk of contamination with pathogens and, obviously, the greater the risk of spoilage.

Usually from the time a product leaves a farm until a consumer purchases it, the agricultural industry is responsible for keeping the product as fresh as possible. If it spoils during this time, the industry takes a loss. Therefore, the food industry is interested in the ways and techniques of keeping the product from spoiling or losing its appeal to buyers. This is why the food industry conducts most of the food research done today. It seeks additional ways to keep food from losing its nutritive value, to make it more appealing to potential purchasers, to enable a longer shelf life and to enhance its flavor, texture, and color.

FOOD PRESERVATION METHODS

Food preservation in some form or another has been largely responsible for human survival in areas that have definite seasons. Food long has been preserved during periods of abundant growth for use during periods of drought and winter or to support people in their movements over the face of the earth when they could not pause long enough to grow food. Today a large metropolitan population could not be maintained if we were dependent entirely upon a daily supply of fresh foods.

The art of preserving foods requires knowledge of bacteria and the effect of the environment on microorganisms. Practically all the methods used pre-date any knowledge of microorganisms but still utilize sound biological procedures. Modern innovations include the perfection of vacuum, filtration, pressure canning, and radiation preservation processes. The primary objective of food preservation is to prevent food from acquiring injurious properties during preparation, shipment, or storage. The principal methods with which we are concerned here are temperature control (including pasteurization, cooking, canning, refrigeration, freezing, and drying), chemical treatment, and fermentation.

Temperature Control

The requirements for microorganism growth outlined in Chapter 2 are important to understanding food quality control. If pathogens are present, the body's defenses might be able to withstand a small number if they all contracted during the log phase. On the other hand, a large dose of toxins from bacteria in the log or resting phase could be sufficient to cause disease or even death. That is the basis for the statement "Keep it hot, keep it cold, or don't keep it long." Public health-wise, the two guiding principles in preserving food are as follows.

1. The beginning product should be as clean, fresh, unadulterated, and wholesome as possible so the food might be used before gross multiplication of microorganisms could bring about deterioration or increase the number of pathogens present.

2. The preservation process should be applied as soon as possible and be sufficient to inhibit or destroy the microorganisms. Refrigeration temperatures should be low enough to maintain the inhibiting effect. Heat in canning, cooking, or pasteurization should be sufficient to destroy organisms that would cause disease.

Cold

Cold inhibits or hinders bacterial activity. Low temperatures may, but do not always, kill bacteria; however, they retard the multiplication of most of them. As a rule, pathogenic bacteria do not grow or multiply appreciably at low temperatures, but many of the saprophilic bacteria and molds will grow at 0° C (32°F) or below. Two ways to keep food cold are refrigeration and freezing.

Refrigeration

Most foods contain a large variety of microorganisms, both harmless and harmful. To prevent potentially harmful microorganisms from multiplying, food should be refrigerated. With normal refrigeration temperatures (36° to 45°F) bacterial growth does not cease entirely but is very much retarded. After long periods of refrigeration, **psychrophilic** (cold-loving) bacteria will multiply and eventually spoil the food.

Recalling the phase diagram (in Chapter 2), one sees that if food can be refrigerated while in the log phase, when few bacteria are present and their multiplication has been retarded, the food will keep much longer. The bacteria have not reproduced rapidly, so their numbers should

be small. Therefore, the possibility of consuming the bacteria and thus contracting disease is equally small. If the food was not refrigerated or if the refrigeration temperature was not low enough, however, bacteria may have multiplied to the point that the body's defenses will not overcome them and the consumer will become ill. One also must be careful with foods that have been cooked, refrigerated, set out for serving, and then refrigerated again, because the food may have become contaminated while on display.

Food should be stored in small, shallow, and, if possible, individual containers. Large containers with great quantities of food are to be avoided because the center of the food bulk essentially remains insulated from refrigeration. The required low temperature must reach all parts of the food. Many food poisoning outbreaks have occurred as a result of large quantities of food having been stored in large containers.

Freezing

For the most part, pathogenic bacteria withstand freezing temperatures. As with all ways of killing bacteria, the time element is essential in freezing. The longer the food is frozen, the fewer the number of live pathogens.

If the temperature is kept low and constant for a long time, freezing will kill some animal parasites in meats and other foods. Temperature should be maintained at subfreezing constantly, though. Power or mechanical failure occasionally causes food to thaw and sometimes even reach incubation temperature. When this happens, bacteria will multiply and, after having been refrozen, the food is potentially hazardous to the consumer. Again, freezing the food while it is in the log phase is important because freezing does not necessarily kill the pathogen.

Care should be taken in thawing frozen meat. It is best to place it in a refrigerator to thaw until time to cook the meat. This eliminates the possibility of its reaching incubation temperature.

Heat

Heat is utilized several ways in the preservation of food. These include cooking, pasteurizing, and canning.

1. *Cooking.* Cooking will stop bacterial growth and kill pathogenic and other organisms. It will not destroy staphylococcal toxins, however. Proper recooking will kill the staphylococcal organism and destroy the toxin of botulism. Therefore, food suspected of being recontaminated should be recooked immediately to kill the organism before it produces a toxin.

2. *Pasteurizing.* **Pasteurization** is a time-temperature process that, if performed properly, destroys the pathogenic organism without destroying the taste, digestibility, or nutritive value of food and milk. Pasteurization time-temperature relationships for milk are as follows:

   145° F (62.7°C) for 30 minutes in vat pasteurizer

   161° F (71.6°C) for 15 seconds in HTST pasteurizer

   194° F (90.0°C) with no set time in vacreators

   Because the high temperature kills certain thermophilic organisms, these temperatures are favored. Thermophiles are not of much public health significance, but they do cause some cleaning difficulties.

3. *Canning.* Canning is practically synonymous with sterilizing when the proper temperatures and time schedules are applied. Oversimplified, **canning** involves sealing a can of food with the microorganism potentially in it and heating the can to kill the organism. No more organisms can get in to the can, so the food will keep for a long time. If, however, organisms manage to penetrate the can or if those initially in the food were not killed during the canning process, spoilage will occur. The formation of gas, which leads to expansion or swelling of the can, may accompany spoilage. This is a sure indicator of improper canning. Done

properly time-wise and temperature-wise, canning is a safe and useful way of preserving food.

Drying (Desiccation)

Moisture is necessary for bacteria to survive. **Drying** simply removes the moisture from a product to kill the bacteria. The product then is kept dry to prevent reinvasion of bacteria. This must be a rapid process.

For centuries, humans have made use of solar heat to preserve their food by drying. The introduction of more rapid vacuum-drying techniques has not changed the principle but has merely widened the variety of products that may be processed effectively. Some of the food products currently preserved by drying are fruits, vegetables, eggs, meats, and milk. In conjunction with the loss of water through evaporation, spoilage may continue slowly. Milk, eggs, and other products may become rancid in time after **desiccation**.

Chemical Treatment

Two chemical methods used to preserve food are osmotic balance disturbance and pH reactions. Table 11.1 gives the approximate pH of some common substances.

Osmotic Balance Disturbance

In **osmotic balance disturbance**, liquids pass into or out of bacterial cells by the process of **osmosis**. This is governed according to whether the cell interior has more or less dissolved solids than the surrounding environment. Bacteria have a tendency to tolerate moderated changes in osmotic conditions, but they cannot withstand sudden changes or high concentration of the dissolved solid.

Bacteria placed in a strong sugar solution will die as a result of **plasmolysis**. Utilizing this technique, fruits and vegetables can be preserved for long periods. Cooking in sugar syrups is most effective. The cooking kills the bacteria, and the syrup prevents the growth of bacteria that may be introduced during repeated opening of the container.

Pickling in salt (brine) is one of the older known methods of preserving food. This process, like that of sugar preservation, pulls the water out of the bacteria. The bacteria become dehydrated and die. The chloride ion from salt acts as a germicide, removing oxygen and inactivating the proteolytic enzymes, thereby aiding death. When brine is used, a concentration of from 18% to 25% salt should be maintained to assure good plasmolysis.

Bacteria must have a favorable pH (hydrogen ion concentration). Pickling also takes advantage of this phenomenon. Acids, usually vinegar (acetic acid) have a low pH, and pathogenic bacteria do not grow under such conditions. Bacteria in a solution with a pH lower

TABLE 11.1 Approximate pH of Some Common Substances

Substance	pH	Substance	pH
Apples	2.9–3.3	Limes	1.3–2.0
Apricots	3.6–4.0	Magnesia, milk of	10.5
Asparagus	5.4–5.7	Milk, cow	6.4–6.8
Beans	5.0–6.0	Milk, human	6.6–7.6
Beers	4.0–5.0	Molasses	5.0–5.4
Beets	4.9–5.6	Olives	3.6–3.8
Blackberries	3.2–3.6	Oranges	3.0–4.0
Bread, white	5.0–6.0	Peaches	3.4–3.6
Cabbage	5.2–5.4	Pears	3.6–4.0
Carrots	4.9–5.2	Peas	5.8–6.4
Cherries	3.2–4.1	Pickles, dill	3.2–3.5
Cider	2.9–3.3	Pickles, sour	3.0–3.5
Corn	6.0–6.5	Pimiento	4.7–5.2
Crackers	7.0–8.5	Plums	2.8–3.0
Dates	6.2–6.4	Pumpkin	4.8–5.2
Flour, wheat	6.0–6.5	Raspberries	3.2–3.7
Ginger ale	2.0–4.0	Rhubarb	3.1–3.2
Gooseberries	2.8–3.1	Salmon	6.1–6.3
Grapefruit	3.0–3.3	Sauerkraut	3.4–3.6
Grapes	3.5–4.5	Shrimp	6.8–7.0
Hominy (lye)	6.9–7.9	Spinach	5.1–5.7
Human blood plasma	7.3–7.5	Squash	5.0–5.3
Human duodenal		Strawberries	3.1–3.5
(intestinal) contents	4.8–8.2	Sweet potatoes	5.3–5.6
Human feces	4.6–8.4	Tomatoes	4.1–4.4
Human gastric		Tuna	5.9–6.1
(stomach) contents	1.0–3.0	Turnips	5.2–5.5
Human saliva	6.0–7.6	Vinegar	2.4–3.4
Human spinal fluid	7.3–7.5	Water, distilled	
Human urine	4.8–8.4	(CO$_2$ free)	6.8–7.0
Jams, fruit	3.5–4.0	Water, mineral	6.2–9.4
Jellies, fruit	3.0–3.5	Water, sea	8.0–8.4
Lemons	2.2–2.4	Wines	2.8–3.8

than the optimum for that specific bacteria will die. Bacteria recontaminating food also would be killed by the unfavorable pH (see Table 11.1).

Fermentation

Fermentation is used in the preparation and preservation of many foods and beverages such as cheese, sauerkraut, vinegar, beer and wine. It involves the action of specialized bacteria or yeast. Fermentation produces byproducts (alcohol or acids) that prevent the growth of flora after the fermentation process. For example, members of the lactobacilli group are responsible for the fermentative process in which the end-product of cabbage is sauerkraut. These organisms produce lactic and other organic acids. Because acid inhibits growth, bacteria other than those desiring an acid medium cannot adapt to the acid medium.

FOOD ADDITIVES

In the past, some industries had little consideration for the potential danger of the chemicals used in food preparation to consumers' health. Foods were being sold with additives that never had been checked for consumer safety and palpability. The foods were shipped interstate, making this a federal problem, and the federal government stepped in. The result was creation of the Food and Drug Administration (FDA) in 1931. Overly simplified, the FDA's laws state that no additives that will produce a detrimental effect on the consumer may be placed in food. The FDA requires that new additives be tested — for example, in laboratories on animals — to be sure the additives will not harm consumers.

The Food Additives Amendment, Public Law 85–929, was signed into law on September 6, 1958. It became fully effective for all new chemicals on March 9, 1959, with an additional year allowed to complete tests of chemicals in use prior to January 1, 1958, in the absence of any reason to believe the chemical was unsafe.

Appraising the situation in the mid 1950s, FDA scientists knew that several hundred potentially hazardous additives were being used.

They knew also that some of those in use had not been tested thoroughly for safety. Under the law prior to September 1958, it was necessary to prove in court that the chemical was poisonous or deleterious. This is not difficult for chemicals that cause immediate or acute illness, but today the big problem is the long-term effect on a person's health.

The Food and Agricultural Organization and World Health Organization (WHO) define a **food additive** as a nonnutritive substance added intentionally to food, generally in small quantities, to improve its appearance, flavor, texture, or storage properties. Some of the additives used in foods are identified below.

- *Vinegar* is used to lower the pH, thereby inhibiting the growth of microorganisms.

- *Sugar* is used to enhance taste and nutritive value and to kill bacteria by plasmolysis (shrinking of the bacterium cytoplasm as a result of loss of water).

- *Salt* is used to enhance taste and nutritive value. It also induces plasmolysis.

- Salt has *potassium iodide* added to prevent simple goiter.

- *Nitrates* give a rich color to meats. They are allowable in concentrations less than 200 parts per million (ppm), but in larger doses they reduce the ability of hemoglobin to carry oxygen and produce methemoglobinemia. Nitrates also may react to produce neurosamines, which cause concern about cancer.

- *Formaldehyde,* formerly used as a preservative for milk and occasionally other foods now is prohibited by the laws of practically all nations.

- *Salicylic acid,* formerly used extensively in jams, juices, and other sweets as a preservative, now is prohibited in the United States.

- *Potassium permanganate* is used on the surface of meat to hide evidence of decomposition.

- *Benzoic acid and benzoate of soda* are weak germicides used in tomato catsup. They are allowable in concentrations up to 0.1 percent in certain foods.

- *Borax and boric acid,* formerly used to preserve meats, milk, butter, oysters, clams, fish, sausage and other foods, are no longer allowed.

- *Sulfites,* which act as an antiseptic and color preserver in red meats, are prohibited but frequently are found on ground meat or dusted lightly on wrapping paper and meat blocks.

- *Cinnamon cloves* and *mustard* have antiseptic powers and are used as preservatives, as well as seasoning and flavoring.

- *Additives used for seasoning and flavoring* include ginger, pepper, nutmeg, and garlic, among many others.

- *Propionates* retard mold growth in bread.

- *Nutrient supplements* are vitamins and minerals added to foods to improve their nutritive value. For example, thiamine (Vitamin B_1), riboflavin (Vitamin B_2), niacin, and iron must be added to bread if it is to be called "enriched."

- *Bleaching and maturing agents.* Freshly milled flour has a yellowish color caused by small quantities of pigments. Bleaching agents change the yellow pigment to white.

- *Sulfur dioxide* is allowable for bleaching if it is labeled properly. It is not a preservative.

- *Benzoyl peroxides* are used for bleaching agents.

- *Coloring agents.* Today's consumer expects food to have a characteristic and appetizing color. To obtain this, substances may be added to correct the color change undergone during processing.

- *Carotene,* an extract from carrots, often is added to products such as margarine to give the desired color.

- *Synthetic colors* are used frequently in soft drinks, cordials, frozen desserts, puddings, meat casings and many prepared mixes. A number of synthetic colors and dyes have been banned from use by the FDA.

- *Leavening agents* are substances used to make foods light in weight.

- *Yeasts* produce carbon dioxide by fermentation; thus, holes occur in breads and other yeast products.

- *Baking soda,* when heated, releases carbon dioxide, which forms holes in bread and other baked products.

- *Baking powder* contains baking soda, an acid salt, and starch. When water is added, the acid reacts with sodium bicarbonate in the soda to produce carbon dioxide. The starch then absorbs the water.

- *Antioxidants* prevent an undesirable change in food when exposed to the air. An example is fresh sliced apples, which will turn brown upon being exposed to oxygen. Lemon, orange, and pineapple juices contain sorbic acid (Vitamin C) and are good antioxidants. Therefore, one can dip sliced apples in these juices to keep the apples from turning brown as readily.

  The darkening of some fruits and vegetables results from a type of oxidation known as "enzymatic browning." If these foods are bruised or cut and subsequently exposed to air, the tissue turns dark. Therefore, many times antioxidants are added to retain the natural color. Fats and oils become rancid as a result of oxidation. Butylated hydroxyanisole, sugar dioxide, propyl gallate, and thiodiproprions acid are a few examples of antioxidants. They may not exceed 0.005 percent of total food content.

- *Emulsifiers* often are added to attain consistency. For example, water and oil will not mix, but if an emulsifier is added, they will mix and stay mixed. Some examples are diglycerides from the glycerolysis of edible fats or oils, monosodium phosphates, and propylene glycol.

- *Stabilizers* in small amounts account for the smooth, uniform texture and flavor of many foods. Stabilizers are added to chocolate milk to prevent the chocolate particles from settling to the bottom, and to peanut butter to prevent separation. They also are used in ice cream to increase the viscosity of the ingredients and help prevent the formation of crystals. Some examples of stabilizers are agar-agar, carob bean gum, and guar gum.

- *Thickeners* form a gel. Some fruits contain enough natural thickeners to form a gel — for example, berries and apples from which we make jams and jellies. Pectin and gelatin are good examples of thickeners.

- *Sequestrants.* The word "sequester" means to set apart or to separate. Many fats and oils contain traces of iron or copper. The sequestrants keep these elements inactivate or allow their removal. Sequestrants also play a role in the soft drink industry, tying up calcium, magnesium, and the like, preventing them from precipitating out in the beverages.

- *Humectants* are used to keep moisture in foods. Before humectants were known to exist, people had to buy a coconut, for example, and use it immediately. Now we can buy soft, fluffy, shredded coconut.

- *Nonnutritive sweeteners* are of great benefit to persons who must limit their intake of ordinary sweets. They add only sweetness, not calories or other food value. Saccharine is a good example.

An egg is a good example of a multi-purpose additive. It serves as a thickener in custards, as a leavening agent to incorporate air in baked goods, as a catalyst in candies, and as an emulsifier in solids. Eggs add color, richness, and flavor to many foods, yet eggs are made of only natural elements. Liquid pasteurized eggs are recommended because raw eggs contain *Salmonella enteritis* in the yolk when they are laid.

Population growth and our modern way of life have made food additives necessary. If regulated and controlled, food additives are not harmful. Thanks to the official enforcing agencies, we now can eat our food knowing that the additives have been tested and proven nontoxic to humans in the concentrations in which they are added.

FOOD QUALITY MANAGEMENT

Food is required for humans to survive. Yet the food we must consume also can transport the causative agents of disease. The causative agents are classified as biological (pathogens), chemical, or physical. Because these causative agents can be spread in food, we have to maintain surveillance over food from the farm to the consumer, as shown in Figure 11.1.

1. *Farm.* To prevent chemical contamination, federal, state, and local regulatory agencies approve chemicals that may be used on crops to control pests and undesirable plants. Chemicals that the plant will absorb and those that will be consumed by and harmful to the public should not be used on crops. An example is the pesticide Aldicarb sulfoxide (ASO), used on California melons in 1985. After eating the treated watermelons, 1,350 people became ill. The pesticide was not registered for use on melons in the United States.

    Physical agents such as radiation can contaminate food. One of the underlying reasons for the ban on testing nuclear weapons above the ground is that P^{32}, SR^{90}, I^{131} and other radioactive isotopes can be transported on food from radioactive fallout. Cattle can pass along the fallout from grass to the consumer through milk. Thus, preventing the contamination of pastures, fruits, and vegetables is necessary.

    Biological agents can contaminate food on the farm. Disposing of human waste in a

---

Farm → Harvest → Transporting → Processing → Storing → Preparing → Consumer

---

FIGURE 11.1 Food production and distribution chain.

sanitary manner prevents food contamination. Pathogens such as salmonella in eggs can be introduced into food if chickens have access to improperly disposed human excrement.

2. *Harvest.* Harvesting food into contaminated receptacles can spread causative agents of disease. Farm workers can contaminate food with pathogens, chemicals, and physical agents. Therefore, farm workers, including migratory workers, must have a safe water supply, sanitary sewage disposal, adequate housing, and an environment free of communicable diseases.

3. *Transporting.* During transportation, food can be contaminated by people, storage containers, and so on. For example, lettuce should not be transported in a boxcar, when the boxcar has been used to transport turkeys, unless the car is cleaned and disinfected. Likewise, using a tanker to transport a concentrated insecticide, then milk, would be unacceptable. Surveillance is necessary during transportation.

4. *Processing and storage.* Most of the principles and practices of food processing and storage have been covered already. Where food is processed and stored, approved water supply, sewage disposal, and solid waste disposal systems must be in place. Rodents, insects (such as roaches), and other vermin should not be in the area of food processing, storage, or preparation, because of their ability to spread disease.

5. *Food preparation and consumption areas.* Restaurants, cafeterias, mess halls, kitchens, bars, and dining rooms can be conducive to growing and spreading pathogens, as well as chemical and physical agents of disease. Hence, special attention must be directed to these areas to create an unfavorable environment for the growth of biological agents of disease and the spread of chemical and physical agents of disease. Health departments and environmental agencies have programs to assist food personnel in preventing the spread of disease. These programs involve licensing and inspecting food establishments as well as education services. The best way to discuss these services is to present a typical inspection form (see Figure 11.2) and explain the various items.

If an establishment does not meet the requirements on the form, it does not qualify to sell food to the public and, therefore, will not receive a permit because of the possibility of the food harming, rather than enhancing, the health of consumers.

Structural Items

Floors, walls, and ceilings should be constructed with a nonabsorbent, easily cleaned material that is in good repair. Doors should open outward and be screened, unless another means of keeping out flies, such as fly repellents or air curtains, is utilized. Windows that open also should be screened. Outer doors should be self-closing. All rooms must be relatively free of odors and condensation, which usually necessitates mechanical ventilation. Where mechanical ventilation is used, the fans, filter, and surfaces should be maintained so as to prevent a buildup of grease, which, among other things, can be a fire hazard.

Lighting standards vary. Generally speaking, more light (100 footcandles) is required in food preparation areas than other areas, to promote cleanliness and safety. An example of a kitchen layout for a cafeteria is shown in Figure 11.3.

Water

An approved potable water supply adequate to serve the operation of the food establishment is required. Toilet facilities should be conveniently located, with hot and cold running water. The restrooms must be in good, clean condition and well-ventilated with self-closing doors. There should be no cross-connection where contamination can enter the water supply. Hand washing lavatories must be convenient, with hot and

INSPECTION FORM FOR EATING and DRINKING ESTABLISHMENTS

Form approved.
Budget Bureau No. 68-R023.4.

Sources

Milk, cream ....

Cream-filled pastries ....

....

Shellfish ....

Type ....

Number served
daily ....

Any kitchen maintained
elsewhere? ....

....
(City, county, or district)

NAME ....   ADDRESS ....

SIR: An inspection of your premises has this day been made, and you are notified of the defects marked below with a cross (x). Violation of the same item on two successive inspections requires immediate degrading [1] or suspension of permit. All menu cards or boards shall display grade [1] .... notice.

Item No. [1]

(1) **Floors.**—Easily cleanable construction, smooth, good repair ( ); clean ( ); cleaned only after closing or between meals ( ), by dustless methods ( ).. ( )

(2) **Walls and ceilings.**—All: clean, good repair ( ); kitchen: light color ( ), walls smooth, washable to level of splash ( )...................................... ( )

(3) **Doors and windows.**—Outer openings with effective screens and outward-opening, self-closing doors, or fly-repellent fans, or flies absent............................ ( )

(4) **Lighting.**—Natural or artificial light equivalent to 10 foot-candles on working surfaces (except in dining room), 4 in storage rooms............................ ( )

(5) **Ventilation.**—All rooms (except cold storage) reasonably free of odors and condensation........................ ( )

(6) **Toilet facilities.**—Comply with plumbing code ( ); adequate, conveniently located for employees ( ); good repair, clean, no flies ( ); well lighted, outside ventilation ( ); in new establishments, no direct opening ( ); self-closing doors ( ); washing sign for employees ( ); privies, if used, comply State standards ( )........ ( )

(7) **Water supply.**—Running water accessible as required ( ); supply adequate ( ); safe, complies State standards ( ).. ( )

(8) **Lavatory facilities.**—Adequate, convenient ( ); hot and cold running water ( ); soap ( ); approved sanitary towels ( ); hands washed after toilet ( ).. ( )

(9) **Construction of utensils and equipment.**—Easily cleanable construction, self-draining, no corrosion ( ); good repair, no open seams, no chipped or cracked dishes ( ); no cadmium or lead utensils ( )... ( )

(10a) **Cleaning of equipment.** — Clean cases, counters, shelves, tables, meat blocks, refrigerators, stoves, hoods ( ); clean cloths used by employees ( ) ( )

(10b) **Cleaning of utensils.**—Single-service cups, plates, straws, caps used only once ( ); eating and drinking utensils thoroughly cleaned after each use ( ); other utensils cleaned each day ( ); suitable detergent used ( ); no cyanide or other poisonous compounds ( ).................................. ( )

(10c) **Bactericidal treatment of eating and cooking utensils.**—Approved bactericidal treatment after cleaning: Immersed 2 minutes in 170° F. water, or one-half minute in boiling water, or 2 minutes in approved chlorine rinse; or kept in steam cabinet 15 minutes at 170° F. or 5 minutes at 200° F.; or in hot-air cabinet 20 minutes at 180° F. ( ); cabinets have thermometer in coldest zone ( ); large utensils adequately treated with live steam, boiling water, or chlorine spray or swab ( ); dish-washing machine properly operated ( ). Utensils comply bacterial standard ( ); drying cloths, if used, kept clean and used for no other purpose ( ) ( )

Item No. [1]

(11) **Storage and handling of utensils.**—Stored above floor in clean place protected from flies, splash, dust, etc., inverted or covered when practicable ( ); no handling of contact surfaces ( ); single-service cups, straws, etc., purchased in sanitary cartons, kept in clean dry place, and properly handled ( ); dispensing spoons, dippers kept in hot or running water ( ).. ( )

(12) **Disposal of wastes.**—Liquid wastes into public sewer or as approved by State ( ); no back-siphonage into water supply from toilets, washing machines, sinks, etc. ( ); garbage stored in tight, non-absorbent, washable receptacles, covered pending removal ( ), removed frequently and receptacles washed to prevent nuisance ( )................ ( )

(13) **Refrigeration.**—Readily perishable foods (including cream-filled pastry, meats, milk, etc.—*see* Code) stored at 50° F. or less ( ); ice stored and handled in approved manner ( ); drip enters open trapped drain or pan ( ).................................. ( )

(14a) **Wholesomeness of food.**—Wholesome, clean, no spoilage ( ); prepared so safe for human consumption ( ); cream-filled pastry rebaked unless filling adequately cooked, and promptly cooled ( ) ( )

(14b) **Wholesomeness of milk products.**—Milk, fluid milk products, frozen desserts from approved sources ( ); milk, etc., served in original individual bottles or from approved bulk dispenser ( ).......... ( )

(14c) **Wholesomeness of shellfish.**—Shellfish from approved sources ( ); shucked shellfish kept in original containers ( ).. ( )

(15a) **Storage of food and drink.**—No contamination by overhead leakage or submerging ( ); not on floors subject to flooding from sewage backflow ( ).. ( )

(15b) **Display and serving of food and drink.**—Minimum manual contact with food and drink ( ); no open displays ( ); no animals or fowls ( ); flies, roaches, and rodents under control ( ); no uncolored poisonous pesticides ( )........................ ( )

(15c) **Ratproofing.**—Structure ratproofed............................ ( )

(16) **Cleanliness of employees.**—Clean outer garments, used for no other purpose ( ); hands clean ( ); no spitting, no tobacco used where food prepared ( ).. ( )

(17) **Miscellaneous.**—Premises kept neat and clean ( ); no operations in living or sleeping rooms ( ); clean, adequate lockers for employees' clothing, not in kitchen ( ); soiled linens, coats, aprons kept in containers ( ).. ( )

(Sec. 9) **Disease control.**—No person at work with any communicable disease, sores, or infected wounds ( ); Section 9 posted in all toilets ( ); employees' health certificates (if required locally) ( )....... ( )

REMARKS: ....

Date ....

....
Inspector.

FIGURE 11.2 Example of an inspection form.

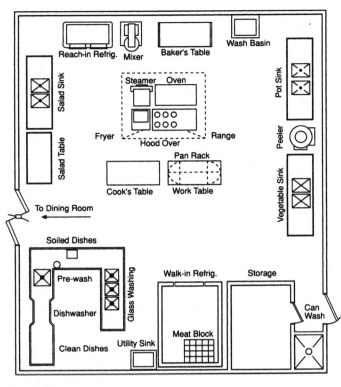

Source: U.S. Public Health Service Training Manual

FIGURE 11.3 Layout of a modern cafeteria kitchen.

cold water adequate to serve the employees and the public. Sanitary towels and soap dispensers are required.

Equipment and Supplies

Food-contact equipment and utensils should be free of cracks and seams where food can build up. This equipment should be kept clean and should be constructed of materials that will not leak toxic substances, such as copper, into the food. No cyanide (commonly used to clean silver) or other poisonous compounds are to be used for cleaning or other purposes in the vicinity of food. Cleaning materials are to be stored in a designated place separate from food. Also, insecticides and rodenticides have no place

where food is displayed, served, or stored but always should be stored in a designated area separate from food.

Equipment that comes in contact with food, and the food itself, must be stored properly in a place unaccessible to flies, rodents, roaches, or dust. This also should be a place where it will not be subjected to "fallout" from above or contact with the floor. If food or food equipment comes in contact with the floor, it may contact contaminants from the people who walk through, as well as the sewage from an overflowing toilet or plugged floor drain, or splash from mopping the floor. Thus, the storage recommendation is that it be at least 6 in. (15 cm) above the floor to prevent contamination and enhance cleaning under storage areas.

Sanitizing of Dishes

Eating and cooking utensils must be cleaned and sanitized after each use. Sanitization can be accomplished through several bacteriocidal methods. To make sure that disease is not spread by forks, spoons, and other tableware, the utensils may be immersed in a chemical rinse, in hot water at least 170°F (76.6°C), or run through a dishwasher with the water at least 180°F (82.2°C).

Generally, dishes are sanitized in food establishments by using a dishwashing machine and a detergent applied through an automatic dispenser and having a wash period of not less than 40 seconds with washwater under pressure at 140 gallons per minute, or 9.2 gallons per rack at a temperature of 150°F. This is followed by a clear water rinse of 10 seconds duration at a temperature not less than 180° F and with a flow of not less than 1.73 gallons per rack at 20 pounds per square inch or 1.5 gallons per rack at 15 pounds per square inch. This is in accordance with the recommendation of the National Sanitation Foundation standard number 5. Because of the possibility of spreading disease, dishwashing is extremely important.

No single antimicrobial agent is "best" or "ideal." This is not surprising in view of the variety of conditions under which agents may be used and the many types of microbial cells to be destroyed. An ideal antimicrobial agent — a disinfectant — would have to possess a formidable array of specific characteristics. A single compound possessing these properties may never be found. Nevertheless, the specifications below can be the goal in preparing new compounds, and they should be considered in evaluating disinfectants made available for practical use.

1. *Toxicity to microorganisms.* The substance must have the capacity to kill microorganisms. It should have a broad spectrum of activity and be microbicidal in high dilution (low concentrations).

2. *Solubility.* The substance must be soluble in water or in tissue fluids to the extent necessary for effective use.

3. *Stability.* Changes in the substance that result from standing should not cause loss of germicidal action.

4. *Nontoxicity to humans and animals.* The compound should be extremely toxic to microorganisms and noninjurious to humans and animals.

5. *Homogeneity.* The preparation must be uniform in composition. Pure chemicals are uniform, but mixtures of materials may lack homogeneity.

6. *Capacity to avoid combination with extraneous organic material.* Many disinfectants have an affinity for proteins or for some other organic material. When these disinfectants are used in situations where there is considerable organic material besides the bacterial cells, little, if any, of the disinfectant will be available for action against the bacteria.

7. *Toxicity to microorganisms at room or body temperatures.* In using the compound, the temperature should not have to be raised beyond that found normally in the environment where it is to be used.

8. *Capacity to penetrate.* Unless the substance can penetrate through surfaces, its germicidal action is limited solely to the site of application. In some instances, of course, surface action is all that is required.

9. *Noncorrosiveness and nonstaining.* The disinfectant should neither rust nor otherwise disfigure metals or stain or damage fabrics.

10. *Deodorizing ability.* Deodorizing while disinfecting is desirable. Ideally, the disinfectant itself should be either odorless or have an odor with aesthetic appeal.

11. *Detergent capacities.* A disinfectant that is also a detergent (cleaning agent) accomplishes both objectives, and the cleansing action improves the effectiveness of the disinfectant.

12. *Availability.* The compound must be available in large quantities at a reasonable price.

Waste Collection

Refuse and other wastes should be stored, collected and disposed in a sanitary manner, as discussed in Chapter 7. It should be stored in adequate fly-tight containers and collected at least twice a week to break the insect breeding cycle. Containers should be kept clean and stored above the ground. (In warmer areas, it is recommended that "garbage rooms" be refrigerated.)

Refrigeration

Refrigeration in food service areas is extremely important in preventing the spread of diseases and in preserving food. Most foods contain a large variety of microorganisms, both harmful and harmless. Therefore, they should be refrigerated to prevent multiplication. At normal refrigeration temperatures of 36° to 45°F (2.2° to 7.2°C), bacterial growth does not cease but is very much retarded. Foods will spoil, though, after a long period of refrigeration, through slow bacterial reproduction of psychrophiles.

Food Purchase, Display, and Serving

Food should be obtained from an approved source and, wherever possible, served in the original container to reduce the chance of contamination. Oysters and other readily perishable foods must be purchased from an approved source and kept under refrigeration until prepared and served. Food canned at home should not be served in restaurants. Display and serving of food should be done in such a manner as to minimize human contact with the food. For example, sneeze guards should be available where food is displayed and served to prevent the public from coughing and sneezing on the food in the serving lines. Surveillance must be maintained over the food and drink to ensure health and safety.

FOODBORNE DISEASES

Foodborne diseases are of two main types: (a) foodborne infections and (b) chemical food poisoning. In foodborne infections, an organism invades the tissues of the host. Generally, fever accompanies foodborne infections. In food poisoning, a chemical, such as the preformed toxin of the staphylococcus does the damage. Fever does not accompany food poisoning.

Some of the most common foodborne diseases are discussed in terms of their causative agents, symptoms, incubation period, conditions of occurrence, body site(s) affected, sources of infection, and methods of control. Foodborne diseases including salmonellosis, typhoid fever, cholera, amebiasis, shigellosis, and brucellosis are discussed in Chapter 3 and are repeated in this chapter with emphasis on the favorable environment and method of control as they apply in food versus water, fomites, and vectors.

Foodborne Infections

Salmonellosis

Causative Agent: Gram negative, rod-shaped bacillus. *Salmonella sp.* is common in all parts of the world. There are 2,000 different strains or serotypes of the organism, and additional ones are being discovered constantly.

Symptoms: Fever, severe abdominal pain, nausea and vomiting, anorexia, weakness, dehydration.

Incubation Period: Symptoms appear 6 to 48 hours after ingestion. Illness usually occurs in 12 to 24 hours and may last from 3 days to 3 weeks.

Conditions of Occurrence: Cases occur throughout the year, with the greatest number reported between July and September.

Body Site(s) Affected: Usually invades and localizes in the gastrointestinal system. In extreme instances it may invade other systems, causing pneumonia, meningitis, pyelonephritis, endocarditis, and pericarditis.

Sources of Infection: Animals serve as the main reservoir of infection — pet dogs, pet turtles, and animals whose flesh serves as food, such as turkeys and chickens. Foods that support growth and multiplication of salmonella are: whole eggs and egg products, poultry, meat and meat products, commercially processed meats and poultry, pies, sausages, unpasteurized whole milk and milk products. Animal feed and mixes are primary sources of salmonella (made from waste animal byproducts).

Methods of Control:

- Thoroughly cook all foodstuffs from animal sources.
- Avoid recontamination of food after cooking.
- Do not eat raw, undercooked, dirty, or cracked eggs.
- Pasteurize milk and milk products.
- Refrigerate foods properly.
- Educate food handlers and homemakers in the importance of adequate refrigeration of foods, hand washing before food preparation, maintaining a sanitary food area, and protecting food from rodent and insect contamination.
- Ensure meat and poultry inspection by trained personnel with supervision of abattoirs, as well as federal inspection of animals (cattle, sheep, goats, swine, horses), interstate shipment with the purpose of excluding diseased animals, and handling of meats.
- Be sure animal feed is cooked or heat-treated.
- Protect foods from exposure to rat or mouse feces and from contact with houseflies.

Typhoid Fever

Causative Agent: Gram-negative bacillus. *Salmonella typhi.* Description: Mobile, flagellated.

Symptoms: Fever, malaise, anorexia, slow pulse, enlargement of spleen, diarrhea or constipation.

Incubation Period: From 1 to 3 weeks, but usually 2 weeks after ingesting contaminated food or water. Patients discharge typhoid bacilli in their feces from the first week of illness throughout convalescence. Often carriers may go for periods of time with feces free of the bacilli, after which they start shedding them again.

Conditions of Occurrence: In 1900, 350,000 cases were reported, in the United States, with 35,000 deaths. In 1933, 65,000 cases were reported, with 10% case fatality rate. Today an occasional case or a small, limited outbreak occurs in some areas. Fortunately, with fewer cases, typhoid fever carriers are not developing in sufficient numbers to offset the loss by death of present older carriers. By the end of the century, if typhoid fever cases and outbreaks continue to be prevented and controlled, all chronic carriers will have died, eliminating the last reservoir of infection in the United States.

Body Site(s) Affected: Early in the disease, typhoid bacilli are found in the blood. After the first week they appear in the feces, and occasionally in the urine.

Sources of Infection: Raw or inadequately cooked foods, and those that require no cooking, such as raw vegetables and fruits, salads, pastries, unpasteurized milk and milk products, and shellfish from areas polluted by sewage. Contamination of food is usually by the fecal-soiled hands of a carrier. Flies are another source of spread, by transferring typhoid from contaminated sewage to food. Water supplies, particularly from wells polluted by sewage from a neighboring cesspool containing the bacilli, have been incriminated in outbreaks. Humans are reservoirs.

Methods of Control:

- Dispose of human excreta in a sanitary manner.
- Protect, purify, and chlorinate the water supply.
- Control flies by eliminating fly-breeding places such as exposed garbage.
- Pasteurize milk and milk products.

- Periodically inspect and provide sanitary supervision of establishments where food is processed, prepared, and served.
- Prohibit the collection and sale of shellfish except from approved sources.
- Instruct patients and chronic carriers in personal hygiene, with emphasis on sanitary disposal of excreta and hand washing after defecation.
- Discover and supervise chronic typhoid carriers, and prohibit them from working as food handlers.
- Educate the general public and food handlers about foodborne diseases, sources of infection, and modes of transmission.
- Vaccinate contacts and persons subject to unusual exposure.

Cholera

Causative Agent: *Vibrio cholerae*. Description: Comma-shaped bacilli.

Symptoms: Sudden onset of violent purging, vomiting, cramps, subnormal temperature, extreme dehydration, and circulatory collapse. Fatality rate ranges from 30% to 80%, with death sometimes occurring within a few hours after onset.

Incubation Period: Brief, from several hours to 3 days.

Conditions of Occurrence: During the 19th-century pandemic, cholera spread repeatedly from its origins in Bengal and other parts of India to most parts of the world. Since 1960, the disease has been recognized as an increasingly serious endemic and epidemic problem in many countries of South Asia and the Western Pacific. People living in endemic areas often acquire immunity to cholera through minute infections that do not become apparent. Patients should be isolated during the acute stage of cholera.

Body Site(s) Affected: Cholera is an acute intestinal disease.

Sources of Infection: The disease is spread when the feces or vomitus of patients or convalescent carriers contaminate food, milk, or water; water is the chief means of infestation. Eating fruits and vegetables washed with contaminated water may convey the disease. It may be spread by direct contact with patients or by flies.

Methods of Control (similar to those of typhoid fever):
- Dispose of patients' feces and vomitus in a sanitary manner.
- Have a protected and purified water supply.
- Pasteurize milk and other foods.
- Control fly populations.
- Educate the public in personal hygiene and hand washing.

Amebiasis

Causative Agent: *Entamoeba histolytica*, a protozoan.

Symptoms: Asymptomatic or mild with abdominal discomfort, distension, and diarrhea alternating with constipation. In severe cases, diarrhea may be more severe, with blood and mucus, dehydration, and blood loss.

Incubation Period: From 5 days to several months; commonly 2 to 4 weeks.

Conditions of Occurrence: Amebiasis occurs in people living under poor hygienic conditions, in institutions, mental hospitals, orphanages, and prisons. In the United States, amebiasis may occur among any group of people, but its highest incidence is in rural areas among lower socioeconomic groups and in crowded areas.

Body Site(s) Affected: Amebiasis is a disease of the large intestine.

Sources of Infection: Found in human excreta. Spread is by contamination of foods by hands soiled with fresh feces. Also, water contaminated with human feces. Flies also can spread the disease.

Methods of Control:
- Provide for sanitary disposal of feces.

- Protect public water supplies against fecal contamination.
- Educate the general public, as well as food handlers, in hygienic measures such as hand washing after defecation and before preparing food.
- Inspect and supervise sanitary practices in public eating establishments.
- Protect food from fly contamination.

Shigellosis (Bacillary dysentery)

Causative Agent: *Shigella bacilli*

Symptoms: Acute infection of the bowel; diarrhea, fever, vomiting, cramps, and tenesmus (ineffective efforts at defecation). In severe cases the stools may contain blood, mucus, and pus.

Incubation Period: 1 to 7 days; usually less than 4 days.

Conditions of Occurrence: In all parts of the world. Occurs most frequently in the tropics and especially in areas of overcrowding, poor sanitary conditions, and malnutrition. Outbreaks have occurred in institutions for children, in jails, in mental institutions, in military bases, and on reservations.

Body Site(s) Affected: Intestines and bowels, resulting in dysentery.

Sources of Infection: Humans are its reservoir; domesticated animals also may harbor and disseminate organisms. Fecal-oral transmission from an infected person; transmitted indirectly by objects spoiled with such feces; by eating contaminated foods or drinking contaminated water or milk; by flies; also, direct contact.

Methods of Control:
- Ensure sanitary disposal of human feces.
- Protect and purify water supply.
- Pasteurize milk and dairy products.
- Supervise the processing, preparation, and serving of foods according to sanitation guidelines.

- Educate mothers in the hygiene of breast-feeding and the preparation of formulas, with emphasis on boiling milk and water.
- Wash hands after defecation and before handling food.
- Control flies through screening and other measures.

Streptococcal Food Infection

Causative Agent: *Streptococcus faecalis* (gastrointestinal tract) and *Streptococcus pyogenes* (respiratory system, sore throat, scarlet fever).

Symptoms: *S. faecalis* — nausea, vomiting, diarrhea, abdominal cramps; *S. pyogenes* — sore throat, headache, pains.

Incubation Period: *S. faecalis* — 2 to 18 hours; *S. pyogenes* — 1 to 3 days; may be transmitted to others for about 10 days.

Conditions of Occurrence: Both occur throughout the world. Because of the many different types of *S. pyogenes*, a person can get the disease again and again.

Body Site(s) Affected: *S. faecalis* — gastrointestinal tract; *S. pyogenes* — respiratory tract.

Sources of Infection: *S. faecalis* — foods such as beef croquettes, sausage, ham, bologna, turkey dressing, coconut cream pie, and whipped cream. *S. pyogenes* — transmitted to respiratory system by intimate contact with patients or carriers, through inhalation of droplets containing the organisms, or by ingesting milk or other foods. Humans are reservoirs.

Methods of Control:
- Educate the public in modes of transmission and complications.
- If milk is not pasteurized, boil it.
- Do not use or sell milk from cows with mastitis.
- Exclude food handlers and others with respiratory infections or other septic conditions from preparing or serving food.

- Prepare foods that favor the growth of streptococci (such as deviled eggs) just before serving or refrigerate at 41°F or below.

Escherichia coli Diarrhea

Causative Agent: *Escherichia coli*

Symptoms: Severe diarrhea, abdominal pain, nausea, vomiting, occasionally fever. Potentially high fatality rate (up to 40%). Illness lasts from 1 to 3 days.

Incubation Period: 12 to 72 hours after infection.

Conditions of Occurrence: Occurs worldwide, especially in Latin American countries. Affects travelers usually within a few days of their arrival in a new area (known as "traveler's diarrhea").

Body Site(s) Affected: Intestinal tract.

Sources of Infection: E. coli is natural flora in intestinal tract of humans and animals. Meat-packing workers are exposed by cattle and swine. Foodborne and waterborne outbreaks occur in communities with inadequate sanitation, through fecal contamination of food or water.

Methods of Control: Preventive measures are like those for typhoid fever and other diseases spread by the fecal-oral route.

Staphylococcal (food) poisoning

Causative Agent: *Staphylococcal aureus*. Forms a toxin in food that is thermostable (not destroyed or altered by heat).

Symptoms: Severe nausea, cramps, vomiting, diarrhea, prostration; often subnormal body temperature and sometimes markedly lowered blood pressure. Deaths are rare. Duration of illness is usually 1 to 2 days.

Incubation Period: Interval between eating food and onset of symptoms is 1 to 6 hours, usually 2 to 4 hours.

Conditions of Occurrence: Widespread and relatively frequent; one of the main acute food poisonings in the United States.

Body Site(s) Affected: Gastrointestinal tract (attacks the intestinal tissues).

Sources of Infection: Pastries, custards, salads, chopped and sliced meats, ham, bacon. Food may be contaminated with pus from a food handler's infected finger or abscesses on an exposed part, or by nasal secretions. Organisms may be present even on hands with intact skin. Contaminated milk from a cow with mastitis (an infected udder). Reservoir in most instances is humans, occasionally cows. For a case or an outbreak of staphylococcal food poisoning to occur, the following conditions must be present: (a) the food is contaminated with enterotoxin-producing staphylococci; (b) the organisms multiply and produce the toxin; (c) the contaminated food is kept for a suitable time period at temperatures compatible with growth of the organism.

Methods of Control:

- Promptly refrigerate food (especially custards and cream fillings) to avoid multiplication of staphylococci introduced accidentally.
- Immediately dispose of or promptly refrigerate leftover foods.
- Temporarily exclude persons who have pyogenic skin infections.
- If you are handling food to be consumed by others and you have a respiratory infection, use a face mask.
- Educate food handlers about strict attention to sanitation and cleanliness of kitchens, including proper refrigeration, hand washing with attention to fingernails, and the danger of working while having a skin or throat infection.
- Emphasize the importance of refrigeration of food. Food prepared a number of hours before it is eaten either should be rerefrigerated at a temperature below 7.2°C (45°F) or should be kept heated above 60°C (140°F). The maximum time that cooked food may be kept between these temperatures is 3 hours.

Botulism (poisoning)

Causative Agent: *Clostridium botulinum*. A harmless saprophyte, but the toxin it produces is one of the most potent neurotoxins known to mankind. Description: rod-shaped, spore-forming, anaerobic bacillus.

Symptoms: Acute digestive disturbances (nausea, vomiting, constipation) occur within 12 to 24 hours after ingesting contaminated food. May be accompanied by weakness, dizziness, headache, and muscular incoordination; soon followed by signs of paralysis of cranial nerves with diplopia (double vision), belpharoptosia (narrowing of slit between eyelids), mydriasis (dilation of pupils), hoarseness with difficulty in speech and swallowing. Fatality rate is about 65% and higher when large amounts are ingested.

Incubation Period: Illness may occur within 12 to 24 hours after eating food containing the toxin. Incubation period may be considerably shorter in more severe illness, with death occurring within 3 to 6 days if the ingested food contains a high concentration of toxin. If the dose of toxin is minimal, symptoms may not appear for several days.

Conditions of Occurrence: Few cases throughout the world. Today, botulism is a relatively rare disease.

Body Site(s) Affected: Gastrointestinal tract and cranial and other nerves.

Sources of Infection: Improper canning of vegetables, meats, and meat products, fish and seafood, and other protein foods. The heat often used in cold-pack canning may not be sufficient to kill the spores and inactivate the toxin. Pressure cooker method is recommended. A temperature of 120° C for 10 minutes is necessary to destroy both spores and toxin. Reservoir — soil, water, and intestinal tracts of animals, including fish.

Methods of Control:
- Educate home canners about safe canning methods in timing, pressure, and temperature required to destroy botulinus spores and the necessity of boiling all home-canned vegetables for 10 minutes before serving. Botulism is very rarely caused by commercially canned or processed foods.
- When in doubt, throw it out.

Clostridium perfringens (food poisoning)

Causative agent: *Clostridium perfringens*. Description: gram positive, short, plump, rod-shaped, spore-forming bacillus, occurring singly or in pairs; capsulated and nonmotile; spores are heat-resistant and capable of surviving boiling.

Symptoms: An intestinal disorder characterized by sudden onset of abdominal colic followed by diarrhea. Nausea is common but vomiting usually is absent. Generally a mild disease of short duration, 1 day or less, and rarely fatal in healthy individuals.

Incubation Period: The incubation period of clostridial food poisoning is 8 to 22 hours, usually 10 to 12 hours.

Conditions of Occurrence: Widespread and relatively frequent in countries with cooking practices that favor multiplication of clostridium.

Body Site(s) Affected: An intestinal disorder, *C. perfringens* is part of the normal flora of the intestinal tract and must be consumed in large numbers to cause illness.

Sources of Infection: Reservoir is the gastrointestinal tract of humans and animals (cattle, pigs, vermin) and soil. Almost all outbreaks are associated with meat — sometimes with fresh meat not cooked thoroughly but usually stews, meat pies, reheated meat, and gravies made of beef, turkey, or chicken. Outbreaks are traced to food-service industries such as catering firms, restaurants, and cafeterias.

Methods of Control:
- Serve all meat dishes hot immediately after cooking.
- Cool cooked food quickly, and adequately refrigerate it until it is served.

- Reheat stored food rapidly before serving.
- Adequately cook large cuts of meat.
- Educate food handlers as to the risks inherent in large-scale cooking, especially of meat dishes.

Fungus Poisoning: Ergotism

Causative agent: *Claviceps purpurea*

Symptoms: First symptom is an excruciating burning sensation. When ingested in bread, it causes contractions of the muscular coat of the arteries, cutting off circulation to the extremities and resulting in gangrene of fingers and toes, and occasionally the ears and nose. In severe cases, neurologic symptoms such as convulsions and hallucinations may occur, sometimes resulting in death. Preceding onset of the gangrene, symptoms are weakness, headache, and convulsive depression.

Incubation Period: The onset is insidious, occurring after ingestion of several meals of diseased bread or meal.

Conditions of Occurrence: Greatest occurrence was during the Middle Ages. The most recent outbreak occurred in 1951.

Body Site(s) Affected: Attacks muscular coat of arteries and can result in gangrene to various body parts.

Sources of Infection: Grows on rye and other grains used in making bread. Infection occurs from ingesting ergot-infested grains.

Method of Control:
- Avoid ergot-infested grain.

Fungus Poisoning: Mycetismus

Causative Agent: *Amanita phalloides* and *Amanita muscara*

Symptoms: Abdominal pain, blood-tinged vomitus, diarrhea, extreme dehydration, salivation, excessive thirst, damage of the liver resulting in jaundice, and damage of the central nervous system with confusion,

collapse and coma. Mortality is from 50% to 90% if untreated.

Incubation period: Several minutes to 6 hours.

Conditions of Occurrence: Areas where poisonous mushrooms grow and are ingested.

Body Site(s) Affected: Stomach, intestines, liver, central nervous system.

Sources of Infection: Ingestion of Amanita species that grow from spring to fall in the woods, by the roadside, and on cultivated lands.

Methods of Control:
- Recognize and avoid poisonous mushrooms.
- Don't eat wild mushrooms.

Poisonous Plants

More than 600 species of plants are known to cause illness and death. Following is an overview.

Berries and seeds

Children have been poisoned, fatally in some instances, after eating brightly colored or unripe berries such as *Daphne mezerion*, Nightshade, and *Latana cancra*. Rosary pea seeds are made into necklaces and sold to tourists as souvenirs; a single seed, if chewed, may kill a child. Necklaces made with caster beans contain resin and are toxic to children.

Garden plants

Among the garden plants that have been found to be poisonous are the seeds of larkspur, flesh of monkshood roots, leaves and flowers of lily-of-the-valley, autumn crocus bulb, underground stem of the iris, parts of azaleas, and leaves of foxglove. Berries from daphne, jessamine, lantana, and yews may be lethal to children. Native Delaware Indians used mountain laurel to make suicide potions. Rhododendron flowers produce a toxic honey. The seeds and leaves of jimson weed will cause stramonium poisoning, characterized by abnormal thirst, distorted vision, delirium, incoherence, and coma.

Field Plants

Some plants growing in the fields should not be consumed. Buttercups produce juice that causes gastroenteritis. Nightshade causes intense digestive and nervous symptoms that can be fatal. We have all heard of hemlock, a potion that killed the ancient Greek philosopher Socrates.

Houseplants

Some houseplants can cause nausea, vomiting, diarrhea, and even death. The leaves and branches of oleander contain a deadly heart stimulant so powerful that, if eaten, may kill a child. People have died merely from eating steak that has been speared on oleander twigs and roasted. Poinsettia, if eaten by a child, can cause illness, as it contains a lethal acrid-burning juice. Children and adults have died after eating mistletoe berries and drinking tea made by brewing the berries.

Trees

Twigs and foliage of the cherry tree and peach tree release cyanide, which, if eaten, cause gasping, excitement, and prostration. Apricot seeds also contain cyanide and should not be eaten. Acorns are food for squirrels, but children are made ill with renal system problems from chewing them.

Preventive Measures

- Keep all plants away from young children who may nibble on them.
- Teach children never to eat or put in their mouth any plants or berries not used as food.
- Refrain from making medicinal concoctions or teas from plants unless you are sure of their safety. Do not chew plant stems.

Natural Food Poisons

Some natural foods contain toxic chemicals, but in most instances the natural toxicants do not threaten our health because they are present in such small quantities that the protective mechanisms of the body can deal with them. The following toxicants are found in some natural foods.

1. Oxalic acid: interferes with the body's absorption of calcium.
2. Tannin: a poisonous and possibly carcinogenic chemical.
3. Nitrate: is capable of causing severe gastroenteritis.
4. Arsenic: a powerful poison.
5. Solanine: an alkaloid neurotoxin that interferes with the transmission of nerve impulses.

Foods that contain small quantities of toxic chemicals produced by nature are:

- Potato: skin of green potatoes and sprouts contain solanine.
- Tomato: foliage and vines contain solanine.
- Rhubarb and spinach: contain 1% oxalic acid, which may crystallize in the kidneys if eaten cooked or raw in large amounts, and can cause convulsions and even death.
- Cabbage, brussels sprouts, soybeans, mustard, onion: may contain chemicals capable of causing goiter by preventing the body from absorbing adequate amounts of iodine.
- Sweet potatoes, peas, cherries, apricots, lima beans: all have chemicals related to the poison cyanide.
- Coffee: contains caffeine, to which some of us are addicted.
- Spices: a number of spices contain safrol (from sassafras root), which in large amounts may cause cancer of the liver.

We may be alive because the toxicants in a number of foods are inactivated by heating. To completely avoid natural toxicants in foods, however, is not possible. Even though harmless in the concentrations in which they appear in food, these toxicants may be hazardous if we consume excessive quantities of any of these foods. People should eat a balanced diet and avoid concentrating on any one food, because small amounts of poison may be tolerated whereas large quantities may cause disease.

Chemical Poisoning

Sources of Infection: Gastroenteritis may be caused by ingesting toxic chemicals present in food or drinks. Chemicals may be ingested in several ways:

1. Ingestion of fruits and vegetables with residual insecticide on their surfaces.
2. Use of utensils for cooking or storing food or drink from which toxic chemicals may leach out.
3. Mistaken use of a toxic chemical in the preparation, seasoning, or sweetening of food.
4. Deliberate and malicious contamination of food by a person for some irrational reason.
5. Ingestion by children believing them to be drinks.
6. Pollution of water while treating farmland or spraying fruit trees.

Symptoms: In most instances the triad of gastroenteritis — vomiting, abdominal cramps, and diarrhea — are the predominant symptoms. Vomiting rids the stomach of the food or fluid containing the irritating chemical.

The chemicals most frequently encountered are:

Sodium Fluoride: An insecticide used for eliminating cockroaches. It has been mistaken for flour, sugar, baking soda, and salt in the preparation of food.

Sodium Nitrite and Sodium Nitrate: Used in curing and preserving meat; can be mistaken for salt. Causes cyanosis, a bluish discoloration of the skin resulting from deficient oxygenation of the blood.

Metallic Poisoning: Caused by cooking acid foods such as apples, and storing sour drinks (lemonade, orange juice) in certain types of pots, trays, or pitchers. If gray cooking enamelware is used, antimony present in the enamel may leach out and cause poisoning. Acid foods cooked in copper pots may leach copper. Drinking water running through lead pipes and acid foods kept in lead vessels will leach out quantities of the metal and cause lead poisoning. Infants may poison themselves by gnawing lead paint from window sills, particularly in old houses.

Pesticides: Chemical insecticides are lethal to insects and also are harmful to humans if ingested. Some of them, when fed to laboratory animals, have been found to be carcinogenic and others teratogenic (capable of causing abnormalities in the fetus). Leafy vegetables should be washed before ingestion.

Silver Polish: A number of silver polishes contain cyanide. If not washed sufficiently to remove residues of the polish, eating with these utensils may result in gastroenteritis

SOME NATURALLY OCCURRING FOOD POISONS

- Favism is a disease caused by eating fava beans. The fava bean (*Vicia fava*) is a main diet item in Mediterranean countries, grown and consumed by people of Italian descent. The danger stems from a nucleoside (vicine) that causes hemolysis. Blood in the urine is a symptom.

- After insufficient cooking, lima beans, sweet peas, kidney beans, Jack beans, navy beans, and soybeans have been found to contain hemagglutinin, capable of agglutinating red blood cells.

- During the warm months, when the plankton Convaulax grows copiously, it turns the water red. Mussels that feed on these diatoms become poisonous. During "red tide" the plankton contain a strong alkaloid so poisonous that a few milligrams may prove fatal to humans within 5 to 30 minutes.

- Certain fish are poisonous as they contain a naturally occurring neurotoxin — not to mention mercury, and other poisons, from polluted water. Several types of fish are capable of causing poisoning in humans.

with cold perspiration, cyanosis, mental confusion, and exhaustion.

Nicotinic Acid: To restore the natural color to meats of inferior quality, dealers add nicotinic acid or sodium nitrate to it. Cooking does not destroy nicotinic acid.

Methods of Control:

- Exercise care in storage and use of chemicals.
- Store chemicals separately from food products and keep them out of children's reach.
- Use colored dyes in toxic products to minimize their being mistaken for useful nutritive items.
- Avoid kitchen utensils, pots, trays, and containers of questionable quality. Stainless steelware, although more expensive, is the most desirable and safest ware.
- Thoroughly wash all fruits that are not peelable and all leafy vegetables.

GENERAL PRINCIPLES FOR THE PREVENTION OF FOODBORNE DISEASES

Foods as a class are perishable. Meats begin to deteriorate shortly after slaughter. Fish start spoiling as soon as they are removed from their natural habitat. Fruits and vegetables become impaired after harvesting. Foods must be handled, processed, and stored so as not to promote further spoilage, to prevent multiplication of any organisms the food may contain and to preclude the additional introduction of pathenogenic agents. Attending the following principles will go a long way in preventing foodborne diseases.

1. Sanitary methods in handling.
2. The application of heat to destroy any living organisms that may be present.
3. Refrigeration at adequately low temperatures to arrest microbial growth.

Sanitation

Most foodborne outbreaks are a result of the unsanitary handling of food. No doubt, a considerable number of cases of gastroenteritis would have been avoided if the people who prepared or served the incriminating foods had taken the time to wash their hands after using the toilet and before handling the foods. In addition individuals with skin infections, upper respiratory infections, and gastroenteritis should refrain from preparing food.

Heat

Although cooking cannot be relied upon to destroy toxins and chemicals responsible for food poisoning, it will destroy pathenogenic organisms present in food. The center of food should attain a temperature of 73.9° to 76.6°C (165° to 170°F). Leftover food should be reheated to at least 73.9°C (165°F) before it is served. A table where uncooked meats have been placed should not be used to slice or serve cooked meats and chicken.

Refrigeration

Every food-handling establishment must have adequate refrigeration facilities so perishable foods may be stored in the range of 0°C to 4.4°C (32°F to 40°F) to prevent growth of toxins. Foods should not be kept at temperatures between 7.2°C and 60°C (45°F and 140°F), as that range favors incubation and multiplication of pathogens. Foods should be refrigerated as promptly as possible after preparation. If food is to be frozen, its center must be reduced to a temperature of 232°C (0°F) or lower.

MILK SANITATION

Milk has been described as nature's most nearly perfect food for humans and microorganisms. Thus, extreme care must be taken to prevent it from spreading the causative agents of disease — biological, chemical, and physical.

On the farm, in the milk barn, in the pasteurization plant to where milk is stored and consumed, the following should be present: a potable water supply, sanitary sewage disposal, proper refuse sanitation, the absence of rats and mice, control of flies, mosquitoes, roaches, and other arthropods, application of heat and refrigeration principles of food preservation, and a safe and sanitary environment, including good personal hygiene. Like other foods, milk requires the application of environmental health principles to create an unfavorable environment for microorganisms.

Milk from a healthy cow is sterile, but if the cow has brucellosis, tuberculosis, or mastitis, the milk can transport these organisms to the consumer. To prevent the spread of these organisms, dairy herds are inspected and tested. They must be totally free of brucellosis and tuberculosis. If a cow has mastitis, the milk cannot be sold while she has the disease or for a stated period of time after she receives antibiotic treatment. Thus, theoretically, if only milk from disease-free cows were used, we still have to be concerned about post-mammary gland contamination. Unfortunately, one cannot be sure that milk is only from healthy cows, so all milk should be pasteurized as a secondary precaution. In summary, we try to get the milk from a healthy cow or other milk-producing animal and ensure that it is not contaminated after it leaves the mammary glands. To accomplish this

goal, we pipe the milk from the cow to the consumer. This is accomplished as portrayed (Figure 11.4).

Milkers are placed on the cow's teats. The first squirt of milk from each teat of the cow is not sold but, rather, is disposed of because microorganisms may penetrate a small distance up into the teats if the cow stands in a pond, for example. The milk then is piped into the refrigerated milk tank on the dairy farm. A pipe from the milk truck is hooked to the refrigerated tank, and the milk is piped to a similar tank on the truck.

When the milk truck reaches the pasteurization plant, the milk is piped from the truck into a bulk milk tank. When it is time to pasteurize the milk, it is piped through the pasteurizing unit, through a cooler, and finally into containers. The sealed containers then are placed in a refrigerated room for shipment to grocery stores, homes, restaurants, and other users, where the milk is consumed. Because it is not feasible to pipe sanitary milk directly into every grocery store, restaurant and home, the aforementioned process is used to prevent the introduction of microorganisms and chemicals, by flies, roaches and humans.

The temperature diagram in Figure 11.4 indicates that milk should be cooled quickly after milking and kept cool until it is pasteurized and subsequently consumed. The reason for refrigeration is to control the growth of

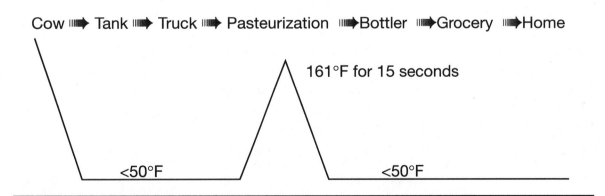

FIGURE 11.4 Path of milk from source to consumer showing desired temperatures.

organisms — pathogens and psychrophiles (cold-loving organisms). For milk, as for other environmental programs, the key is prevention. For example, if milk is not cooled quickly and staphylococcal organisms are present, the organisms will multiply and emit toxins that are heat-stable and will not be destroyed by the pasteurization process. How can staphylococcal organisms get into milk? From people coughing and sneezing into it or from an infected finger. Mastitis also is caused by staphylococci and streptococci invading the udder and causing infection, and thereby can contaminate the milk.

The quality control of milk on the farm has to be maintained during pasteurization and storage. Thus, various tests are run on raw and pasteurized milk to determine its quality. Table 11.2 outlines some of the most important tests run on raw and pasteurized milk together with their purposes.

Pasteurization renders most milk safe. The goal of public health supervision of milk

TABLE 11.2 Laboratory Quality Control Test

Raw Milk	
Test	**Purpose**
Sediment Test*	To determine amount of debris, etc., in milk
Cryoscopic Test	To determine amount of water in milk
Lactometer Test*	To determine amount of water in milk
Standard Plate Count	To determine bacteriological quality of milk
Direct Microscopic Test	To determine bacteriological quality of milk; also, the test will detect dead organisms, red blood cells, and white blood cells
Resazurin Test*	To determine bacteriological quality of milk
Methylene Blue Test	To determine the bacteriological quality of milk
Butter Fat	To determine the percentage of butter in milk (usually should be 3.25°%)
Acidity	To help determine the age of milk
Ring Test	To detect brucellosis in the herd
Antibiotic Test	To determine if antibiotics are in the milk
Pasteurized Milk	
Cryoscopic Test	To determine the water content of milk
Lactometer Test*	To determine the water content of milk
Standard Plate Count	To determine the bacteriological quality of milk
Phosphatase Test	To determine if milk is pasteurized properly
Coliform Test	To determine if milk has been contaminated after pasteurization
Butter Fat	To determine if the % butterfat is present as advertised
Thermoduric Test	To determine if equipment is cleaned properly
Psychrophylic Test	To determine if the sample is old; higher counts are indicators of old milk

*Psychrophylic. Not used much in the United States, but still used in developing countries

Environmental Health

suppliers, however, is to assure a good raw milk supply, with pasteurization as a safety factor. Good raw milk means healthy cows, clean barns, good milking methods, and equipment and healthy personnel to handle the milk.

Because milk is a nearly perfect medium for the growth of microorganisms and it is the main food for infants, milk has been monitored carefully by governmental agencies and the milk industry. As the tests in Table 11.2 reveal, milk producers' ratings will be degraded or they will be prevented from selling milk entirely if the milk does not meet the rigid standards. Milk production and milk standards, except for actual distribution and marketing, are under the jurisdiction of the U.S. Department of Agriculture.

Much of the monitoring of milk on the farm is done by the pasteurization plant. If it purchases a poor product, it places a greater burden on industry to have a product that will meet the standards of the regulating agencies, such as the Agriculture Department and Public Health Service.

SUMMARY

The same food that is a necessity of life can lead to deterioration of life through disease-causing agents. Thus, food quality management is an important component of public and environmental health programs, and preventing the entrance of foodborne pathogens is of major concern. It involves monitoring food from its agriculture origin through harvest, processing and storage, transportation, to food preparation and consumption.

Foodborne diseases are of two main types: foodborne infections and chemical food poisoning. Preventive measures include sanitary handling, the application of heat, and refrigeration. Food preservation methods include temperature control (pasteurization, cooking, canning, refrigeration, freezing), drying, chemical treatment (osmotic balance disturbance and pH reactions such as in pickling) and fermentation, the process used in making cheese, vinegar, and sauerkraut.

Food additives are placed in foods intentionally to improve appearance, flavor, texture, or storage properties. These include vinegar, sugar, salt, nitrites and nitrates, sulfites, and coloring agents, among many others. The entities largely responsible for monitoring foods are the U.S. Department of Agriculture (particularly milk) and Public Health and Environmental Health Agencies (restaurant inspection).

REFERENCES

Food and Drug Administration. *What Consumers Should Know About Food Additives.* (Leaflet No. 10). Washington, DC., n.d.

Longree, Karla. 1996. *Quantity Food Sanitation.* 5th ed. New York: John Wiley and Sons, New York.

Longree, Karla, and Gertrude G. Blaker. 1971. *Sanitary Techniques in Food Service.* John Wiley and Sons, New York.

Potter, Norman N. 1986. *Food Science.* 4th ed. AVI Publishing, Westport, CT.

Public Health Service. 1995. *Food Service Code.* Government Printing Office, Washington, DC.

_____. 1965. *Grade A Pasteurized Milk Ordinance.* U.S. Government Printing Office, Washington, DC.

Tartakow, Jackson, and John H. Vorperian. 1981. *Food-borne & Water-borne Diseases.* AVI Publishing, Westport, CT.

Taylor, R. J. 1980. *Food Additives.* John Wiley and Sons, New York.

Shelter Environments

Key Terms

Asbestos
Carbon monoxide
Exchange
Exothermic
Favorable environment

Friable
Humidity
Lead
Metabolism

Physiological needs
Pollution
Sick building syndrome
Volatile organic compounds (VOCs)

Objectives

- List several physiological needs in shelters.

- List several psychological needs in shelters.

- List 10 communicable diseases that can be spread in shelters.

- List six diseases caused by chemicals that can be contracted in shelters.

- Discuss sick building syndrome.

- Discuss the effects of formaldehyde on the body.

- Discuss radon control

- List the diseases transmitted by indoor air.

One of the major global public health concerns of the 20th century is pollution. In simple terms, **pollution** can be defined as contamination of the environmental air with substances/items that have adverse effects of human health. Shelter and protection against unfavorable elements in the environment are a basic need of humans. Extremes in temperature, ionizing radiation, animals, insects, noise, sun rays, and wind are examples of unfavorable elements in the environment against which humans must be protected. Shelters include private homes, hotels, hospitals, nursing homes, jails, prisons, motels, mobile homes, ships, mental institutions, schools, universities, military bases, camps, and housing for migrant workers and senior citizens. Housing or shelters should minimize the risk of accidents and the spread of disease while keeping humans safe, happy and productive. **The four fundamental needs that housing (shelters) should provide are: (1) fundamental physiological needs, (2) fundamental psychological needs, (3) protection from causative agents of disease, and (4) protection against accidents** (discussed in Chapter 2).

FUNDAMENTAL PHYSIOLOGICAL NEEDS

By altering the environment, putting on and taking off clothing, people can live in very cold and very hot environments. The first modern endeavors to alter the environment included opening windows, designing draft systems, and burning wood in fireplaces. Now sophisticated air-conditioning systems have been developed to cool the indoor environment when it is too hot, creating an environment that permits adequate heat loss. In many places the fireplace has been replaced by elaborate, convenient, heating systems that protect the body from undue heat loss.

Temperature and Humidity

These systems usually control humidity as well as temperature. **Humidity** control is important in maintaining a comfortable environment. For example, one might be comfortable in a room that is 78°F (25.5°C) with 50% humidity, whereas with 90% humidity the same room at 78°F (25.5°C) would be uncomfortable. Hence, the American Public Health Association's Committee on the Hygiene of Housing has recommended temperatures and humidity levels. A temperature of 65°F (18.3°C) is recommended for working and sleeping areas. Temperature readings should be made 18 inches (45.7 cm) above floor level. If young children are playing on the floor, that temperature should be 70°F (21.1°C) at 18 inches (45.7 cm) above the floor. Hot and humid environments cause one to feel sluggish. Dry, cooler environments stimulate people. Low humidity (less than about 20%), however, can cause nosebleeds and chills because the body's mucous linings dry out as a result of loss of moisture to the dry air, which predisposes one to communicable disease. That is why between 40% and 60% humidity is desirable.

Ventilation

An unventilated room when occupied by people will undergo changes. The temperature will increase because the body is **exothermic** and radiates the excess heat to the environment, thus warming the air. The body loses excess heat by conduction, convection, radiation, and evaporation. If one sits on a block of ice, the body will lose heat as the ice absorbs it. Heat flows from hot to cold. When hot and perspiring, we like to stand in the breeze and lose heat by convection. This is what happens when we create a draft by a fan. The body loses some heat by radiation. When the body cannot lose the excess heat in the above mentioned ways, we perspire (sweat). If the body does not lose the excess heat, the body temperature will become elevated, with associated problems, and even brain damage in extreme cases. Thus, to exchange air and prevent drafts, air movement is recommended to be less than 500 feet per minute at the dust exit.

Second, an unventilated room will increase in humidity. The body loses moisture by perspiration and by breathing. When air is pulled into the lungs, it picks up moisture. This phenomenon plus radiated body heat accounts for a room that was at first comfortable eventually becoming too warm and humid. It is recommended that a room's air be exchanged every hour.

Third, an unventilated room will retain odors. In food establishments, the main reason for ventilation is to remove food odor. Other changes taking place in an unventilated room may be a decrease in the amount of oxygen and an increase in the amount of carbon dioxide and possibly carbon monoxide, as humans breathe in O_2 and exhale CO_2.

Favorable Environment

Protection against unfavorable elements so as to maintain or enhance health is necessary in all types of shelters, where creating an environment favorable for habitation is tantamount. By **favorable environment**, we mean adequate space, a safe water supply, approved means of sewage and solid waste disposal, the absence of pests, such as insects and rodents, the absence of excessive noise and ionizing radiation, a favorable thermal environment, a means of protecting

Environmental Health

the food supply, the absence of indoor and outdoor air pollution, a structural design that will reduce the likelihood of injuries, and the absence of toxic materials.

Proper lighting is a need of humans. If light is insufficient, eye strain and fatigue may result. Proper lighting can be accomplished by using either natural or artificial lighting. Those who recognize the need for energy conservation advocate the use of natural light and natural ventilation as much as possible.

Protection against excessive noise is another human need. Housing in noisy environments requires soundproofing materials to reduce the noise. Hearing the neighbor's television while you are studying or doing work that requires concentration is annoying. Housing regulations should require soundproofing in all multi-unit dwellings. (Noise is discussed further in Chapter 15.)

Regardless of the type of shelter, be it a house or a penal institution, adequate space is a basic physiological need. Opportunities for physical exercise and recreation, for adults and children alike, are essential for physical, mental, and social well-being. In planning shelter environments, the provision of recreational space often is omitted because of cost, shortage of space — and many times a lack of understanding as to the role of exercise and recreation in maintaining health. Housing projects, prisons, nursing homes, schools, day care centers, and so forth, should provide adequate space activity. At least 22 square feet should be provided for each student in a classroom. For physiological and psychological needs, houses should provide at least 10 square feet per person, with one room having at least 150 square feet. To reduce the spread of communicable disease, approximately 400 cubic feet of space is needed.

FUNDAMENTAL PSYCHOLOGICAL NEEDS

To many people, the word "home" signifies the place where they can isolate themselves from the world. Privacy is a basic need, and adequate housing should provide a means of fulfilling that psychological need. In rural areas this need is not as great, because people can find privacy. In cities, however, the home is a refuge from the noise, tension, crime, and other stress-producing agents of a crowded environment. For psychological and sociological health, housing authorities recommend that a house have a living room where youth can meet and socialize with different age groups and sexes.

Psychiatric opinion holds that children over age 2 years should have a sleeping room separate from their parents'. The need for privacy in bathrooms and bedrooms is also a psychological and social requirement of housing. It is recommended that only children of the same sex sleep in a bedroom after they reach 8 years of age. Also, most standards are based on no more than two people per bedroom.

Because of the psychological and social values that result from participating in normal community life, family housing should be in a community that permits easy access to basic institutions of culture, commerce, and employment. Community facilities that should be convenient to the home areas include schools, churches, shopping centers, entertainment facilities, libraries, medical care facilities, and recreation. Unfortunately, "normal community life" is not possible in some large, crowded areas that are plagued with problems associated with overcrowding. Drugs and crime force some people to live behind locked doors. Society tries to correct this problem by putting those causing the problem behind the locked doors of prisons.

A psychological, as well as physical, need for humans is the provision of facilities that will maintain cleanliness of the dwelling and the person. Baths, showers, and lavatories are needed for keeping the body clean. Some shelters have mop sinks, vacuum systems, and other facilities to promote cleaning. These systems require running water and electricity. Some homes, however, do not have electricity and running water; brooms, mops, and standpipes (a water spigot in the yard) are used and water is heated on the stove. In some countries a standpipe serves several homes and a central community shower (bathhouse) fulfills the need for personal cleanliness.

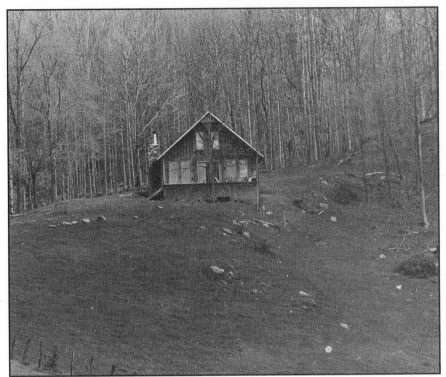

A cabin in the mountains provides a favorable environment, away from noise, congestion, and other stress-producing agents.

PROTECTION AGAINST CAUSATIVE AGENTS OF DISEASE

Communicable Diseases

In Chapter 2 we discuss the causative agents of disease. Chapter 3 groups the communicable diseases by their mode of transmission. A potable water supply, as discussed in Chapter 4 should be provided to prevent the spread of waterborne infectious diseases. Plumbing should be constructed to prevent cross-connections where the water supply can be contaminated by sewage, chemicals, or other contaminants. Adequate toilet facilities should be provided to prevent the spread of communicable disease. In areas where, for geological or financial reasons, flush toilets are not available, pit privies may be used. Toilets and privies should be constructed as discussed in Chapter 6, to prevent the spread of disease by flies, roaches, water, or direct contact.

Another basic need for housing is to exclude of vermin from the shelter. Rats and other vermin spread disease, in addition to destroying property, as discussed in Chapter 8. Hence, "building them out" is desirable. This can be accomplished (as described in Chapter 8) by screening doors and windows and using hardware cloth over openings.

Adequate space for each person housed in a facility is necessary to prevent the spread of respiratory diseases. For example, in barracks and dormitories. This translates to more than 6 feet (1.82 m) between the center of adjoining cots or a space of more than 50 square feet (4.64 m) per bed. Approximately 400 cubic feet (1–1.3 m) per occupant in sleeping areas is desirable. If ventilation is inadequate, more space should be provided.

Asbestos

The presence of **asbestos** is undesirable in shelter environments. Asbestos is a mineral mined

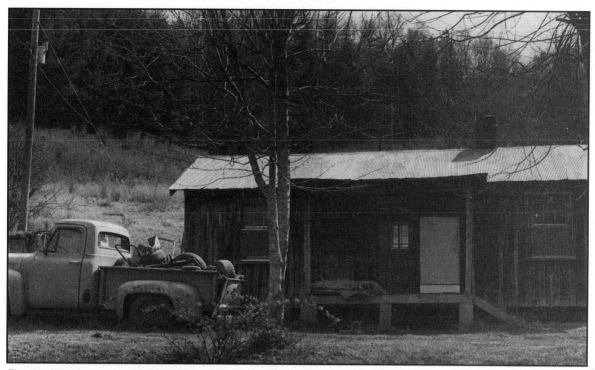

The shelter environment should be adequate, safe, and free of refuse, insects, and rodents.

in much the same way as other minerals. However, asbestos crystals are fiber-shaped rather than crystal-shaped like those of table salt. Three common varieties of asbestos are: chrysotile, amosite, and crocidolite. All three varieties are resistant to chemicals, making them popular for a variety of industrial and commercial uses. Asbestos has been used in more than 3,000 products.

The three major health problems associated with asbestos are asbestosis, lung cancer, and mesothelioma. Asbestosis was first recognized in the 1920s, but no maximum allowable concentration for safety was determined. In 1986, the Occupational Safety and Health Administration (OSHA) set the occupational exposure limit at 0.2 fibers per cubic centimeter. Asbestosis-related lung cancer was detected during the 1930s and 1940s, and mesothelioma (a crocidolite and amosite asbestos-related lung disease) was reported in the 1960s.

Exposure to airborne asbestos continues to be a major area of occupational health concern.

Material containing asbestos has been used widely for thermal insulation, fireproofing, sound absorbents, and aesthetic purposes. Friable materials such as insulation, fireproofing, and decorative materials containing asbestos can endanger employees if they are damaged, exposed, or disturbed in some way. A material is considered **friable** if it can be crumbled, pulverized, or reduced to a powder by hand. Generating any amount of airborne asbestos is significant because of the serious potential health hazard posed to any person exposed to it. The hazard is long-range or chronic and may not manifest itself for as long as 25 to 40 years after exposure.

Generally, the amount of asbestos that may be present in materials used for fireproofing or insulating ranges from 10% to 80% of total dry weight. Friable asbestos insulation can be found in any structure regardless of the year of construction or type of insulation.

If asbestos is present, special procedures and precautions must be followed to protect employee health and comply with OSHA and

EPA regulations. Regardless of the amount of asbestos-containing materials removed, EPA notification is required. If insulation or other material containing asbestos is damaged, handled, demolished, or removed, appropriate procedures must be followed to ensure adequate employee protection and compliance with government regulations.

Asbestos minerals are classified as one of two groups: serpentine and amphiboles.

1. The *serpentine* group has only one member, chrysotile, which constitutes about 90% of the asbestos used in the United States. Chrysotile comes primarily from Quebec, Canada, but deposits in British Columbia also are a source. Arizona has a deposit that is superior for electrical uses, and chrysotile also has been mined in Vermont and California.

2. The *amphiboles* group has three members of commercial importance: crocidolite, amosite, and anthophyllite. Tremolite and actinolite also are members of the amphiboles group, but these occur primarily as contaminants in other minerals. Although their chemical and physical properties differ, all amphiboles are crystalline, fibrous, and noncombustible. Amosite and crocidolite come primarily from South Africa, although materials from Bolivian sources have been used in the United States. Anthophyllite derives from several deposits in Georgia. Tremolite occurs as an impurity in commercial talc and other minerals.

An important property of asbestos, especially chrysotile, is fiber length. All asbestos is graded by fiber length, depending on the amount passing three screens — half-inch, 4-mesh, and 10-mesh. Chrysotile has the finest fibers and is more flexible so that it can be most easily spun and woven into cloth. The amphiboles minerals differ from one another, but, unlike chrysotile, they are all acid-resistant. Although all types of asbestos can cause the lung disease asbestosis, they differ in their ability to cause cancer, particularly mesothelioma. All asbestos varieties are heat-resistant, with a melting point of 1200 to 1500 R.

R = Rankine = absolute temperature on Fahrenheit scale.

Asbestos can be made into weavings, yarn, cloth, tape, and braided tubes. Because of its excellent thermal and electrical resistant properties, asbestos textiles have been used for a diversity of fire- and heat-resistant applications: clothing, welding blankets, high-temperature insulation coverings, and many others.

The largest use of asbestos in tonnage has been in asbestos cement. Because of its superior strength, asbestos cement has been used for roofing, wallboard, drainage pipe, pressure pipe, laboratory hoods, ventilation ducts, and many other products. Although amounts vary, most final products using asbestos cement are only 10% to 25% asbestos. The second most common use of asbestos, after cement, has been in friction products — disk brakes, drum brakes, jaw and band brakes, and dry and oil clutches.

The fibrous mineral nature of asbestos makes it appropriate for sealants and gaskets, and, like other fibrous materials, it can be made into paper. As an electrical resistor, asbestos has been used as roving or braid around electrical wires, as a board in electrical apparatus, and as the strengthening agent in high-pressure laminates. Asbestos used as a filler is found in roofing compounds, gasket cement, floor tiles, and plastic products.

In the past, asbestos was mixed with a variety of rubbers to make gasketing materials. It has been used as paper, cloth, and raw fiber to form the gaskets and sealants that can be made to resist any material for high-pressure or high-temperature use. For thermal insulation, asbestos has been used as a spray, magnesia block, calcium silicate block, and Marinite. Sprayed asbestos is characterized by its homogeneity, seamless surface adherence to any surface, ability to be formed, and capacity to improve acoustic properties of walls and ceilings.

A special use of crocidolite, anthophyllite or amosite asbestos was in the acid-resistant construction material Haveg, used for pipes, tanks, valves, reaction vessels, acid towers, and pump housing. It consisted of asbestos with a penthol of furane resin and hardening agent. Virtually all uses of asbestos, of course, are being phased out in the United States.

Carbon Monoxide

Carbon monoxide is a colorless, odorless, tasteless gas produced from the incomplete burning of fuels containing carbon. Exhaust from the internal combustion engine is the principal contemporary anthropogenic source of carbon monoxide. Motor vehicle exhaust falls into this category.

Other manmade sources of carbon monoxide include industrial processes, agricultural burning, fuel combustion in stationary sources, solid waste disposal and cigarette smoking. Natural sources include volcanic activity, natural occurrence in the ground, and photochemical degradation of certain organic compounds. Rising carbon monoxide levels are undesirable because they affect human health adversely. To explain how carbon monoxide harms health, some basic physiological processes are explained below.

The human respiratory and cardiovascular systems, working together, normally transport oxygen from the atmosphere to the various tissues of the body at a rate sufficient to maintain tissue **metabolism**. Oxygen in ambient air is inhaled into the lungs, where it is absorbed by the bloodstream. The oxygen becomes bound to the hemoglobin in red blood cells and may be transported from the lungs to the extrapulmonary tissues.

Carbon monoxide harms health by competing with oxygen for binding sites on the hemoglobin molecule. Because the affinity of hemoglobin for carbon monoxide is more than 200 times that for oxygen, carbon monoxide, even at low partial pressures, can impair the transport of oxygen from the blood into body tissues. When the gas combines with hemoglobin, it forms a compound called carboxyhemoglobin, which prevents oxygen from being transported to and utilized by the body's cells.

Adverse physiological effects begin at carboxyhemoglobin levels of approximately 2.5%. Exposure to air with 50 ppm of carbon monoxide for 90 minutes, or 15 ppm for 10 hours, is enough to reach this level. Carbon monoxide exposure producing carboxyhemoglobin levels as low as 3% was found to result in adverse effects on complex mental functions such as concentration and memory. Epidemiological evidence also has linked the incidence of myocardial infarction to the concentration of carbon monoxide in the air. The current EPA standard for carbon monoxide is justified mainly on the basis of preventing adverse effects in persons with cardiac and peripheral vascular disease.

Manifestations of carbon monoxide poisoning include brain functioning impairment, irregular heart functioning, dizziness, blurred vision, headache, seizures, vomiting, and coma. Skin color of the affected person varies from normal (in more than half of the cases) to flushed, cyanotic (bluish) or cherry-pink. Blisters and bullous lesions also may occur. After apparent recovery, persistent neurologic complications are common. At very high concentrations (such as 1500 ppm for 1 hour), death may occur. Fetuses and the very young are especially susceptible to the

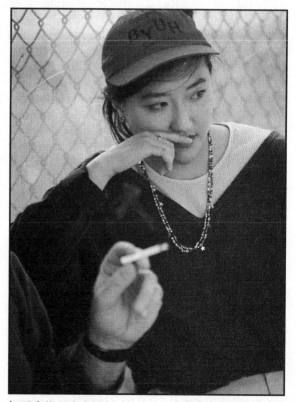

Legislation to protect nonsmokers' rights is being stepped up.

toxic effects of carbon monoxide and the resulting lower oxygen saturation.

In treating carbon monoxide exposure, high concentrations of oxygen are administered. This hastens elimination of the carbon monoxide gas from the body.

Although outdoor carbon monoxide concentrations are a cause for concern, indoor concentrations may be even more important. Not only does the average person spend most of his or her time indoors, but high carbon monoxide levels indoors generally are not diffused readily into the atmosphere. Most buildings today have been weather-proofed, or sealed tightly. These buildings do not allow adequate air exchange between the indoor and outdoor environments. In attempting to make homes and other buildings energy-efficient, we may be exposing ourselves to dangerous levels of carbon monoxide, as well as other pollutants.

Some possible sources of indoor carbon monoxide production are cooking appliances such as gas stoves, space heaters, furnaces, fireplaces, wood-burning stoves, and cigarette smoking. An inadequate supply of air for combustion — that which occurs in "airtight" wood-burning stoves and improperly maintained gas stoves and gas and oil furnaces — greatly increases the rate of carbon monoxide emission. If set wrong, flues and dampers restrict the flow of carbon monoxide and other combustion products to the outside, causing a potentially harmful buildup indoors.

Two types of indoor environments that are more likely to have higher than normal carbon monoxide concentrations are (a) indoor garages and buildings with attached indoor parking areas, and (b) residences with improperly ventilated space-heating equipment. These settings often maintain carbon monoxide concentrations as high as 100 ppm. Cigarette smoking also can produce high concentrations of carbon monoxide. Mainstream cigarette smoke contains up to 40% carbon monoxide.

Because of the potential for serious health problems resulting from carbon monoxide exposure, measures should be taken to decrease indoor levels. One method to stabilize indoor carbon monoxide levels is to remove the source of contamination. Preferably, the garage is separated from the house. Combustion appliances can be replaced with cleaner devices that perform the same function. For example, electric appliances or solar heating systems can be used in place of combustion appliances such as gas stoves. A source may be altered by a change in design. An example of this is using an electric ignition rather than a gas pilot light in gas stoves. Spatial confinement also may be utilized to decrease carbon monoxide exposure in a home. This can be accomplished by placing combustion appliances in isolated rooms. Oil and gas combustion heating units may be placed outside of the house. Timing the production of contaminants to periods of nonoccupancy also reduces carbon monoxide exposure.

One simple and effective method of decreasing carbon monoxide exposure is to avoid cigarette smoke — not to smoke and to stay away from those who are smoking. People are justified in not allowing smoking in their home and insisting on the separation of smokers and nonsmokers in their place of employment. Most businesses and public agencies now have smoking policies.

Ventilation or general air exchange between inside and outside air is another uncomplicated method of reducing indoor carbon monoxide levels. A local ventilation device such as a simple exhaust fan can be used for combustion appliances.

The general public is largely unaware of the dangers of carbon monoxide exposure, especially indoor concentrations. People need to be educated as to what produces carbon monoxide within their own homes and how to prevent dangerous levels from forming. Regulation of combustion appliances such as gas stoves and kerosene heaters is helpful, but they must be properly installed and maintained to prevent them from becoming health hazards. CO detectors might be used in sleeping areas of shelter environments.

The two main factors that could help us all breathe a little easier are increased public education and enforcement of regulations (such as building codes and consumer-product requirements).

Sick Building Syndrome

Of the air most individuals breathe, 80% to 90% is indoor air. The air, sometimes clean, sometimes polluted, is modified in composition because of confinement. With the onset of the energy crisis in the 1970s, buildings (commercial, nonresidential, and residential) in advanced countries were constructed to be energy-efficient with less air exchange between them and their surroundings. Among the problems that arose in these buildings as a result of this energy efficient mindset were

— retention of higher temperatures
— higher humidity levels
— decreased ventilation
— increased odor retention.

The advent of higher temperatures and increased humidity levels in buildings gave birth to the proliferation of microorganisms in indoor environments. In addition, certain synthetic materials used to construct the buildings, as well as some furnishings, were found to produce volatile organic compounds, all of which have adverse effects on human health. These factors have created indoor air pollution, a term used interchangeably with the term adverse indoor air quality.

The EPA estimates that 6,000 cancer deaths are caused by indoor air pollutants yearly. This estimate may be a reason for indoor pollution-control ballooning into a billion-dollar-a-year business.

The average holding time for airborne substances is of the utmost importance in indoor pollution. The air in a room must be exchanged with an open atmosphere via open doors, windows, a variety of leaks, and by ventilating fans and ducts. **Exchange** is measured by the time required for full replacement of air. Half an hour to 5 hours is the average turnover time for residential buildings. Houses built by conventional standards show values of 50 to 100 minutes, excluding conditions created by unusual winds or extreme contrasts in temperature. Larger buildings have required forced ventilation by design.

An ancient source of particulate additions to indoor air was *combustion*. Today, most combustion products are vented directly outdoors by way of a chimney or hood. More fires, although tiny, burn unvented. They are produced by cigarettes. These tiny fires burn at a mean rate of about one per U.S. household.

A study done in India of the typical kitchen with a housewife or cook demonstrated particulate concentrations more than two dozen times the U.S. open-air standard for 24-hour exposure. Even the most inefficient natural-gas stove is less noxious than that.

Direct analysis of even a small sample of houses displays wide sources of contamination. Vapors and degradation products result from pesticides used to preserve wood structure, organic sprays, and solvents. The concentrations of these organic air contaminants are low but appear to be higher in summer than in winter. This finding is contrary to the belief that open windows and doors (in the summer season) are effective in decreasing the concentrations because of more circulation and outside air transfer. The higher vapor pressures and higher reaction rates of warm weather more than make up for the better summer ventilation.

Fatal lung cancer incidents are rising in direct relation to smoking. The factor is a 10% to 12% increase among pack-a-day smokers. The effect of smoke on nonsmokers has yet to be established. One research study showed that

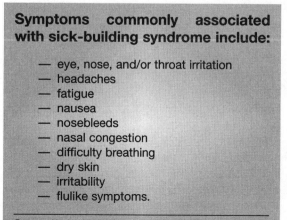

Symptoms commonly associated with sick-building syndrome include:

— eye, nose, and/or throat irritation
— headaches
— fatigue
— nausea
— nosebleeds
— nasal congestion
— difficulty breathing
— dry skin
— irritability
— flulike symptoms.

Source: Medical Laboratory Observer, 1996

a couple of smokers in a modest room may be able to raise particulate counts close to or beyond legal standards for outside air. Another study showed that Boston children and adult French women who lived in a household among smokers had a poorer measured lung function than those who did not. Other studies of non-smoking women married to heavy smokers, showed a doubled rate of lung cancer.

Air pollution, biological hazards, and toxic chemicals, if not ventilated properly, contribute to many maladies suffered by workers in new and old office buildings (see Table 12.1). The World Health Organization has estimated that as many as 30% of new and old renovated office buildings emit various toxic substances.

INFECTIOUS DISEASES TRANSMITTED VIA INDOOR AIR

Obligate pathogens	Opportunistic pathogens
Bacterial	*Bacterial*
Anthrax	Legionnaire's disease
Brucellosis	Pontiac fever
Streptococcal pneumonia	*Legionella* sp.
Tuberculosis	*Pseudomonas* sp.
Viral	
Common cold	*Viral*
Chicken pox (Varicella)	Herpes I & II
Influenza	Shingles (Zoster)
Measles	
Rubella	*Fungal*
Hantavirus	Aspergillosis
	Cryptococcosis
	Candida sp.
Fungal	Mucormycosis
Blastomycosis	Phycomycosis
Coccidioidomycosis	
Histoplasmosis	*Protozoal*
	Cryptosporidiosis
	Pneumocystis
	Pneumonia

Source: Medical Laboratory Observer, 1996

Volatile organic compounds (VOCs) can be found in the air of new buildings in concentrations as much as 100 times higher than those found outdoors, and they can remain elevated for 6 months after construction. Pollutants classified as VOCs are found in cleaning solvents, glue, and paint. (Outdoor sources of VOCs include automobile exhaust and vapors from engine refueling.) In a study conducted by the EPA, the most common VOCs were benzene, toluene, chloroform, acetone, styrene, and ethylene oxide. The 1982 study was prompted by increasing reports and complaints of **sick building syndrome.**

Fifty building materials were studied for emission of one or more target chemicals. The highest emitters were molding and carpet adhesives, latex caulks and paints, and vinyl rubber moldings. Proper ventilation systems can control the emission of these particulates. Heating, ventilation, and air conditioning (HVAC) systems often are linked to respiratory ailments and complaints when they do not function consistently. The systems, sometimes invaded by mold, mildew, and bacteria, must be serviced and cleaned to maintain function. Other particulates include airborne fibers from common fabrics such as cotton, wool, nylon, and rayon.

Sick building syndrome is not created solely by the structure itself but, for the most part, from the activities of its occupants. Sources of sick building syndrome include tobacco smoke, use of appliances, power equipment, equipment chemicals, bacteria and other organisms in the air, wear and tear of structural materials, radon, chemicals in building material, and intrusion of outside chemicals. These sources, many of which are inevitable, magnify a problem when there is improper ventilation. National Institute of Occupational Safety and Health research studies indicate that about 50% of all sick building syndrome problems are the result of inadequate ventilation. Consequently, the first step in rectifying the phenomenon is to check the ventilation system and proceed accordingly.

Most indoor pollutants are invisible and odorless. They tend to be emitted at low levels, which makes them hard to track down. Once the culprit is identified, however, the remedy is usually straightforward. Remedies include cleaning ventilation systems, replacing carpets, and replacing and segregating office machines in a single, well-ventilated room. If the problem comes from the outside, outdoor air-intake ducts may be moved away.

Formaldehyde

Formaldehyde is a gas with a pungent smell that is water-soluble and colorless at room temperature. Frequently it is marketed in the form of an aqueous solution labeled "formalin." Formaldehyde has a wide variety of industrial uses. It often is used in the manufacture of plastics and resins, photographic chemicals, paints and glue, rubber, synthetic textiles, explosives, and various types of building materials and insulation. Formaldehyde is a component of cigarette smoke, automobile exhaust, diesel exhaust, photochemical smog, and out-gases from some urea foam insulation, particle board, and other building materials. The average person may come into contact with these quite frequently.

The extensive use and presence of formaldehyde in everyday occupational, recreational, and domestic activity has received quite a bit of attention recently because of its irritant effect on the respiratory tract, eyes, and exposed skin surfaces. Much concern has been raised over the potential carcinogenic effects of formaldehyde, as well as its effects on actual lung function and neurological changes. The most common complaints of people frequently exposed to formaldehyde or formalin are

— irritation of the upper airway

— burning of eyes and nasal passages

— skin irritation and rashes

— chronic bronchitis

— shortness of breath.

TABLE 12.1 Examples of Building-Related Illnesses

Disease	Cause
Pontiac Fever An acute self-limited, febrile, nonpneumonic illness with an incubation period of 36 hours. Attack rate: 90%–100%	*Legionella* sp. (bacteria)
Legionnaire's Disease Life-threatening bronchopneumonia with an incubation period of 2–10 days. Attack rate: 5%–10%	*Legionella pneumophila* (bacteria)
Hypersensitivity Pneumonitis Acute extrinsic allergic alveolitis. Chronic form may have characteristics of an interstitial fibrotic pneumonitis. Genetics may influence attack rate.	Fungi, bacteria, organic dust, organic chemicals aerosolized protein, etc.
Humidifier Fever A type of hypersensitivity pneumonitis characterized by an acute febrile attack accompanied by malaise, cough and dyspnea. Chronic form is called humidifier lung. Genetics may influence attack rate.	Fungi, bacteria, protozoa, microbial endotoxins, mycotoxins, arthropods.

Source: Medical Laboratory Observer, 1996

In addition, headache, chest tightness, nausea, irritability, memory dysfunction, and anorexia have been linked to prolonged exposure to formaldehyde. In many instances where lung function test have been performed in direct association with formaldehyde exposure, a slight decrease in lung function has been found with short-term, acute exposure, which usually is transient in nature. A much more significant decrease is found with prolonged, repeated exposure. This, too, usually can be reversed with absence of exposure for several weeks. Carcinogenic effects, particularly nasal cancer, are being studied. To date, no direct cause-and-effect relationship has been documented.

Various occupations with high exposure rates to formaldehyde or formalin include wood workers, workers in plants producing acid-curing paints, workers in an industry producing phenol-formaldehyde-plastic components of fiberglass, histology technicians, and funeral service workers. People living in homes insulated with urea formaldehyde foam also are at high risk.

A 1980 study examined the effect of formaldehyde on workers in a wood product manufacturing plant that produced kitchen cabinets coated with veneer that was glued on with a urea resin. The hardening process and subsequent processes released formaldehyde, to which employees were directly exposed. Researchers measured exposure, studied lung functions, conducted spirometric tests and interviewed workers. (The researchers used a control group of non-exposed workers in whom factors such as smoking and age were taken into account.) The study established a dose-response relationship. Slight impairment of lung function, as well as upper airway and mucous membrane irritation, occurred after only one 8-hour shift, but the effects were transient. A 5-year follow-up study of these same exposed workers revealed a significant decrease in lung function that would reverse itself after 4 weeks of non-exposure.

Complaints of histology technicians at hospitals in Los Angeles and a request for inquiry into the effect of solvents and fixatives used in their laboratories led to a study involving 76 women who were histology technicians in hospitals and laboratories in that city. Researchers used a control group of the same number of clerical workers and secretaries in the same hospitals. The researchers studied the effect of formaldehyde and xylene exposures on respiratory and neurobehavioral symptoms. They found that disturbances of memory, mood, equilibrium, and sleep occurred simultaneously with headache and indigestion. The women working in histology who were exposed daily to xylene, toluene, and other agents incurred irritation of eyes, upper airway and trachea much more often.

Studies done to determine the effect of residing in homes insulated with urea formaldehyde showed results similar to those done in industrial settings. The most significant symptoms by the homeowners were eye irritation, upper airway irritation, headaches, and skin rashes. Lower airway and lung function impairment showed a correlation. A dose-response relationship was demonstrated. The support for a causal relationship between impaired health and living in urea-formaldehyde foam-insulated residence was established to be moderately strong. The demonstrated adverse effects, however, were considered to be generally minor in nature.

Another case stated that residents at a formaldehyde concentration of 1 part per million and above voiced health complaints. Conclusions were that 4 ppm, as targeted by the U.S. Department of Housing and Urban Development, may not be suitable or adequate to protect occupants from the discomfort and acute effects of formaldehyde.

OSHA states that the permissible limit for 8-hour, time-weighted, average exposure to formaldehyde is 3 parts per million. The acceptable ceiling concentration established by OSHA in the mid-1970s is 5 parts per million. Judging from recent research, these levels may be slightly high, suggesting a need for adjustment.

The EPA was created many years ago to serve the United States as a controller of outdoor air pollution. Twenty years later, the concern of greater import is indoor air pollution, which studies have shown can be twice the acceptable level of its outdoor counterpart.

The average white-collar worker may be exposed to benzene from cleaning solutions, toluene from rubber-cement solvent, ozone from copying machines, hydrocarbons from typewriter correction fluids and copy papers, bacteria and fungi from ventilation systems, and insecticides. Most office workers have no reaction to these substances, but as many as 10% could be chemically sensitive. The symptoms can be mild and flulike or debilitating, respiratory attacks.

Radon

Radon is a colorless, odorless, tasteless, naturally occurring radioactive gas that is a product of uranium decay. Uranium tends to concentrate in rock formations and deposits such as granites and shales. When these rocks are heated in the presence of a liquid, the uranium flows with the liquid until it cools. This accounts for the widespread distribution of uranium soils and rocks across the United States. When uranium begins to decay, it gives off a lower atomic weight radioactive element — radon gas. Because radon is a gas, it tends to enter the atmosphere. It rises from the soil beneath buildings and enters these structures through their foundations. The gas is still radioactive when it enters the building. Radon remains radioactive until it decays in a sequence that includes a number of radionuclides, finally reaching a stable isotope of lead. Before becoming stable, radon decays to radioactive particulate substances that attach themselves to particulate matter in the air. These combined particles, if inhaled, concentrate in the lungs, where they become inactive isotopes of lead, which can lead to lung cancer.

Radon emits alpha particles, which are more damaging biologically than beta particles or gamma radiation. Therefore, the risk of cancer increases in the presence of radon. Radon tops the list of indoor hazards, along with accidents from falls and fires. Because radon occurs naturally, it also is considered more dangerous than asbestos, pesticides, and other pollutants. The EPA has estimated that 20,000 deaths have been caused by radon.

Radon tends to be more lethal to men than to women, and also more lethal to smokers than to nonsmokers. Many scientists believe that smoke-damaged respiratory tracts cannot clear the alpha particles effectively, permitting longer time for the cells to be exposed to the carcinogen. According to Jacob Fabrikant of the University of California at Berkeley, a person who spends 12 hours a day in the presence of excess radon levels increases his or her risk of lung cancer by 50%.

Radon is more dangerous indoors than outdoors because diffusion within the air dilutes outdoor radon. Outdoor radon measures approximately 0.2 picocuries per liter of air. Outdoor levels vary widely depending on geographical location (and thus geology), permeability of the soil, energy-efficiency of the building, presence of a water well, and the use of stone building materials. The EPA has set a guideline for indoor radon levels at 4 picocuries per liter. An estimated 8 million homes in the United States have radon levels high enough above the guideline to cause lung cancer.

The radon rising from the earth tends to be pulled into the house because of less pressure inside the home. This vacuum action is stronger when the house is more energy-efficient and lacks ventilation. The most effective way to reduce this vacuum is to reverse the air flow. This can be achieved by drilling through the basement floor and installing a system to diffuse the air away from the house. This system costs up to $2,500, plus electricity to operate the system. Cheaper methods include sealing walls and floors, which should be tried first.

Radon concentrations usually are highest in the basement, attic, and closed-in places with little ventilation. Radon also rises with groundwater tables. Therefore, if the water supply originates from a well, the gas may enter through the plumbing, causing a high concentration in closed-in shower stalls.

Testing

Radon concentration in the home is about 60% higher, on the average, in the winter when windows and doors are likely to be closed. Therefore, when testing for radon, the test kit should be set up in one of these potentially high-concentration areas, and testing should be done in winter.

The EPA recommends that all homes be tested. If radon levels exceed 20 picocuries per liter, the test should be repeated.

One of the most common tests is the alpha track detector. Alpha radiation is given off as radon breaks down. These alpha particles etch tracks across the film in the test kit. The radon level is determined by counting the marks left on the film, which is done professionally. Another common test involves use of a charcoal canister. In this test, the alpha particles are absorbed by the activated charcoal and then analyzed by professionals to determine radon levels.

Reliable tests usually require 2 to 3 days. The EPA warns consumers to beware of test kit vendors who promise quick results.

Preventive Measures

If the test results show a high level of radon, preventive measures should be taken. These include sealing cracks in the foundation and walls, increasing ventilation by opening a window or installing vents, installing a fan to create cross-ventilation, and putting in gas drains. If these measures do not decrease the radon levels to within desired limits, a more sophisticated system may be installed to diffuse the gas away from the house.

Lead

Lead is everywhere around us. Although some lead comes from natural sources, most is caused by human activities. Lead has been used in making batteries, pottery, solder, pesticides, cooking utensils, plumbing, and — what has received so much recent attention — household paint. Another source of lead in the environment has been leaded gasoline.

The amount of lead, even in remote areas such as Greenland, has been increasing since about 800 B.C, when people began mining and using lead. The amount of lead in the environment increased sharply during the industrial revolution and even more with the coming of the internal combustion engine. The latter increase occurred because manufacturers began putting lead in gasoline as an anti-knock additive.

Lead is one of the oldest known toxic materials. Some historians believed it hastened the fall of the Roman Empire. During the Romans' reign, many people in the ruling class suffered from stillbirths, sterility, and brain damage — attributable, it is believed, to lead poisoning from lead cooking pots, wine vessels, and drinking water that came from waterlines that contained lead. The high concentration of lead found in the bones of some ancient Romans support this theory. Probably many house painters, as well as artists such as the Spanish painter Goya, died of lead poisoning. Some painters put the brushes in their mouths to shape them — thus ingesting lead.

Before 1940, lead was used in house paint in the United States. Later, and largely as a result of children ingesting paint, lead poisoning became a national concern. In 1971 the Lead Poisoning Prevention Act was passed, setting permissible levels of lead for paint.

Children are particularly vulnerable to lead poisoning because they are more likely to swallow things that contain lead. Examples are ingesting paint chips and lead-laden dirt, inhaling or eating street dust, color magazines, newspaper, wallpaper, wrapping paper, and snow and icicles containing lead. Also, children may lick their hands after playing in the streets where auto exhaust has deposited lead. Approximately 15,000 children are treated for lead poisoning each year.

Lead is a cumulative poison. Except when exposed to high levels, such as in lead smelters and battery plants, lead usually is excreted from the body in the urine. Small amounts, however, are deposited in bones, replacing calcium. Cortisone therapy can cause a release of lead into the blood at toxic levels. The United States has had the highest levels of lead in the world except Japan — because of automobiles releasing lead into the air. Unleaded gas is alleviating that problem.

HOUSING REQUIREMENTS

The federal government entered the housing arena when it passed the first Federal Housing Law in 1934, creating the Federal Housing Authority. By offering low-interest rates for FHA and GI loans, the federal government has helped to improve housing in the United States. Before those loans can be obtained, the houses must meet electrical, structural, plumbing and other standards, in addition to having an approved water supply and an approved sewage disposal system.

SUMMARY

The advent of higher temperatures and increased humidity levels in buildings gave birth to the proliferation of microorganisms in indoor environments. Also, certain synthetic materials used in building construction and furniture were found to have organic compounds with adverse effects on health by creating indoor air pollution.

Houses should be designed to allow for fundamental **physiological needs** such as advantageous lighting, ventilation, soundproofing, and space, as well as psychologically enhancing features such as privacy and proximity to community facilities. The control of communicable diseases is a major goal of housing design and maintenance.

Some chemical and physical agents of disease are in the earth or in the building material. Pollutants that have been addressed specifically through legislation and testing procedures include asbestos, carbon monoxide, and lead.

REFERENCES

Am. Ind. Hyg. Association Tech. Committee on Indoor Environmental Quality. 1993. *The Industrial Hygienist's Guide to Indoor Air Quality Investigations.* ed. P. J. Rafferty, Am. Ind. Hyg. Association, Fairfax, VA.

American Public Health Association. 1954. *Basic Principles of Healthful Housing.* New York.

American Society of Heating, Refrigerating and Air-Conditioning Engineers. 1989. "Ventilation for Acceptable Indoor Air Quality." ASHRAE Standard 62–1989, Atlanta.

Apter, A., A. Bracker, M. Hodgson, J. Sidman, and W. Y. Leung. 1994. "Overview: Epidemiology of the Sick Building Syndrome." *Journal of Allergy Clinics Immunology*, 94(2):277–88.

Batterman, S. A. and H. Burge. 1995. "HVAC Systems as Emissions Sources Affecting Indoor Air Quality: Critical Review." *HVAC & Refrig. Res.* v. 1 n. 1, pp. 61–80.

Blum, Steven. "Pesticides in Urban Housing." *Journal of Housing and Community Development.* Sept–Oct 1995. v. 52 n. 5. pp. 38.

Brief, R. S., and T. Bernath. 1988. "Indoor Pollution: Guidelines for Prevention and Control of Microbiological Respiratory Hazards Associated with Air-Conditioning and Ventilation Systems." *Appl. Indus. Hyg.* v. 3 n. 3 pp. 5–10.

Burge, H. A., and M. E. Hoyer. 1990. "Indoor Air Quality." *Appl. Occup. Env't. Hyg.* v. 5 n. 2, pp. 84–93.

Clayton, G., and F. Clayton. 1978. *Patty's Industrial Hygiene and Toxicology.* John Wiley and Sons, New York.

Godish, T. 1995. *Sick Buildings: Definition, Diagnosis and Mitigation.* Lewis Publishers, Boca Ration, Fl.

Greene, Robert E., and Philip Williams. 1996, October. "Indoor Air Quality Investigation Protocols." *Journal of Environmental Health.* v. 59 n. 3.

Hansen, S. J. 1991. *Managing Indoor Air Quality.* Failmont Press, Lilburn, GA.

Hicks, J. B. 1984. "Tight Building Syndrome: When Work Makes You Sick." *Occupational Safety & Health.* v. 53 n. 1, pp. 51–56.

Jones, J. R. 1994. *Solving Indoor Air Quality Problems: The Work Environment.* Vol. 3, ed. D.J. Hansen, Lewis Publishers, Boca Raton, Fl.

Kohuth, Barbara, and Boyd Mansh. 1974. *An Education Guide for Planning an Improved Human Environment.* Inner Circle Press, Hudson, OH.

Kreiss, K. 1989. "Epidemiology of Building-Related Complaints and Illness." *Occup. Med.,* v. 4 n. 4, pp. 575–92.

Lane, C. A., J. E. Woods, and T. A. Bosman. 1989. "Indoor Air Quality Procedure for Sick and Healthy Buildings." *ASHRAEJ.* v. 31 n. 7, pp. 48–52.

Light, E. N., and N. Presant. 1994. "Investigation of Indoor Air Quality Complaints." *Immunol. Aller. Clinics N. Am.* v. 14 n. 3, pp. 659–78.

Lippy, B. E., and R. W. Turner. 1991. "Complex Mixtures in Industrial Workspaces: Lessons for Indoor Air Quality Evaluations." *Environmental. Health Perspective.* v. 95, pp. 81–93.

Mariso, L. 1994. "Cleaning the Air: IAQ Emerges as a Major Health Issue of the 90's." *The Synergist.* v. 5 n. 10, pp. 8–9.

Melius, J., K. Wallingford, R. Keenlyside, and J. Carpenter. 1984. "Indoor Air Quality: The NIOSH Experience." *Annals Am. Conf. Gov't. Ind. Hyg.* v. 10, pp. 3–7.

Mobile Home Manufacturers Association. 1960. *Mobile Home Park Sanitation.*

Morey, P. R., M. J. Hodgson, W. G. Sorenson, G. J. Kullman, W. W. Rhodes, and G. S. Visvesvara. 1984. "Environmental Studies in Moldy Office Buildings: Biological Agents, Sources and Preventive Measures." *Annals Am. Conf. Gov't. Indus. Hyg.* v. 10, pp. 21–35.

National Safety Council. 1983. *Fundamentals of Industrial Hygiene,* Chicago.

Passon, Theodore Jr., James W. Brown, and Seth Mante. 1996, July. "Sick-Building Syndrome and Building-Related Illness." *Medical Laboratory Observer.* v. 28 n. 7.

Public Health Service. *Environmental Engineering for the School.* Government Printing Office, Washington, DC.

Quinlan, P., J. M. Macher, L. E. Alevantis, and J. E. Cone. 1989. "Protocol for the Comprehensive Evaluation of Building-Associated Illness." *Occup. Med: State of the Art Rev.* v. 4 n. 4, pp. 771–779.

Tamblyn, B. T., and S. Khandekar. 1994. "IAQ: An Operation and Maintenance Perspective." *ASHRAEJ.* v. 36 n. 7, pp. 37–42.

U. S. Environmental Protection Agency. 1991. *Building Air Quality* (EPA/400/1–91/003). Washington, DC.

U. S. Public Health Service. 1976. *Basic Housing Inspection.* Government Printing Office, Washington, DC.

Environmental Safety

By Trenton G. Davis, Dr.P.H.
East Carolina University

Key Terms

Epidemiology

Injury

National Electronic Injury Surveillance System (NEISS)

Years of potential life lost (YPLL)

Objectives

- Understand the magnitude of the accident problem.

- Recognize the historical basis for environmental safety programs.

- Identify the major accident hazards in homes, recreational activities, and transportation.

- Identify major federal laws that relate to environmental safety programs.

- Discuss what individuals can do to reduce the risk of accidents.

Injuries continue to constitute a significant public health problem in the United States. Compounding the problem, safety and accident prevention programs tend to be underfunded in relation to the magnitude of the impact of injuries on public health and safety programs generally do not have the same level of public support as many other public and environmental health programs. The public seems complacent when ranking the importance of injuries, possibly because the risk of injury often is accepted as a voluntary one for which the hazards are known.

Another factor may have to do with the public's perception of accidents as being random events over which they have no control. Most people do not understand that injuries are preventable. Injuries are considered to be accidents, and the term "accidents" implies that these events are not predictable or preventable. To the contrary, research has shown that injuries are just as predictable and preventable as illnesses such as mumps, heart attacks, and lung cancer.

One example of the predictability and preventability of injuries that has been studied in some detail centers on motor vehicle injuries. One of the most important determinants of motor vehicle injury is driving after drinking alcohol. Drivers who have been drinking are much more likely to be involved in crashes than drivers who have not been drinking. Because people who drink and drive are more likely to do this at night and on weekends, more motor vehicle injuries occur at night and on weekends. If people could be prevented from drinking and driving, the motor vehicle injury death rate might be cut in half. Therefore, motor vehicle injuries are preventable. By getting drunk drivers off the road, the roads could be made safer for all drivers.

This way of thinking about injuries is not very different from the way we think about preventing measles or polio by immunizing children. Although preventing drinking and driving may not be as easy as giving immunizations, it is no less important.

Injuries may be intentional or unintentional. Intentional injuries include homicide, assault, suicide, child abuse, rape, and other acts of violence. Unintentional injuries are those that frequently are referred to as accidental injuries because they do not involve someone attempting to inflict harm on another person. This chapter focuses on unintentional injuries that occur outside of workplace environments.

For years, the category of "unintentional injuries" has been the leading cause of death in the United States for individuals below the age of 44 and the fourth leading cause of death overall. Recently, however, acquired immunodeficiency syndrome (AIDS) has become the leading cause of death among Americans in the 25–44 age groups, dropping unintentional injury to second place for that age group. This in no way reduces the importance of unintentional injuries as a public health problem.

More than 60 million Americans incur nonfatal injuries each year. Non-fatal injuries are those usually defined as being severe enough to cause a person to seek medical treatment or to be unable to perform usual activity for a day or longer.

Another way to consider the magnitude of injury mortality is to review data pertaining to **years of potential life lost (YPLL)** published by the Centers for Disease Control and Prevention,

National Center for Health Statistics. YPLL before 65 is a measure of mortality that reflects deaths occurring before age 65. In 1988, unintentional injury was the leading cause of YPLL before age 65, accounting for 2,319,400 years of life lost, or 18.9% of the total years of potential life lost. This is followed by cancer at all sites (14.7%), diseases of the heart (11.9%), suicide and homicide (11.1%), and congenital anomalies (5.5%). YPLL before age 65 caused by AIDS has become a leading cause of years of potential life lost, especially in some age groups, and may impact the leading causes of YPLL in the near future.

SAFETY CONCEPTS

Over the years, many investigators have contributed to greater understanding of injury causation and prevention. In 1961, J.J. Gibbons observed that all injury events involve the harmful effects of only five agents which are all forms of physical energy:

1. kinetic or mechanical energy,
2. chemical energy,
3. electricity,
4. radiation,
5. thermal energy.

Injury thus is physical damage to the body that results when energy is transferred to the body in amounts greater than it can withstand, such as fires or poisons, or when the body is deprived of sufficient energy, such as oxygen or heat. Because the absence of needed energy also may lead to physical damage to the body, drowning is considered to be an injury, as is suffocation. Any number of events potentially can transfer energy to the body. All of the human and environmental components thought previously to be the agents of injuries now are recognized as either vehicles or vectors — enabling factors for the real agents.

John E. Gordon wrote, in 1948, that application of **epidemiology** techniques was an appropriate way to increase understanding the causes of injury, and thus prevent or reduce accidents. He suggested that injuries involve much more than the agent; rather, they involve a combination of forces from at least three sources: the host, the agent, and the environment in which host and agent find themselves. Strategies to prevent injuries can be directed at any of the three factors.

Table 13.1 gives specific injury prevention strategies directed at the host, the agent of energy exchange, and the environment, for the three leading causes of unintentional childhood injury death in North Carolina.

In 1963, William Haddon, Jr. divided the injury event into three phases. During the pre-injury or pre-event phase, the energy source goes out of control. In the injury phase, the amount of energy released and the nature of its transfer to tissues determine whether injury occurs and its severity. Finally, during the post-injury or post-event phase, personal homeostatic mechanisms and external factors, including the timing, quantity, and quality of emergency and rehabilitative care, contribute largely to the final outcome. Definition of the three phases made it evident that an injury event is not a simple occurrence in which a harmful outcome can be avoided by preventing the initial event. Strategies to prevent injuries can be directed toward preventing events that may cause injury (pre-event-phase strategies); or toward protecting individuals against injury if a mishap occurs (event-phase strategies); or toward minimizing the consequences following an injury through prompt and skilled emergency services and medical care. Table 13.2 indicates how strategies from all three phases can be used to control selected injuries.

TABLE 13.1 Prevention Strategies for Motor Vehicle Injuries, Fires, and Drownings

	Host	Agent	Environment
Motor vehicle Injuries	Persuade people to use seatbelts and child safety seats	Provide safety features such as airbags in automobiles	Modify roadways to include features such as guardrails, adequate lighting, and separate areas for cars, bicycles, and pedestrians
House fires	Teach families to develop and practice escape	mandate fire-safe cigarettes (cigarettes that are less likely to ignite house fires)	Provide smoke detectors to alert household members of a fire
Drownings	Teach parents never to leave children unattended in the presence of water	Put child-resistant latches on toilet seats to prevent curious toddlers from falling in	Build a fence around swimming pools, with self-closing and self-latching gates

Source: Saving Children's Lives: Preventing Childhood Injuries, by J. D. Moore, and L.W. Gardner, North Carolina Public Health Forum, 1994, Vol. 3, No. 1, p. 14.

TABLE 13.2 Injury Control Strategies, by Relationship to Event

Relationship to event	Purpose of Strategies	Examples	
		Drowning	Intentional Self-poisoning
Pre-event phase	To prevent events that may cause injuries	Four-sided fencing for pools	Diagnosing and treating depression
Event phase	To prevent injury when event occurs	Personal flotation devices	Limiting total amount of medication prescribed
Post-event phase	To prevent unnecessary severity or disability when an injury has occurred	Cardiopulmonary resuscitation	Removing toxic substance from the body by lavage or dialysis

Source: *Saving Children: A Guide to Injury Prevention*, by M. H. Wilson, S. P. Baker, S. P. Teret, S. Shock, and J. Gabarino. Oxford University Press, 1991

CONSUMER PRODUCT SAFETY COMMISSION

In 1972, the U.S. Congress passed the Consumer Product Safety Act, which created the Consumer Product Safety Commission (CPSC) because "an unacceptable number of consumer products which present an unreasonable risk of injury are distributed in commerce." Before then, thousands of products intended for use by consumers were not regulated by any agency. These products were responsible for more than 20 million injuries in the United States each year in and around the home, more than 30,000 of which resulted in death.

The Consumer Product Safety Act authorizes the CPSC to ban hazardous consumer products, to initiate recalls for products that pose imminent or substantial hazards to the public, and to establish mandatory performance standards and warning and instruction requirements for consumer products. The act requires that a mandatory safety standard be "reasonably necessary to prevent or reduce an unreasonable risk of injury associated with such products." The CPSC also is responsible for administering and enforcing the Federal Hazardous Substances Act, the Poisoning Prevention Packaging Act, the Flammable Fabrics Act, the Refrigerator Safety Act, and the Child Protection and Toy Safety Act.

The CPSC was granted broad authority to issue and enforce standards over more than 10,000 consumer products — from toasters to cribs to lawnmowers. Exempted from the CPSC's authority are firearms, food, drugs, cosmetics, economic poisons, airplanes, motor vehicles, and boats, as they are covered by other-regulatory agencies. The CPSC's overall contribution to a safer America has been positive. Consumer product standards have been established for a variety of products including children's sleepwear, bicycles, baby cribs, power mowers, matchbooks, swimming pool slides, and toys with small parts. Age restrictions have been applied to toys with sharp points. Warning labels and instructions have been required for items where misuse would be particularly harmful. And some extreme hazardous sources of injury, such as unstable refuse bins, flammable contact adhesives, and materials containing free-form asbestos have been banned.

A study published in 1981 showed that in the 9 years after the CPSC came into existence, accidental household injuries fell more than 2.5 times faster than they did in the 9 years

Environmental Health

previous to the CPSC. Through the use of a **National Electronic Injury Surveillance System (NEISS)**, the CPSC has improved the state of knowledge of product-injury epidemiology and identified the most dangerous consumer products. The system monitors admissions to selected hospital emergency rooms daily for injuries involving consumer products. Then the CPSC supplements the emergency room data by conducting on-site investigations, after which a hazard index of product categories is published.

Bicycles had the dubious distinction of heading the first list as the consumer product that seemed to pose the greatest threat of injury to the American public. Today, bicycles rank low in the category of sports and recreational equipment because of widespread use of reflective devices to improve the visibility of bicycles at night, and the increased use of helmets by riders. Although accidents involving bicycles continue to occur, the severity has decreased.

In recent years, the effectiveness of the CPSC to function on behalf of the public has been questioned. The Commission's budget has been cut drastically, and the number of highly experienced technical specialists on staff has been reduced significantly. The number of reporting hospitals in the NEISS has been cut in half, thereby weakening the CPSC's major data-gathering activity. Finally, the CPSC has virtually ceased to promulgate regulations or to impose hazardous product bans. One can only wonder whether the public is now being adequately protected from consumer products that present an unreasonable risk of injury.

The CPSC is not the only agency that has responsibility for programs designed to reduce or prevent injuries. At the federal level, the U.S. Department of Transportation and the Division of Injury Control within the Centers for Disease Control and Prevention are involved in activities to develop a coordinated national injury agenda. At the level of state government, injury prevention activities are sponsored by a number of agencies including state health agencies. At the local level, many health departments have taken the lead in developing safety programs in their communities. Many nonprofit agencies and

In 1937, a drug manufacturer decided that the best way to capitalize on the popularity of the new sulfa drugs was to market them in a liquid, nonprescription form. He developed a product called Elixir Sulfanilamide, which combined a sulfa compound with diethylene glycol — a commercial solvent used in making antifreeze and brake fluid.

Because the drug control laws of the time did not require safety testing, the manufacturer was free to put the product on the market, and he did so — with devastating results. Although only 2,000 pints of the elixir were produced and only 93 were consumed, 107 people died from effects of the solvent.

citizen groups, including the National Safety Council, are important contributors to efforts to prevent injuries.

HOME SAFETY

Someone once wrote, "Your home may be your castle, but the enemy is not entirely outside the walls" — a thought-provoking statement, as more accidents occur in and around the home than in any other place.

To verify that the home is a hazardous place, one simply has to review annual statistics on home accidents. A home accident is defined as one that occurs on home premises to members of the family or invited guests. Excluded are individuals who are on home premises during the course of gainful employment, such as repair persons, postal workers, delivery persons, and the like.

A major portion of one's life is spent in and around the home setting. Young children spend nearly 90% of their time in home settings. As children enter school, they spend less and less time in the home environment. During the working years, the amount of time spent at home stabilizes, and with ensuing age, most people spend more of their nonworking hours in the home. In retirement, most people have gone full circle and again spend 90% of their time at home. This means that the youngest and oldest members of our population are at greater risk from home accidents, in part because of the greater number of hours of exposure in home environments.

Falls

Falls are the leading cause of accidental death in the home, outpacing burns and all other causes combined. Among the elderly and children, falls top the home unintentional injuries list.

Children

In children, falls occur under a wide variety of circumstances, but the risk of death or permanent impairment is related strongly to the height of the fall and the nature of the material struck. Falls from windows — an especially serious problem during the summer among children younger than 5 — increase in severity as the height of the window and the hardness of the surface increase. Falls from second-story windows usually are not fatal unless the child lands on concrete or other hard surface.

Many falls from children's furniture occur. Each year some 9,000 injuries are related to cribs, 8,000 to highchairs, and 22,000 to bunk beds. For each of these products, the majority of injuries are caused by falls. Children also fall from bassinets and shopping carts. Most falls down stairs do not have serious consequences, partly because the fall is broken by each step the child lands on. In contrast, when an infant in a baby walker falls down stairs, the fall may be unbroken until the bottom, in which case death or permanent brain injury can result, especially if the floor is concrete.

Many of the serious childhood injuries occurring on stairs are related to walkers. In 1991, of the 27,000 injuries to children up to 15 months of age that were related to baby walkers, 92% were to the head or face. Some experts suggest that because walkers are of no known developmental benefit, their use should be discouraged.

In the case of falls on the same level, sharp corners on furniture, glass coffee tables, and broken glass in play areas are some of the sources of injury.

Caregivers must be vigilant in their supervision of young children and anticipate that the young are interested in exploring their world and are highly active. Efforts must be made to remove hazards in their environment that may increase the risk of injury from falls.

Older Adults

Unlike fall victims who are children, older fall victims are much more likely to die from falls. The difference is that older individuals are unable to absorb as much physical trauma as the young. Children are more resilient and more readily able to recover from injury.

The death rate from falls among the elderly aged 75 and older is nearly 12 times greater than the rate for all other ages combined. The risk of hospitalization is nearly seven times as great.

Visual acuity and depth perception may be seriously diminished with aging. Physical responses become slower, and balance and coordination are impacted adversely to the extent that older adults may not be able to react quickly enough when they commence to fall or slip. The widespread use of drugs and medications by older adults has been associated with increased incidents of dizziness, loss of coordination, and falls.

Preventing Falls

Stairways are the site of more than 750,000 fall injuries each year. Factors involved in these accidents include obscured vision, poor lightning conditions, obstacles on stairs, and slippery tread surface. To reduce accidental falls involving stairways, stairs should be well lighted, handrails should be provided, the height of steps should be no greater than 8.25 inches, tread width should be at least 10 inches, stairways should not be used as storage areas, and stair coverings should be composed of slip-resistant materials.

Falls also occur on floors and walkways and in bathtubs and showers. Efforts must be made to prevent conditions that may lead to slippery floors and walkways. Older adults must be especially cautious in bathrooms — one of the most hazardous areas in the home.

Although not as numerous as stairway accidents or falls on level surfaces, falls from ladders account for more than 100,000 injuries yearly. Falls from ladders can be reduced by selecting the proper ladder for the intended use and then using the ladder properly.

Fire and Burn Injuries

Despite continuing efforts to prevent injuries and deaths from fires and burns, fire still kills about 5,000 people in the United States annually — an average of 13 per day. This is one of the highest fatality rates in the industrialized world.

Fire kills disproportionately. People who are black, poor, old, or very young are two to three times more likely to die in fires than the national average. Most residential fires occur during December through March, a period of colder weather and longer darkness. In 1991, residential fires constituted the second leading cause of injury deaths (after motor-vehicle related injuries) of children aged 1–9 years and the sixth leading cause of such deaths in persons aged 65 years and older.

In 1991, 48% of fire deaths occurred during January, February, March, and December. The three leading causes of deaths of children younger than 5 years, were:

1. Children playing with fire-ignition sources, such as matches (37%)
2. Faulty or misused heating devices (19%)
3. Faulty or misused electrical distribution sources (11%)

For persons older than 70 years, the three leading causes were

1. Careless smoking (33%)
2. Faulty or misused heating devices (19%)
3. Faulty or misused electrical distribution sources (12%).

Despite the 37% decline in rates of residential-fire deaths from 1970 through 1991, the overall rate in 1991 (1.5 per 100,000 persons) exceeded the rate targeted by a national health objective for the year 2000 (reducing the rate of residential fire-related deaths to no more than 1.2 deaths per 100,000 persons). In particular, the rates for children younger than age 5 (3.7 per 100,000 children) and for persons age 65 and older (3.5 per 100,000) — the highest-risk groups — exceeded the age-group specific target goal of 3.3 per 100,000 for each group.

The increased occurrence of fire-related deaths during winter months reflects the seasonal use of portable heaters, fireplaces, and chimneys, and Christmas trees. Fires associated with electrical portable heaters usually result from electrical shortages or device failures rather than from ignition of nearby materials such as draperies. Electrical cords for portable electric-space heaters should be plugged directly into the wall and not linked through an extension cord, kept at least 3 feet from any combustible material, and unplugged when not in use. Fires attributed to the use of kerosene portable heaters usually result from using the wrong fuel, faulty switches and valves, and fuel leaks and spills that subsequently ignite. Kerosene heaters should be used only with K-1 kerosene, rather than gasoline or camp-stove fuel, and should be refueled outdoors after the heater has cooled. Chimney fires usually result from the buildup of creosote, a highly flammable byproduct of wood fires. Chimneys should be cleaned or inspected annually to detect and prevent cresote buildup. A fire screen should be used in front of the fireplace. Wood stoves and fireplaces should burn only seasoned wood, not green wood, trash, or wrapping paper.

Fires related to Christmas trees usually result from electrical problems, such as overloaded electrical circuits caused by using several extension cords in one outlet, or frayed wire and cords. In 1991, of the four leading causes of residential fires, Christmas trees accounted for the lowest number of fires but a substantially higher proportion of deaths than the other types of residential fires. People in households with electric holiday decorations should examine the electric lights periodically and should not place trees near heating sources or fireplaces. In addition, live cut trees should be watered sufficiently to reduce drying.

To reduce the risk of death or injury resulting from fires, a smoke detector should be installed outside each sleeping area on every habitable level of a home, and the battery should be changed at least annually. Occupants should develop escape plans that include identifying two exits from every living area and should practice exit drills and meeting at a designated safe location sufficiently distant from the home. In addition, every home should have a multipurpose fire extinguisher conveniently available for use in extinguishing small fires. If a fire cannot be extinguished within 1 minute, the residence should be evacuated because of the rapid rate of accumulation of heat and toxic gases.

Children playing with fire-ignition sources were the leading cause of fires resulting in the deaths of children younger than 5 years. Therefore, children should be taught not to play with matches or lighters and these items should be stored out of the reach of young children.

Scalding rarely is a cause of death, but it is important because of its high incidence in young children and elderly adults. Hot tap water, coffee, and tea are the most common agents, and boiling water or food is the most damaging. Scalds occurring when children upset containers of hot liquid often affect the face and hands.

Tap water scalds can be reduced by setting thermostats on hot water heaters at a temperature no higher than 120°F in all residences and institutional dwellings. Water heated to 140°F can cause third-degree burns in only 2 seconds. Unfortunately, many hot water heaters are set at this temperature. When the water temperature is turned down to 120°, the same burn takes 5 minutes to occur.

Poisoning

In 1961, poisoning claimed the lives of 450 children under the age of 5. By 1989, that number had dropped to 42. This reduction in the age group at greatest risk is attributable to several factors including child-resistant packaging, better emergency care, more poison-control centers, reformation of some poisonous substances such as lead paint, reduced use of other substances such as kerosene, and parental education.

Despite the progress in reducing the number of deaths from poisoning, non-fatal poisonings still occur in a substantial number of children. Estimates indicate that for every death from poisoning in children younger than age 5, some 80,000 to 90,000 children will go to an emergency room for treatment, approximately 20,000 of whom will have to be hospitalized.

The substances that children ingest most commonly are aspirin, solvents and petroleum products, tranquilizers, and iron compounds. The highest rates are seen in children about 1–2 years of age; boys are at slightly higher risk than girls. Other substances ingested frequently include personal care products such as shaving cream, deodorants, bath oils, nail polish, and pediatric cough syrup.

A study by the CPSC revealed that 23% of oral prescription drugs ingested by children under age 5 belonged to someone who did not live with the children. Overall, 17% of the drugs ingested belonged to a grandparent or great-grandparent. Education of parents, grandparents, babysitters, day care providers, and teachers is imperative if the accidental poisoning rates are to decrease significantly.

Parents and other caregivers must carefully assess the poisoning hazards in homes where young children live and take action to childproof those environments. The American Academy of Pediatrics offers the following recommendations:

- First and foremost, store household products and medicines out of reach of children, and use safety latches on all drawers and cupboards that contain potentially harmful substances.
- Keep products in their original containers. Never put products that can be poisonous in old food or beverage containers.
- Never call medicine "candy."
- Have syrup of ipecac available at home, and use it to induce vomiting if a child ingests a poisonous substance.

- Keep poison control and other emergency phone numbers near the telephone, and call immediately in an emergency.
- Leave original labels on all products.
- Clean out medicine cabinets periodically and discard unneeded and dated medications in a safe manner.

A number of poisonous plants found in and around the home are capable of causing severe itching, burning, and swelling of skin tissues on contact, or nausea and vomiting if ingested. These plants include poison ivy, mushrooms, azalea, oleander, dieffenbachia, rhododendron, and poinsettia. Parents and other caregivers should be knowledgeable about these and other poisonous plants and take the necessary precautions to protect children from accidental exposure.

Firearm Injuries

From 1968 through 1991, firearm-related deaths increased by 60% (from 23,875 to 38,317). Based on these trends, by the year 2003, the number of firearm-related deaths will surpass the number of motor-vehicle-related deaths and firearms will become the leading cause of injury-related death. Firearm injuries usually have been divided into homicides, suicides, and unintentional shootings. This separation has masked the severity of the firearm problem as a major killer of children and young adults. In 1988, gunshot wounds were the eighth leading cause of unintentional injury deaths in all age groups in the United States and the third leading cause among children and teenagers aged 10–19 years. For males aged 10–19 years, the unintentional firearm-related death rate is seven to ten times that for females. Males aged 15–19 years are at higher risk than are males in any other age group. Children and teenagers living in the Southern region of the country are at highest risk for dying from an unintentional gunshot wound; those living in the Northeast are at lowest risk. Within regions, white males aged 15–19 are at greatest risk in the South; in all other regions, deaths are highest for black male

teenagers. Overall, children and teens living in nonmetropolitan regions are more than twice as likely to die from an unintentional gunshot wound as those living in metropolitan areas.

The apparent intent of the shooter in firearm deaths varies with the age of the victim. At ages 0–4 the majority of firearm fatalities are homicides. At ages 5–9, most of firearm deaths are unintentional. At ages 10–14, deaths from guns are almost evenly divided among suicides, homicides, and unintentional shootings. For persons aged 15 and above, suicides and homicides are most commonly the intent.

A multifaceted approach to reduce firearm-related injuries should include at least three elements.

1. Foster changes in behavior through campaigns to educate and inform persons about the risks and benefits of possessing firearms and the safe use and storage of firearms.

2. Direct legislative efforts toward preventing access to or acquiring firearms by specific groups that should not have firearms (e.g., felons and children) and toward regulating the storage, transport, and use of firearms.

3. Make technologic changes to modify firearms and ammunition so as to render them less lethal (e.g., a requirement for childproof safety devices such as trigger locks).

Reduction of morbidity and mortality from unintentional firearm-related injuries among children and teenagers must emphasize limiting access to loaded weapons.

Nonpowder firearms (those using gas, air, or a spring to propel ammunition, including BB guns) cause more than 14,000 injuries annually among children younger than age 15, with boys accounting for over 80% of the injuries. Although nonpowder-firearm injuries generally are less severe than those from powder guns, fatalities and permanent disabilities do occur. Nonpowder firearms should be used only under responsible adult supervision and should be treated in much the same way as other firearms.

Power Lawnmower Injuries

Power lawnmowers (walk-behind and ride-on) continue to be responsible for hundreds of injuries each year, in spite of the CPSC's long-time effort to reduce injuries associated with these labor-saving machines. Commencing in the late 1970s, manufacturers adopted numerous voluntary safety standards designed to reduce the risks, including reducing blade speed on rotary motors, installing blade control systems to prevent the blade from operating unless the operator actuates the control, installing deflector covers over discharge chutes, and using devices that cause the blade to stop within 3 seconds after the control is released.

Operators must recognize that power lawnmowers are extremely hazardous and must be operated safely. Further reduction in injuries through changes in design may not be effective without greater attention to safe operation.

Approximately half of all injuries that happen while using power lawnmowers are to persons under 16 or over 55 years of age. Though rare, deaths do occur from power lawnmower accidents. More than 60% of the deaths are children under age 5 and adults over 65 years of age. This means that the lawnmowing task must not be assigned to young, inexperienced operators or to older adults who may not have the strength or reflexes necessary to operate a power lawnmower safely.

RECREATIONAL SAFETY

Millions of Americans participate in leisure activities each year. These activities range from those that constitute a low risk of injury to those that may constitute a high risk. Among the features that may determine the degree of risk are the activity itself, the participant's age, skill level, and health, and the condition of the environment. No doubt, individuals who are skilled in an activity, who understand the risks, and who adhere to safe practices are at lower risk of being involved in injury-causing accidents.

This section will highlight a few of the leisure activities in which Americans participate.

Swimming

Swimming is one of the most popular recreational activities in the United States, and also one of the most dangerous. Drowning, the fourth leading cause of childhood fatal injuries, is most common in children 4 years of age and males aged 15–19 years. In the latter group, drownings occur in a wide variety of environments and alcohol use is associated with an estimated 40% to 50% of these events. Drowning rates for black children are almost twice those for white children. In three states (Arizona, California, and Florida) drowning is the leading cause of fatal injuries for children 4 years of age. In all states, up to 90% of drownings among this age group occur in residential swimming pools.

In a study of swimming pool drownings in Maricopa County, Arizona, 40% were attributed to a lapse in supervision, 35% to absence of a pool fence (a fence that completely encloses the pool and isolates it from the house and play area), 14% to an inadequate or unclosed gate or latch, 2% to an inadequate fence, and 9% to other causes.

Data from this study suggest that pool fencing, in combination with adequate gates and latches, could have prevented 51% of the drownings or near-drownings reported. Because so many incidents were attributed to a lapse in supervision (the supervisor's attention was diverted or a child was not observed momentarily while the adult performed a chore in the pool area), educating parents and caregivers about constant vigilance at a pool should complement an emphasis on passive barriers to the pool. Other measures may include instruction on the maintenance of gates and latches, cardiopulmonary resuscitation classes, and improvement in the design and placement of pools. Figure 13.1 shows hazard areas in residential swimming pools.

Suction drains in spas, hot tubs, whirlpool baths, and swimming pools are extremely hazardous. They have proven fatal and caused injuries to children who have been sucked against the drain or had their hair drawn into the drain. Some states now require that all newly constructed pools be designed to reduce the risk of suction-drain injuries.

People who swim in natural bodies of water may be at greater risk than those who swim in residential-type swimming pools. Additional hazards include changing environmental conditions such as depth, currents, and weather; insufficient warning signs; murky or cloudy water, close proximity to water craft; and inaccessibility of emergency medical services.

In some states, laws have established basic safety requirements for natural swimming areas, including depth markings and warning signs, lifeguards, life-saving equipment, and first-aid supplies, telephones for emergency use, safety plans, and restrictions on the number of persons allowed in a specific swimming area.

In addition to drowning, many injuries are associated with water activities. The most serious are paralysis resulting from diving into shallow water in a pool, river, or other body of water. Propeller injuries to water skiers are too common and could be eliminated if propellers were shielded adequately. Hundreds of children are injured on swimming pool slides each year.

Recreational Boating

Recreational boating continues to grow in popularity each year, and with it comes a corresponding increase in risk. Recreational boats include canoes, rowboats, duckboats, sailboats, motorboats, yachts, jet skis, and kayaks.

A review of statistics on recreational boating fatalities in recent years indicates that fatalities are highest among the 20–28 age group, and that a high percentage of accidents occur on Saturday and Sunday. June and July are the months in which the greatest number of accidental boating deaths occur. In most cases the watercraft were open outboard motorboats or boats less than 15 feet in length with no motor (excluding sailboats) and with only two persons aboard. The most frequent type of accident is capsizing while boating in nontidal, calm waters, with clear weather conditions and a light wind.

The greatest number of fatalities occur while the boat is cruising, which means that the vessel is proceeding normally and unrestricted, with no drastic rudder or engine changes at the time of the accident. The second largest number of fatalities occur while the boat is being used for fishing. Drifting, in which a vessel is carried along with the tide or wind, is the operational category accounting for the third largest number

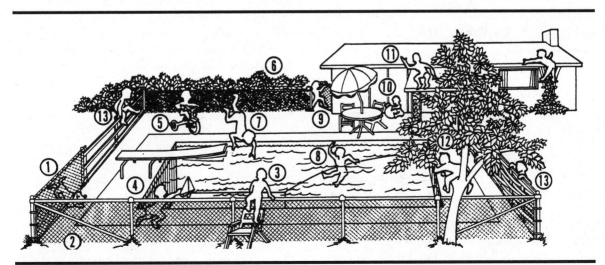

FIGURE 13.1 Each number represents an unsafe act for a swimming pool area.

of fatalities. These three operations account for more than two-thirds of the fatalities each year.

One of the newest and fastest growing recreational boating activities involves personal watercraft or jet skis. These are small, agile boats powered by an inboard engine and a jet pump mechanism. Deaths and injuries involving personal watercraft have increased dramatically since the mid-1980s. In fact, the death rate per 100,000 registered boats is more than twice as high for personal watercraft as for all other types of boats.

Boaters should take the following precautions to reduce the risk of an accident

- Be totally familiar with the boat's operation. This means that young, inexperienced operators should be supervised until they acquire skills necessary to be safe operators.

- Equip boats with approved personal floatation devices for each person, and with fire extinguishers and other safety equipment.

- Be familiar with all of the rules of safe boating.

- Avoid the use of alcoholic beverages. Studies conducted by the U. S. Coast Guard suggest that alcohol may be involved in as many as 60% of recreational boating fatalities.

OTHER RECREATIONAL ACTIVITIES

Each year in the United States an estimated 30 million persons ride horses. The rate of serious injury per number of riding hours is estimated to be higher for horseback riders than for motorcyclists and automobile racers. Falls account for most horseback-riding injuries, and fewer than 20% of riders were wearing a helmet at the time of the fall. Even when riders wear headgear, it may be decorative or secured improperly, thereby providing limited or no protection. Horseback riders should wear properly secured hard-shell helmets lined with expanded polystyrene or similar material.

Horseback riders sometimes are injured when they collide with fixed objects, are dragged along the ground with a foot caught in a stirrup, are crushed between the horse and ground, or are trampled, kicked, or bitten. Equipment problems associated with injuries include improper boot stirrup fit, broken reins, bridles, or stirrup straps, and malfunctions of the stirrup-release mechanism. All equipment must be kept in good repair.

Recreational use of *snowmobiles* is extremely popular in many regions of the country. One study suggests that most fatal snowmobile incidents involve male operators in their 20s, use of alcohol, or excessive speed, and that half the persons killed sustained head injuries. It has been estimated that helmet use could reduce the risk for death among snowmobile users by approximately 42% and could reduce the likelihood of head injury in a non-fatal incident by approximately 64%.

All-terrain vehicles (ATVs) are three- or four-wheeled vehicles designed mainly for recreational or agricultural off-road use. Licensing is not required in most states. Since ATVs became popular in the United States in 1982, more than 1,100 persons have died while operating them, and more than half of these deaths were among children under 16 years of age. In addition, nearly 420,000 non-fatal injuries have resulted nationwide from operation of these vehicles.

ATVs overturn easily, especially on rough terrain. Concern about instability and resulting injuries led to a ban on the sale of three-wheeled ATVs in December 1987.

Data support a strong recommendation prohibiting use of ATVs by children younger than 16 years. Certainly, children younger than 16 should not use adult-size ATVs. Helmets offer protection against head injury and should be required, but helmets cannot prevent spinal cord injury and other injuries associated with ATVs.

Firearm injuries associated with *hunting* appear to affect the young disproportionately. As many as 25% of hunting firearm injuries are fatal. One in seven shooters in hunting fatalities is a male younger than age 15. Hunting injuries could be reduced by encouraging hunters to participate in hunter safety instruction, requiring hunters to wear orange clothing while hunting, and prohibiting children under age 12 from hunting unless accompanied by an experienced adult.

TRANSPORTATION SAFETY INTRODUCTION

Over the past four decades, numerous interventions in motor vehicle and highway safety have contributed to reducing transportation injuries and deaths in the United States. These interventions have focused on a multifaceted, science-based approach to reduce mortality from motor vehicle crashes and have included public information programs, promotion of behavioral changes, changes in legislation and regulations, and advances in engineering and technology. These strategies have resulted in safer vehicles (e.g., the addition of laminated windshields and interior padding), safer driving practices (e.g., reduced occurrence of alcohol-impaired driving and increased use of safety belts), safer travel environments (e.g., construction of safer highways and roads), and improved emergency medical services.

Key elements of the science-based approach include the establishment of a national data-collection system to routinely monitor motor-vehicle-related deaths, identification of modifiable risk factors, design and implementation of preventive measures, and evaluation of the effectiveness of these measures. Since 1966, when the federal government identified transportation safety as a major goal and subsequently established the National Highway Traffic Safety Administration (NHTSA) to help reduce death and injury on the highway, the annual number of motor-vehicle-related deaths in the United States has decreased, even though the annual number of vehicle-miles traveled has increased more than 114%. From 1968 through 1991, motor-vehicle-related deaths decreased by 21%. Despite these considerable efforts and results, motor-vehicle injuries continue to be the leading cause of death (> 40,000 deaths annually) for people from 1 to 34 years of age and are the leading cause of work-related deaths. Of those who die, 15% are pedestrians. Motor vehicle accidents also are the major cause of serious head and spinal cord injuries.

The impact of motor-vehicle injuries on certain groups is illustrated by the following:

- Motor-vehicle crash injuries claim the lives of more than 5,500 teenagers each year.
- More than over 2,200 children ages 0–12, die in motor-vehicle crashes annually.
- More than 40% of the deaths of 16 to 19 year-olds from all causes result from motor vehicle accidents.
- Motor vehicle accidents are the cause of about half of all child deaths from injury.
- Alcohol is involved in about half of all deaths from motor-vehicle crashes.
- Motor-vehicle crashes cause the deaths of more than 5,500 pedestrians each year.
- Motor-vehicle crashes cause 23% of all occupational injury deaths.
- Annually, motor-vehicle crashes are the cause of fatal injuries of more than 6,000 elderly people (65 years of age and older); 65% are passenger-car occupants and 20% are pedestrians.

Child Restraints

Although in recent years the increase in child safety seat use has saved lives of and prevented injuries to infants (children 1 year old and younger) and toddlers (children aged 1–4 years), the leading cause of death in children ages 1–4 years continues to be injuries to motor-vehicle occupants. These injuries account for the largest number of years of potential life lost before age 65 and the highest costs associated with pediatric injury.

In 1990, child safety seats were used with an estimated 83% of infants and 84% of toddlers, compared to 60% and 38%, respectively, in 1983. Despite this high level of use, 500–700 infants and toddlers died each year from 1983 through 1990 in traffic crashes. In 1990, NHTS reported that 624 children younger than 5 years of age were killed in motor-vehicle crashes, of whom 70% were not restrained. The evidence is clear that children who are not restrained may be at greater risk of involvement in a potentially fatal crash. Based on estimates from 1982 through 1990, the use of restraints (both child safety seats and adult safety belts) saved 1,546 lives of young children in passenger-vehicle crashes. Further reductions in child crash fatalities will require education and motivation of parents to use child safety seats and safety belts.

Pedestrian Safety

Pedestrian injuries are the leading cause of death in children aged 4–8, with the peak at age 6. Each year approximately 1,100 pedestrians ages 0–14 years are killed in traffic accidents. In addition, approximately 200 are killed in non-traffic locations such as private driveways, parking lots, and farms. One-year old children are at highest risk. Annually, more than 80,000 children are treated in emergency rooms from injuries sustained in traffic accidents, many of whom require admission to hospitals.

Because of the tremendous force involved and the lack of protective structures surrounding pedestrians, severe multiple injuries are common. Case-fatality rates are very high when head injuries are present and are particularly high for children. Rates of death and serious injury are about twice as high in boys as in girls, and are especially high in urban and low-income areas.

Children are struck by cars when they dart into traffic, especially where parked cars obscure them from the driver's view, cross the street in front of school buses, and walk or crawl near motor vehicles in yards and driveways. Injuries are concentrated in the after-school hours from 3:00 to 7:00 p.m. During the hour after sunset, when visibility is poor, pedestrian deaths are especially likely.

Prevention requires separating children from vehicular traffic, making it easier for children and cars to see one another, slowing traffic in areas where children are apt to be crossing the street, supervising children until they are old enough to make reliable decisions regarding street crossing, and training those old enough to cross alone.

For elderly persons, poor night vision and reduced physical abilities may increase the risk of pedestrian accidents. These people should wear brightly colored clothing or clothing that contains retroreflective materials to increase nighttime visibility.

Motor Vehicles

Human error accounts for more than 80% of all accidents, including motor vehicle accidents. The term frequently used to describe the causes of these accidents is "improper driving." This includes actions such as speeding, failure to yield right-of-way, driving left of center, incorrect passing, and following too closely.

Speed is considered to be the major factor in over 25% of all fatal motor vehicle accidents. Included in these statistics are fatalities resulting from operators driving too fast for road conditions, not necessarily exceeding posted speed limits. Even so, speed is definitely a factor. An estimated 2,000 to 4,000 lives were saved annually during the years when the 55-mph speed limit was in force. There is concern that recent laws that allow states to establish speed limits will lead to increased fatalities on our highways.

Nearly 20% of the annual motor vehicle fatalities involve three types of right-of-way errors: failure to yield, not stopping at a stop sign, and disregarding a signal. Failure to yield accounts for the greatest percentage of these accidents. Defensive driving is the best approach to take in preventing right-of-way accidents. The driver should not assume that the other driver will follow the rules of the road.

The most important factor in fatal motor vehicle accidents is alcohol. Annually, more than half of the motor vehicle deaths in the United States are alcohol-related. Statistical estimates from the NHTSA indicate that two in five Americans will be involved in an alcohol-related crash at some point in their lives. Use of drugs and other chemical agents that impair driving ability also play a role in motor vehicle accidents, particularly when drugs are combined with alcohol use.

Law enforcement personnel and organizations such as Mothers Against Drunk Driving (MADD) have worked closely with legislators and citizens to develop better ways to educate the public about the hazards of drinking and driving.

Environmental factors, both natural and manmade, account for less than 5% of vehicle accidents. When these factors are combined with some degree of human error, however, they become a significant factor in 27% of accidents. Natural environmental factors such as rain, snow, wind, fog, and ice cannot be directly controlled or prevented, but they can be modified to some extent through roadway design. Also, drivers must be educated about the risks associated with driving in adverse weather conditions.

Another factor that must be considered in motor vehicle crashes is vehicle design. Improvements in vehicle characteristics and components such as braking, steering, mirrors, tires, seatbelts and airbags, and vehicle lighting enable the driver to handle the vehicle more safely and efficiently. Motor vehicles are safer for occupants than motor vehicles manufactured prior to 1966, in part because of the publication of Ralph Nader's book *Unsafe at Any Speed*. Nader described numerous hazards to occupants that have been addressed through improved design. As a consequence, vehicles are safer.

Passenger restraints, including seatbelts, reduce the risk of injury in the event of a motor vehicle crash by protecting the passenger from impact with components of the vehicle's interior. Investigations by the NHTSA and other organizations have indicated that the life-saving effectiveness of lap and shoulder belts, when they are worn, is about 50%. Despite the benefits of safety belts and their presence in practically all passenger vehicles, many Americans do not use them regularly. Some studies indicate that almost half of U.S. motorists do not wear seatbelts.

In efforts to reduce injuries and fatalities in motor vehicle crashes, many states have passed mandatory safety belt laws. Also, passive restraints or airbags now are installed in most new passenger vehicles. This should provide greater protection to occupants, especially the driver and front-seat passenger.

Although motor vehicle accidents, the leading cause of accidental deaths, have declined in recent years, much more must be done in the

In 1962, Dr. William Hadden, Jr. developed a list of 10 strategies for injury prevention and control that still are applicable today. These are listed, with examples of current significance in parentheses.

1. Prevent the creation of the hazard. (Ban the production and sale of all-terrain vehicles.)
2. Reduce the amount of the hazard. (Package medicines in small amounts so the entire bottle, if ingested, is not a lethal dose.)
3. Prevent the release of a hazard that already exists. (Manufacture all cigarettes to be self-extinguishing when not inhaled.)
4. Modify the rate or spatial distribution of the hazard. (Require airbags in cars.)
5. Separate, in time or space, the hazard from that which is to be protected. (Use bicycle paths to separate bicycles from cars.)
6. Separate the hazard from that which is to be protected by a material barrier. (Build fences around swimming pools.)
7. Modify relevant basic qualities of the hazard. (Manufacture nonflammable upholstery.)
8. Make what is to be protected more resistant to damage from the hazard. (Prevent osteoporosis, which weakens hip bones and makes them susceptible to breaking.)
9. Begin to counter the damage already done by the hazard. (Provide emergency medical care.)
10. Stabilize, repair, and rehabilitate the object of the damage. (Provide acute care and rehabilitation services.)

Source: Injury in North Carolina

future. Data indicate that too many drivers are driving while impaired, too many drivers exceed safe speeds, too many drivers fail to wear a seatbelt, and too many drivers fail to yield the right-of-way and commit other driving errors.

SUMMARY

Unintentional injuries constitute a continuing public health problem in the United States. Americans are at risk in their homes, on the highways, at work, and while engaging in recreational activities. Much has been learned about the actual causes of accidents through the application of epidemiological sciences to the study of accidents and through other research techniques. Research findings have led to reduction of injuries and fatalities in many categories of accidents.

Although the home environment is, indeed, an unsafe environment, this environment can be made safer for family and invited guests by better understanding the dynamics of home accidents. Adults must assume responsibility for making the home environment safe for members of the family who are at greatest risk: children and older adults.

Many popular recreational activities are extremely dangerous. Young, inexperienced persons seem to be at highest risk and should be supervised closely. Using proper equipment and avoiding alcohol while participating in recreational activities will reduce the risk of injury. Application of the 10 strategies for injury prevention and control presented in this chapter, along with application of the three E's of environmental safety (education, engineering, and enforcement) will help to make the country safer for all citizens.

REFERENCES

Berger, Lawrence R. 1985, Nov./Dec. Childhood injuries. *Public Health Reports*. v. 100, n. 6, pp. 572–574.

Bever, David L. 1992. *Safety: A Personal Focus*. 3d ed. Mosby Yearbook, St. Louis.

Brobeck, Stephen, and Anne C. Averyt. 1983. *The Product Safety Book: The Ultimate Consumer Guide to Product Hazards*. E. P. Dutton, New York.

Centers for Disease Control and Prevention, U. S. Department of Health and Human Services. 1993, May. *Injury Control in the 1990's: A National Plan for Action*, Atlanta.

Centers for Disease Control and Prevention. 1995. Injuries associated with use of snowmobiles — New Hampshire, 1989–92. *Morbidity and Mortality Weekly Report*, v. 44 n. 1 pp. l–3.

Centers for Disease Control and Prevention. 1994. Deaths resulting from residential fires — United States, 1991. *Morbidity and Mortality Weekly Report*. v. 43 n. 49 pp. 901–904.

Centers for Disease Control and Prevention. 1994. Deaths resulting from firearm and motor vehicle-related injuries — United States, 1968–1991. *Morbidity and Mortality Weekly Report*. v. 43 n. 3 pp. 37–41.

Centers for Disease Control and Prevention. 1993. Carbon monoxide poisoning — Weld County, Colorado, 1993. *Morbidity and Mortality Weekly Report* v. 43 n. 42 pp. 765–767.

Centers for Disease Control and Prevention. 1993. Unintentional carbon monoxide poisoning following a winter storm — Washington, January 1993. *Morbidity and Mortality Weekly Report*, v. 42 n. 6 pp. 109–111.

Centers for Disease Control and Prevention. 1992. Suction-drain injury in a public wading pool — North Carolina, 1991. *Morbidity and Mortality Weekly Report*. v. 41 n. 19 pp. 333–335.

Centers for Disease Control and Prevention. 1991. Child passenger restraint use and motor vehicle-related fatalities among children — United States. *Morbidity and Mortality Weekly Report.* v. 40 n. 34.

Centers for Disease Control and Prevention. 1990. Child drownings and near drownings — Maricopa County, Arizona, 1988 and 1989. *Morbidity and Mortality Weekly Report*, v. 39 n. 26 pp. 441–442.

Centers for Disease Control and Prevention. 1990. Years of potential life lost before ages 65 and 85 — United States, 1987 and 1988. *Morbidity and Mortality Weekly Report.* v. 39 n. 2 pp. 20–21.

Chemical Manufacturers Association, Simple steps to improve safety in the home. 1992, May. *Chemecology*, pp. 2–3.

Christoffel, Tom, and Katherine Christoffel. 1989, March. The Consumer Product Safety Commission's Opposition to consumer product safety: Lessons for public health advocates. *American Journal of Public Health.* v. 79, pp. 336–339.

Committee on Trauma Research, Commission on Life Sciences, National Research Council, and the Institute of Medicine. 1985. *Injury in America: A Continuing Public Health Problem*, National Academy Press, Washington, DC.

Gordon, John E. 1949, April. The epidemiology of accidents. *American Journal of Public Health.* v. 39 n. 4, pp. 504–515.

Governor's Task Force on Injury Prevention and Control. 1989, Oct. *Injury in North Carolina.* Raleigh, NC.

Iskrant, Albert P. and Paul V. Joilet. 1968. *Accidents and Homicide.* Harvard University Press, Cambridge, MA.

Moore, Jill D., and Luanne W. Gardner. 1994, Winter. Saving children's lives: Preventing childhood injuries. *North Carolina Public Health Forum*, v. 3 n. 1 pp.10–16.

National Safety Council. 1993. *Accident Facts*, 1993 ed. Itasca, IL.

Rice, Dorothy P., Ellen J. Mackenzie, and Associates. 1989. *Cost of injury in the United States: A report to Congress.* Centers for Disease Control, Atlanta.

South Carolina Department of Health and Environmental Control, *South Carolina Plants May Poison*, Columbia. SC.

U. S. Consumer Product Safety Commission. 1992, Jan/Dec. Baby walker-related injuries. *NEISS Data Highlights*, v. 16.

U. S. Consumer Product Safety Commission. 1991, Jan/Dec. Power mower related injuries 1983–1990. *NEISS Data Highlights*, v. 15.

U. S. Consumer Product Safety Commission. 1990, Jan/Dec. Head injuries. *NEISS Data Highlights*, v. 14.

U. S. Consumer Product Safety Commission. 1985. *Protect Someone You Love From Burns.* Washington, DC.

U. S. Department of Health and Human Services, Centers for Disease Control and Prevention. 1991, Oct. *Preventing Lead Poisoning in Young Children.* Atlanta.

Waller, Julian A., 1985, Nov./Dec. The epidemiologic basis for injury prevention. *Public Health Reports.* v. 100, n. 6, pp. 575–576.

Waller, Julian A., 1980. Injury as a public health problem. In *Maxcy-Roseneu Public Health and Preventive Medicine*, 11th ed. Appleton-Century-Crofts, New York.

Wiant, Chris. 1993, Feb. Injuries are no accident. *Journal of Environmental Health*, v. 55, n. 4, p. 36.

Wilson, Modena H.; Susan P. Baker, Stephen P. Teret, Susan Shock, and James Garbarino, 1991. *Saving Children: A Guide to Injury Prevention.* Oxford University Press, New York.

Air Quality

Key Terms

Anthropogenic
Catalytic converters
Deforestation
Desertification
Electrostatic precipitators

Global warming
Greenhouse effect
Nitrogen oxides
Ozone
Ozone layer

Particulate air pollution
Photochemical smog
Smog
Sulfur oxides
Thermal inversion

Objectives

- 🌐 Identify the components of air.
- 🌐 Identify and differentiate the important air pollutants.
- 🌐 Discuss the historical basis of air pollution.
- 🌐 Discuss the sources of air pollution and describe methods used to control air pollutants.
- 🌐 Identify the causes and effects of acid precipitation.
- 🌐 Identify and describe human diseases associated with exposure to elevated levels of air pollution.
- 🌐 List the primary national laws to control and reduce air pollution.
- 🌐 Identify the causes of depletion of the ozone layer and the impact on human health.
- 🌐 Recognize the impact of deforestation on air quality and the environment.
- 🌐 Calculate a community pollution standard index.

A person may survive many days without food, or a few days without water, but without air a person could not exist long enough to walk 100 feet. The air that humans must have is an odorless, colorless mixture of natural gases, roughly 78% nitrogen and 21% oxygen. The remaining 1% is mostly argon (0.93%), carbon dioxide (0.032%), and traces of neon, helium, ozone, xenon, hydrogen, methane, krypton, and varying amounts of water vapor. When anything else is added, it becomes air pollution.

HISTORICAL PERSPECTIVE

Until the 19th century and the industrial revolution, air pollution was not a problem because pollution was readily diluted in the atmosphere and did not build up over densely populated areas. When humans learned to burn fuel (wood, coal, and others) to convert water into a stream to turn a turbine, they started creating air pollution problems. The belching smoke-stacks brought new wealth to the industrialized nations, but grimy effluents became the price for the desired affluence. Industrialization raised the standard of living while lowering the visibility and causing disease. People sought affluence without regard for the effluent from the affluent society. Only after air pollution disasters were obviously responsible for multiple deaths did people become concerned about air pollution.

During the last week of October 1948, a high concentration of pollutants — then called **smog** by Harold Antoine Des Voeuy at a London Public Health Congress — settled down over the air surrounding Donora, Pennsylvania, and the surrounding area. This particular smog encompassed the Donora area on the morning of Wednesday, October 27, reducing visibility to the extent that native Donorians became lost. On Saturday morning at 2:00 a.m. the first death occurred. The deaths continued until, by Sunday night, 19 people had died, and one became ill and died a week later.

In London, 4 years later, in 1952 an air pollution episode gripped the city for 5 days. The thick yellow smog was so dense that people walked with handkerchiefs over their noses, and visibility was about 4 yards. People walked into each other, and only the blind knew where they were going. The "pea souper" of December 1952 caused the death of 4,000 people in London. These deaths, attributed to the smog, were far in excess of those normally expected to occur during that time of year.

New York City also has had air pollution episodes. The worst, in 1965, caused the death of 400 people. These episodes are not limited to large cities or cities downwind from large cities. Secluded Muse Valley, Belgium, underwent an air pollution episode in 1930 that resulted in 63 deaths and 6,000 illnesses. These and other pollution disasters are listed in Table 14.1. The episodes in the table represented cases where the "dumping ground" (the atmosphere) could not disperse the materials being emitted from natural and manmade sources. As populations grew, power demands to operate machinery, provide transportation, heat homes and other

Date	Location	Deaths: Normal Predictions — Exceeding Mortality
1930	Meuse Valley, Belgium	63
1948	Donora Valley, PA	20
1950	Poza Rica, Mexico	22
1952	London	4,000
1953	New York City	250
1956	London	1,000
1957	London	700–800
1962	London	700
1963	New York City	200–400
1966	New York City	168

TABLE 14.1 Air Pollution Disasters Since 1930 and Associated Death Rates

buildings, prepare food, and so forth, increased, and the ability of the atmosphere to dilute or disperse the pollutant was overcome, causing the air pollution disasters.

SOURCES OF AIR POLLUTION

Some *natural* sources of air pollution are forest fires, dust storms, and volcanic eruptions. Plants such as ragweed contaminate the air with pollen. Decaying leaves and other forms of vegetation release gases that contribute to air pollution and cause a haze.

Anthropogenic air pollution, that produced by humans, also may affect human health adversely. Some sources are smoke from chimneys, gases from septic tanks and house sewer systems vents, odors from cooking food, and fumes, gases, vapors and particles released from paint, household cleaner, hair sprays, and so on. *Industrial pollution* is created by the release of gases, vapors, fumes, and the like, where industry is making the cars, clothing, cleaning agents, furniture, and other products we purchase.

Air pollutants are created in *agriculture* where our food is grown. For example, crop yields are increased greatly when insecticides and herbicides are used to rid the crops of pests.

Environmental Health

At the same time, these insecticides and herbicides add to the air pollution problem.

Transportation contributes to the pollution problem and, according to some sources, accounts for approximately 50% of all air pollution. Carbon monoxide (CO) is a major source of air pollution generated by transportation. In 1983, 70% of the non-natural emissions of carbon monoxide were from highway vehicles. Now catalytic converters installed on automobiles have reduced CO emissions from this source significantly.

CO is the result of incomplete combustion of products; in contrast, complete combustion produces carbon dioxide (CO_2). **Nitrogen oxides** and hydrocarbons are additional byproducts of the combustion of petroleum products. They undergo photochemical reactions to produce what is called **photochemical smog**, a major problem in large cities.

Energy use and production are the major contributors to deterioration of our air quality. When coal or wood is burned to produce electricity or heat, the combustion process releases air pollutants: CO, CO_2, sulfur dioxide (SO_2), nitrogen oxides, heat and particulate matter, depending on the fuel — to name a few. Of particular importance is SO_2. This gas is emitted into air by burning oil and coal, which contain sulfur impurities ($S + O_2 = SO_2$) In the United States, 15% of SO_2 emissions are from industrial plants and 68% is from coal and oil-burning electric power plants. Refuse often is burned to generate heat as electricity, a process called waste-heat recovery, which also generates a small percentage of air pollution.

EFFECTS OF AIR POLLUTION

Health Effects

Epidemiological studies indicate that high levels of air pollutants contribute to or cause a number of respiratory conditions. A Harvard study estimated that as many as 60,000 people die annually from **particulate air pollution**. A phenomenon called **thermal inversion** traps pollutants in layer of cool air that cannot rise to disperse the pollutants (see Figure 14.1). Twenty-eight million Americans with chronic respiratory problems are exposed regularly to harmful levels of smog that worsen their illnesses. Some of these respiratory ailments are the following.

1. *Asthma*, an irritation of the bronchial passages that leads to severe difficulties in breathing, is a growing public health problem nationwide. From 1983 to 1993, its prevalence increased 34%, according to the National Institutes of Health. The nation's urban areas, especially those with high levels of air pollutants, seem to be the most affected. Particulates and SO_2 are among the air pollutants that seem to be linked to asthma.

2. *Chronic bronchitis* occurs when an excessive amount of mucus is produced in the bronchi, which results in a lasting cough. There seems to be a significant correlation between death rates from chronic bronchitis and SO_2 concentrations. Sulfur dioxide may irritate the nasopharynx (mucous membrane) and the bronchi. Repeated exposure to high levels of SO_2 over time may cause the body to produce excessive mucus as a defense.

3. *Pulmonary emphysema* is characterized by weakening of the walls of the alveoli, the tiny air sacs in the lungs. As the disease progresses, the alveoli become enlarged, lose their resilience, and their walls disintegrate. Shortness of breath is a primary symptom. Nitrogen dioxide has been identified as one of the air pollutants that may contribute to emphysema.

Lung cancer and heart disorders also may be caused or exacerbated by exposure to air pollutants.

Other Effects

Sulfur dioxide, carbon monoxide, **nitrogen oxides** and other contaminants not only adversely affect our health, but they also affect our property. Some pollutants damage vegetation, thus

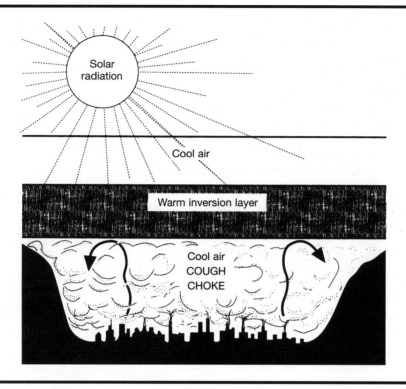

FIGURE 14.1 Thermal inversion.

affecting the landscape. Near Los Angeles, smog is destroying pine trees around the city. Some forms of air pollution directly damage leaves of crops and trees when these gases enter leaf pores (stomata). Chronic exposure to these air pollutants (including NO_2, SO_2, and ozone) breaks down the waxy coating, allowing excessive water loss and damage from disease, pests, drought, and frost. In addition, acid deposition can leach vital plant nutrients such as calcium from the soil and kill essential microorganisms such as the decomposers.

Each year air pollutants cause millions of dollars in damage to various materials. Ozone causes rubber to crack and lose of strength. Sulfur dioxide is responsible for loss of strength and surface deterioration of leather and other natural fabrics. Pollutants can cause the corrosion, erosion, discoloration, and soiling of stone, metals, paint, paper, and glass. Table 14.2 notes the significant impacts of some air pollutants.

AIR POLLUTION CONTROL

Because air pollution affects our health, crops, buildings, and the natural environment, efforts are made to reduce air pollution. **Catalytic converters** are used to improve the burning of petroleum products so as to reduce the amount of carbon monoxide, nitric oxides, and hydrocarbons in the air. More fuel-efficient cars not only save energy but also emit less exhaust.

Coal gasification and sulfur removal of sulfur dioxide are being practiced to reduce the amount of sulfur dioxide in the air, especially during thermal inversions. Coal that is low in sulfur is being burned to help lower the SO_2 in the air. That practice, however, can hurt the economy in coal mining areas that have coal with a higher sulfur content.

Emission control efforts concentrate on the settling chamber, the afterburner — which

Environmental Health

requires a high temperature to ignite and burn particles — and the electrostatic precipitator. First used for fly ash control in 1925, the **electrostatic precipitator** now is used widely in the United States. Operation consists of attaching electric charges to particles, achieved by high-voltage discharges of the particles that give them a charge. The charged particles then are attracted to metal plates called collection electrodes. The particles are intermittently cleaned from the plates.

The bag house method, used for years by the grain mills, cement factories, and the like utilizes fabric bags to capture particles in the air. This method works like a large vacuum cleaner. Now electric utilities are trying to use the bag house method to reduce air pollution in large, power-generating plants.

Pollution control methods are approached from two aspects: input control and output control. Input control concentrates on preventing or reducing the severity of the problem, whereas output control treats the symptoms, by attempting to remove pollutants once they have entered the environment.

Input Control

Some input control methods for reducing the amount of pollution before it reaches the environment are to:

1. Control population growth.

2. Reduce the need for energy.

3. Enhance fuel-dependent units such as gas engines.

4. Recycle resources and prevent loss of metals and chemicals into the environment.

TABLE 14.2 Characteristics of Some Air Pollutants

Name	Formula	Properties of Importance	Significance as Air Pollutant
Sulfur Dioxide	SO_2	Colorless gas, intense choking, odor, somewhat soluble in water to form sulfurous acid (H_2SOA_3)	Damage to vegetation, property, and health
Hydrogen Sulfide	H_2S	Rotten egg odor at low concentrations, odorless at high concentrations	Highly toxic
Nitric Oxide	NO	Colorless gas	Produced during high-temperature, high-pressure combustion. Oxidizes to NO_2.
Nitrogen Dioxide	NO_2	Colored gas, used as carrier	Relatively inert. Not greatly produced in combustion.
Carbon Monoxide	CO	Colorless and odorless	Product of incomplete combustion. Poisonous.
Carbon Dioxide	CO_2	Colorless and odorless	Formed during complete combustion. Possible effects in producing changes in global climate.
Ozone	O_3	Highly reactive	Damage to vegetation and property. Produced mainly during the formation of photochemical smog.

5. Emphasize quality in products (e.g., cars) so they will last longer.

6. Encourage repair of products rather than supporting remove-and-replace practices.

7. Reduce our dependency upon conveniences and our desire for affluence.

8. Reduce our dependency upon fossil fuels.

9. Find new nonpolluting sources of energy (e.g., wind, tidal, and solar energy).

10. Reduce our dependency upon electricity by reducing the use of electric toothbrushes, electric knives, and electric can openers and instead emphasizing simplicity — hand-operated toothbrushes, knives, and can openers.

Output Control

Strong emphasis on input control methods reduces the need for output control, which consists of the following practices:

1. Remove pollutants after combustion by using scrubbers and electrostatic precipitators.

2. Add lime and other materials to raise the pH of lakes, streams, and the soil damaged by acid rain.

3. Support improved methods of emission control.

4. Research new methods of removing pollutants in emissions.

5. Find ways to convert pollutants to a resource.

6. Improve catalytic conversion in automobiles.

Legislation

Four years after the London episode of 1952, Great Britain passed the Clean Air Act, aimed at improving the air by banning the burning of soft coal at home and in industries. The Londoners were unhappy at first, but after seeing the improvement, they welcomed the absence of the thick, yellow smog that had caused some 4,000 deaths.

Federal statutory law addressing air pollution began in the United States with the 1963 and 1967 Clean Air Acts. Although these laws

In Copperhill, Tennessee, coal was used to smelt the sulfur-containing ore and extract pure copper in copper-smelting plants of that area. The high-sulfur coal was burned for years with much SO_2 coming from the smokestacks and falling out around Copperhill and Ducktown, Tennessee. The pollution killed trees, grass, and other forms of vegetation.

With time the pollution spread to Georgia, where the Georgia legislature contacted the U. S. Public Health Service, controlling federal agency at the time. The PHS contacted the Tennessee government and required that the pollution stop, as Tennessee did not have a right to pollute Georgia. Tennessee subsequently contacted the industry and relayed the information.

At that point, the industry started looking for ways to stop or reduce the pollution. It began removing SO_2 from the stack emissions, converting it into a resource, sulfuric acid, and then related products, which the industry sold.

provided broad clean air goals and money for air research, they did not provide for air pollution control throughout the entire United States. In 1970 the Clean Air Act was amended to cover the entire United States, and the U. S. Environmental Protection Agency was created to promulgate the 1970 amendments.

In accordance with a 1977 amendment to the Clean Air Act, the Environmental Protection Agency (EPA), and the Council on Environmental Quality, along with other agencies, developed a Pollutant Standard Index (PSI). The PSI is a national air-monitoring network using a uniform air quality index. The EPA believed it was necessary to devise a method of conveying air quality data to the public in a way that would give people a good understanding of how daily levels of air pollution might be affecting their health. The PSI is given in Table 14.3.

The act was revised most recently in 1990. Under the Clean Air Act, most enforcement power is concentrated at the federal level and is delegated to the states by the EPA. The states must show the EPA that they can clean up the air to the levels required by the National Ambient Air Quality Standards (NAAQS), given in Table 14.4. The main intent of NAAQS is to protect public health and to "protect welfare." Air quality levels are determined as those needed to protect health and welfare (see Table 14.4). The states must have an Air Quality Implementation Plan (AQIP), containing all of the state's regulations governing air pollution control, including local regulations within the state. The EPA must approve the AQIP. Once approved, it has the force of federal law.

SOME AIR QUALITY PHENOMENA
Acid Precipitation

All rainfall is somewhat acidic. Decomposing organic matter, the movement of the sea, and volcanic eruptions all contribute to accumulation of acidic chemicals in the atmosphere. The main contributor is atmospheric carbon dioxide. Manmade pollutants, too, accelerate the acidification of rainfall. Emission of sulfur dioxide (SO_2) and nitrogen oxides transform into acids in the atmosphere. The acid deposition more commonly called acid rain is a misleading term because these acids and acid-forming substances are deposited not only in rain but also in snow, sleet, fog, and dew.

Acid precipitation has become a worldwide problem, first in the Scandinavian countries, then in the northeastern United States and Southeastern Canada, then Europe, Japan and Taiwan. Studies are revealing that what was

TABLE 14.3 Pollutant Standard Index

Index Value	Health Effect Descriptor	General Health Effects	Cautionary Statements
0–50	Good		
51–100	Moderate		
101–200	Unhealthful	Mild aggravation of symptoms in susceptible persons, with imitation symptoms in the healthy population.	Persons with existing heart or respiratory ailments should reduce physical exertion and outdoor activity.
201–300	Very unhealthful	Significant aggravation of symptoms and decreased exercise tolerance in persons with heart or lung disease, with widespread symptoms in the healthy population.	Elderly and persons with existing heart or lung disease should stay indoors and avoid physical exertion and outdoor activity.
301–400	Hazardous	Premature onset of certain diseases in addition to significant aggravation of symptoms and decreased exercise tolerance in healthy persons.	Elderly and persons with existing diseases should stay indoors and avoid physical exertion. General population should avoid outdoor activity.
401–500	Hazardous	Premature death of ill and elderly. Healthy people will experience adverse symptoms that affect their normal activity.	All persons should remain indoors, keeping windows and doors closed. All persons should minimize physical exertion and avoid traffic.

considered pure rainwater is now highly acidic. This precipitation is the product of sulfur oxides and nitrogen oxides produced in the burning process. The **sulfur oxides** come from burning coal and other fuels that contain sulfur. Under certain conditions, the sulfur oxides convert to sulfuric acid in the atmosphere and fall to earth in precipitation. The **nitrogen oxides** are produced from the high-temperature combustion of fossil fuels, such as in cars, in which the nitric oxides are oxidized to nitrogen dioxide, which further oxidizes and dissolves in water droplets to form nitric acid. These acids depress the pH of the soil, lakes, rivers, and other natural resources after precipitation such as rain or snow.

In the northeastern United States the culprit in most of the acid precipitation is sulfuric acid coming from coal-fueled power plants. Prevailing winds blowing from the Southwest to the Northeast dump the sulfuric acid on the northeastern United States and Canada (see Figure 14.2).

Only precipitation that has a pH of 5.6 and below is considered acid precipitation. In some parts of the world, the acidity of rainfall has fallen well below 5.6. In the northeastern United States, for example, the average pH of rainfall is 4.6, and rainfall with a pH of 4.0 — 1,000 times more acidic than distilled water — is not unusual. Figure 14.3 compares acid rain to other products in terms of pH.

TABLE 14.4 National Ambient Air Quality Standards (NAAQS) 1990

Pollutant	Primary (Health-Related) Standard Level		Secondary (Welfare-Related) Standard Level	
	Averaging Time	Concentration	Averaging Time	Concentration
PM_{10}b	Annual Arithmetic Mean	50 μg/m^3	Same as Primary	
	24-hour	150 μg/m^3	Same as Primary	
TSPb	Annual Geometric Mean	75 μg/m^3	Annual Geometric Mean	60 μg/m^3
	24-hour	260 μg/m^3	24-hour	150 μg/m^3
SO^2	Annual Arithmetic Mean	80 μg/m^3 (0.03 ppm)		
	24-hour	365 μg/m^3 (0.14 ppm)	3-hourc	1300 μg/m^3 (0.50 ppm)
CO	8-hourc	9 ppm (10 μg/m^3)	No Secondary Standard	
	1-hourc	35 ppm (40 μg/m^3)	No Secondary Standard	
NO_2	Annual Arithmetic Mean	0.053 ppm (100 μg/m^3)	Same as Primary	
O_3	Maximum Daily 1-hour Averaged	0.12 ppm (235 μg/m^3)	Same as Primary	
Pb	Maximum Quarterly Average	1.5 μg/m^3	Same as Primary	

a. The value in parentheses is an approximately equivalent concentration; the standard is in the first units shown.

b. Until July 1, 1987, total suspended particulate matter (TSP) was the indicator pollutant for the particulate matter standards. In 1987, EPA adopted the PM_{10} standard (for particles less than ten micrometers [μm] in diameter). Until attainment status of all Air Quality Control regions for PM_{10} is determined, and new plans submitted and approved, many State Implementation Plans (SIPs) will continue to address TSP. The PM_{10} annual standard is attained when the expected annual arithmetic mean concentration is less than or equal to 50 μg/m^3; the PM10 24-hour standard is attained when the expected number of days per calendar year above 150 μg/m^3 is equal to or less than one.

c. These standards are not to be exceeded more than once per year.

d. The standard is achieved when the expected number of days per calendar year with maximum hourly average concentrations above 0.12 ppm is equal to or less than one.

Source: 40 CFR Part 50 (1989); U.S. EPA (1990, March), National Air Quality and Emissions Trends Report, 1988, EPA-450/4-90-002, Research Triangle Park, NC

Environmental Health

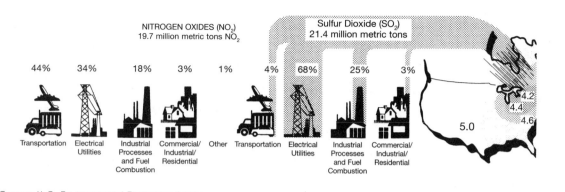

NITROGEN OXIDES (NO₂)
19.7 million metric tons NO₂

Sulfur Dioxide (SO₂)
21.4 million metric tons

44%	34%	18%	3%	1%	4%	68%	25%	3%

Transportation | Electrical Utilities | Industrial Processes and Fuel Combustion | Commercial/ Industrial/ Residential | Other | Transportation | Electrical Utilities | Industrial Processes and Fuel Combustion | Commercial/ Industrial/ Residential

4.2
4.4
4.6
5.0

Source: U. S. Environmental Protection Agency

FIGURE 14.2 Precursors of acid precipitation in northeastern United States.

LONDON'S AIR EXPERIENCE

London used to be a place where the sky was always dingy, where the only birds were pigeons, where people lived in dread of the thick yellow smog that sneaked up on the city and strangled thousands.

By 1972 Londoners lived in one of the cleanest atmospheres in the world. Hawks, wild ducks, and bullfinches, returned to nest in the parks. The sun began to shine brightly again. Even the clothing on the line dried whiter. The reason: Britain's Clean Air Act, which deprived Englishmen of their traditional glowing coal fire for the privilege of breathing fresh air.

The 1956 Clean Air Act was the first legislation of its kind in the world. Its main feature was to ban the burning of soft coal — a move that meant homeowners had to board up their fireplaces and switch to electric or gas heaters. Only the well-to-do could afford the hard, smokeless coal the act required. Lord Kennet said:

> The hearth has always been the focal point of an Englishman's living room. The sight of a glowing coal fire is built very deep in him and people felt very lost at first without it.
>
> But it was the domestic hearth which was the killer. Three fourths of the terrible

concentration of smoke in the air in 1956 came from the chimneys. They were a health horror.

The long-range advantages of the act far outweighed any temporary disgruntlement. Even the most home-loving Englishman conceded a preference for clean air over glowing hearths. The amount of smoke was reduced by 75% in London and 50% countrywide.

The number of chest diseases and heart complaints were reduced greatly. The hours of sunshine increased by 50%. People now could see the dome of St. Paul's Cathedral from Westminster Bridge, several miles away, on a clear morning — something they couldn't in the 1950s.

Whiter buildings and cleaner clothes were other benefits. Plants began to flourish in the parks, and a range of bird species returned to London. "They came back in the hundreds suddenly one spring in the early sixties — as if they had sniffed the air and said, 'It smells good; let's nest in Berkely Square,'" Lord Kennet said. Most important, the killer smogs that had hit London every winter completely disappeared.

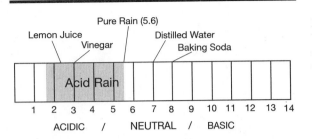

Source: U.S. Environmental Protection Agency

FIGURE 14.3 Comparative pH of acid precipitation.

The pH scale ranges from 0 to 14. A value of 7.0 is neutral. Readings below 7.0 are acidic; readings above 7.0 are alkaline. The more pH decreases below 7.0, the more acidity increases.

Because the pH scale is logarithmic, there is a tenfold difference between one number and the one next to it. Therefore, a drop in pH from 6.0 to 5.0 represents a tenfold increase in acidity, and a drop from 6.0 to 4.0 represents a hundredfold increase.

The extent of damage caused by acid deposition in an area depends on several factors. For example, an area with acid-neutralizing compounds in the soil does not reveal problems as quickly as an area without the neutralizing compounds.

Aquatic ecosystems reveal the effects of acid precipitation more clearly. The acids lower the pH, creating an unfavorable environment for aquatic life. When exposed to acid water, female fish, frogs, salamanders, and other sea creatures fail to produce eggs or may produce eggs that do not develop normally. Some scientists believe that acid water can kill fish and other aquatic life, using as evidence some lakes in areas of high acid deposition, which have been found to be highly acidic and lifeless.

The effect of acid precipitation on land, crops, forest, and other vegetation is unknown. Some believe that "dieback" (unexplained death of whole sections of once-thriving forest) is caused by acid precipitation. Present concerns have been expressed in regard to trees dying in Germany and in the Appalachian Mountains of the United States.

We do not know the effect, if any, of acid precipitation on human health. We do know that acid water can leach out as well as other chemicals from pipes. The effects of inhaling air that contains sulfur dioxide and nitrogen oxides are not known at this time.

Some methods of controlling acid precipitation are the following.

1. Reduce population growth, and thus the number of people driving cars and needing energy. Prevent unwanted pregnancies and restrict immigration.

2. Reduce the need to travel by using communication methods such as phones, faxes, and e-mail.

3. Engage in carpooling to work, school, and other trips, whenever possible.

4. Use energy more efficiently. Over 50% of energy used in the United States each year is wasted. Use energy-efficient heat pumps to provide space heating rather than burning oil.

5. Convert coal to gaseous fuel or a liquid to remove sulfur and to reduce emissions of sulfur oxides from burning solid coal.

6. Shift from fossil fuels to a mix of energy sources such as solar, tidal, nuclear, geothermal, hydroelectric, refuse, and biomass energy.

7. Shift to low-sulfur coal (less than 1%) for power plants, homes, and so on, and convert high-sulfur coal to gasoline.

8. Remove sulfur from coal, even if expensive, rather than pay high prices for foreign oil.

9. Design better and more efficient automobiles, heating units, and coal- and oil-fueled power plants.

10. Increase the efficiency of scrubbers and electrostatic precipitators.

11. Reduce the need for energy by emphasizing recycling and conservation and by deemphasizing "keeping up with the Joneses."

12. Plant trees and other plants to remove carbon dioxide and produce more oxygen for better burning.

The Greenhouse Effect

The earth's temperature remains relatively constant because some of the solar energy absorbed by earth eventually is radiated back into space. Since the 1800s, however, the heat is not being radiated back into space as much as it once was, and thus the earth is undergoing a warming trend. This warming is caused by CO_2 and water vapor in the air, as well other substances.

With the discovery that coal could be burned to convert water into steam to rotate a turbine that turns wheels on trains, pulleys on machinery, paddles on river boats, and generators in electricity-producing plants, the potential to add CO_2 to the air increased greatly. This fossil-fuel burning began producing carbon dioxide in huge quantities.

CO_2 can be removed from the atmosphere in two ways:

1. By green plants using it in the process of photosynthesis

2. By dissolving in the oceans, where it may be converted to dolomite (calcium magnesium carbonate).

The capability of these two systems is severely limited, however. As humans remove forests and pollute oceans, the need for CO_2 from the air decreases. At the same time, the world produces more CO_2 each year as the population grows. Thus, more CO_2 remains in the air each year. Studies reveal that about half of the CO_2 now emitted into the air remains in the air.

The sun radiates heat into space in every direction and has been reaching earth ever since its genesis. Some of the radiation is reflected back into space or absorbed by the earth itself. **Ozone** (O_3) in the upper atmosphere absorbs some of the short-wavelength range of ultraviolet light, X-ray, and gamma radiation, preventing it from reaching the earth's surface. At levels lower than the **ozone layer**, dust particles suspended in the air, clouds, and the earth's surface reflect about 3% of the incoming radiation back into space. About 20% is absorbed by water droplets, water vapor, and dust in the air and some 50% reaches vegetation, seas, snow-covered land and ice-covered seas that can reflect it back into space.

Burning fossil fuels in automobiles, coal-fired electric plants, and the like produces more CO_2 and, consequently, more remains, in the atmosphere. Research has shown that water vapor and CO_2 absorb radiation. Hence, more and more radiation is absorbed and trapped in the atmosphere. This causes an increase in the earth's temperature, termed the **greenhouse effect**. A greenhouse lets in sunlight through its glass. The light warms the inside, and the glass prevents the heat from escaping. Like the glass, CO_2 and water vapor in the atmosphere absorb the long-wavelength heat radiated by the earth.

The greenhouse effect causes much concern because of the possible repercussions of **global warming**. A National Academy of Sciences committee of experts estimated a global temperature increase of 3° C with a doubling of the CO_2 content of the atmosphere. A normal sample of air contains approximately 0.03% CO_2 or 320 ppm. According to the committee, from 1880 to 1980 the CO_2 level increased by 10% to 12%, contributing to a mean global temperature increase of 0.4°C. The temperature increase resulted in melting of some of the polar icecaps and glaciers, and the global ocean level increased by 5.4 inches (14 cm) in that time span.

A 1983 report by the National Academy of Sciences indicated a general consensus among 70 atmospheric scientists that, based on computer models of atmospheric processes, a doubling of the 1980 carbon dioxide levels in the atmosphere would raise the average global temperature of the atmosphere between 1.5°C and 4.5°C (2.7° and 8.1°F) and two to three times this temperature increase at the earth's polar regions. A 1985 model of the atmosphere suggested that global warming from CO_2 buildup may be only half as great as these earlier projections because the denser and wetter clouds containing more CO_2 should reflect more sunlight into space. Other studies, however, indicate that dozens of other gases such as chlorofluorocarbons (CFCs) found in trace amounts in the atmosphere could produce a global warming at least as great as that caused by carbon dioxide alone.

Global warming has two possible harmful effects:

1. Distribution of rainfall and snowfall over much of the earth could change. This change would mean that the world's major food-growing regions (such as those in much of the United States) would shift northward to areas of Canada and other northern countries where the soils tend to be poorer and less productive.

2. Glaciers and icefields in polar regions would melt, causing a projected rise in the average sea level of about 2.4 meters (8 feet) by 2100 — thus possibly causing flooding of coastal cities and industrial areas.

Ozone Layer Depletion

The main cause of the depletion of the ozone layer is chlorofluorocarbons (CFCs). The chlorofluorocarbons are propellants used in products such as hair spray, bathroom cleaners, and other aerosol products. Chlorofluorocarbons can be found in the production of foam coffee cups, egg cartons, furniture cushions, and building insulation. Hospitals use a nonflammable gas made of chlorofluorocarbons for sterilization of medical equipment.

Early in 1989, scientists were surprised that the ozone layer above the Antarctic had become thinner. David Hofman of the University of Wyoming discovered this by conducting tests with balloon-borne instruments. The Antarctic ozone "hole" in 1989 was almost twice the area of the Antarctic continent.

The Arctic ozone layer also has been researched. Scientists from Norway concluded that weather conditions over the Arctic are too dark for chlorine to destroy the ozone layer. They say, however, that destruction will come later because of an increase in sunlight. These scientists concluded that the "polar stratospheric clouds," together with the sun, promote chemical reactions that turn pollutants into ozone-depleting chemicals.

CFCs

Chlorofluorocarbons (CFCs) have become suspect in depletion of the ozone layer. Thomas Midgley developed CFCs in 1930 to replace the poisonous ammonia used in refrigerators during the 1920s. CFCs were considered safe because they did not react with other substances or break down easily. Although CFCs did not break down below the stratosphere, their inventor did not see their reaction in the stratosphere.

CFCs contain chlorine. When the CFCs reach 10 to 20 miles into the atmosphere, chlorine is released when the chloroflourocarbon's molecular bonds break down. Once released, the chlorine takes a molecule from an atom of ozone. Ordinary oxygen, which has no sun-blocking properties, is left.

Some researchers suspect the bromine also destroys the ozone layer. A study of bromine levels in the Arctic by Walter W. Berg, a scientist for the National Center for Atmospheric Research, and other scientists found a substantial amount of bromine in the Arctic atmosphere — a level 10 times higher than normal and about the same level found in a heavily polluted environment. Berg suggests that the two major contributors to depletion of the ozone layer are long-range manmade air pollution and red algae, which produces large quantities of bromine-contaminated compounds in the water under the Arctic ice. Other scientists agree that the major source of bromine is marine but question the mechanism for releasing the bromine into the atmosphere. The significance of the bromine is believed to be its synergism with the chlorine chains, which could aid in destruction of the ozone layer at lower altitudes in the stratosphere and under dark conditions — the opposite of what is done by chlorine.

The major concern with depletion of the ozone layer is that the increase in ultraviolet light will reach the surface, increasing the incidence of skin cancer and cataracts. It also could affect plants and the food chain in some undetermined way.

Not withstanding all the research, experts disagree as to the severity of ozone depletion.

Research must continue to understand the problems fully.

Solutions

According to many researchers, the best answer to the ozone problem is a new breed of CFCs that are less likely to harm the environment. One compound already on the market is 95% less destructive to the ozone layer than standard CFCs. Although this compound, called HCFC-22, costs up to 50% more than its predecessors, it is gaining popularity as a coolant for commercial and residential air-conditioning systems. In December 1987, the Food and Drug Administration approved HCFC-22 for use in containers used by the fast food industry.

One drawback to HCFC-22 is that it is less versatile than many of the ozone-depleting CFCs. It is a poor candidate for building insulation and for use in automobile air conditioning systems. It has poor insulating qualities and a high boiling point, and it requires higher pressure for air conditioning systems.

Chemical companies have developed other alternative CFCs. These have caused problems in the waste products they give off during the manufacturing process. Years of toxicity testing are necessary before these compounds can be marketed commercially.

The National Aeronautics and Space Administration (NASA), the National Oceanic and Atmospheric Administration, the Federal Aviation Administration (FAA), the World Meteorological Organization, and the United Nations Environment Program have studied ozone depletion using ground-based and satellite instrumentation. They concluded that from 1969 to 1986, the decline in annual average of ozone was from 1.7% to 3% in the Northern Hemisphere. They also found losses of 95% between altitudes of 15 and 20 kilometers.

By far the main focus of research seems to be developing a new form of CFCs that will not harm the environment, especially the ozone layer. After years of denying the adverse effects of CFCs, manufacturers now recognize the problem. They have begun using CFC replacements as well as curbing CFC production. Manufacturers of foam food containers also are involved in researching substitute compounds.

The control measures being taken are simple: an outright ban on CFCs, reduction in CFCs, and development of alternatives. Europe has recognized the CFC problem and has made a proposal to ban all CFCs by the end of the century. The United States seeks a ban on all CFCs by the year 2000 and already has banned CFCs in aerosols. Dupont, the largest producer of CFCs, has indicated that it will phase out these compounds by the end of the century if its replacement is ready by then.

DEFORESTATION EFFECTS

Although they may seem peaceful, forests are places of intense activity. Countless animals, plants, and microorganisms grow and reproduce, there, and in the process they filter the air and water, regulate stream flow, store water, and reduce soil erosion. Removing trees changes the ecology in several ways. For example, if even a small plot of tropical forest is cut, the temperature of the region fluctuates from extremely high during the day to cool temperatures at night.

Deforestation can change weather patterns, as it has in Panama, where rainfall in areas where deforestation occurred 50 years ago has decreased by 1 cm every year (50 cm for the 50 years) compared to adjacent uncleared land. Forest soil filters the polluted rainfall and cleanses it before it reenters the surface or groundwater supply. Forest vegetation and soil also purify the air. Many environmental pollutants stick to leaves and branches and are removed. Environmental pollutants also are removed by leaves, detoxified by microorganisms, and taken up by plant roots. Hence, air is cleaner when it leaves the forest than when it enters.

Desertification is a problem related to deforestation. When trees are removed and the land is overgrazed or cultivated, it effects the ecosystem. That is evidenced by the drought

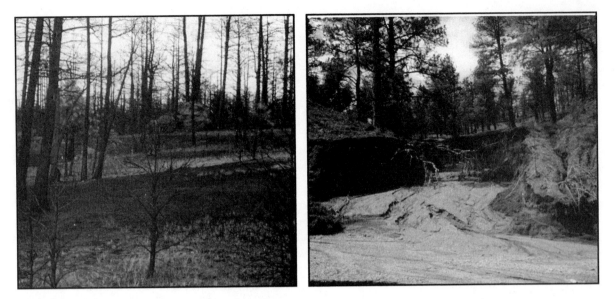

It takes years to restore a forest after a forest fire. With fewer trees, erosion is the result. © Fred Milenovich

that killed tens of thousands of people in the Sahel region of Africa in the early 1970s. In many developing countries, desertification is accelerated by deforestation where wood is burned for fuel and the land is overused. This was evidenced around Khartoum, Sudan, where the acacia tree no longer grows.

Soil erosion and flooding are direct results of deforestation. Where clear-cutting of trees (cutting everything) occurs, soil erosion follows. Also, when all of the trees are cut, more water runs off and flooding ensues. This happens because the trees that once held water on their trunks, limbs, and leaves are no longer there to hold water after a rain during peak runoff. Some of the water retained on the trees before they were cut reentered the hydrologic cycle by evaporation, thus not adding to the peak flow and causing floods. Also, forests have a "sponge effect"; they soak up rainfall during wet weather and release it during dry weather.

Another effect of deforestation is the loss of the oxygen generating "factories." By depleting the forest, we reduce the means of converting carbon dioxide at a time when there is a greater need for oxygen.

Finally, plants use carbon dioxide and give off oxygen. By depleting the forest, we reduce the means of converting carbon dioxide at a time when there is a greater need for oxygen.

SUMMARY

Health effects of air pollution can be serious, including asthma, chronic bronchitis, pulmonary emphysema, lung cancer, and heart disorders. Air pollution has been classified by its major sources. Examples of *natural* sources of air pollution are forest fires, dust storms, and volcanic eruptions, as well as pollen-laden plants that irritate the mucous membranes. *Anthropogenic* air pollution — that which is produced by humans — includes things such as smoke, paint vapors and particles, and gases from septic tanks and house sewer systems.

Industrial pollution is created wherever industry releases gases, vapors, fumes, and the like from the manufacture of cars, clothing, furniture, and so on. *Agricultural* pollutants are created where our food is grown, particularly where insecticides and herbicides are used.

Environmental Health

Transportation is probably the major contributor to air pollution, accounting for approximately half of all air pollution, although catalytic converters in automobiles have drastically reduced pollution from carbon monoxide emissions. A final source is *energy* use and production.

Some air quality phenomena are acid precipitation, the greenhouse effect, and ozone layer depletion.

A 10-year study by EPA suggests that urban air quality is improving. The study shows that since 1984:

- smog (ground-level ozone) dropped 12%

- lead decreased 89%
- sulfur dioxide fell 26%
- carbon monoxide declined 37%
- nitrogen dioxide dropped 12%

In addition, particulate levels decreased 20% from 1998 to 1993.

These findings are encouraging and motivate us to continue to make improvements that will protect the health of millions of Americans who live, work, and play in areas where air pollutant levels are still too high.

REFERENCES

National Tuberculosis and Respiratory Disease Association. Air Pollution Primer. 1969. New York.

Chiras, Daniel D. 1988. *Environmental Science: A Framework for Decision Making.* Benjamin/Cummings Publishing, Menlo Park, CA.

Faith, W. L., and Arthur Atkisson, 1972. *Air Pollution.* John Wiley and Sons, New York.

Miller, G. Tyler, Jr. 1988. *Environmental Science: An Introduction.* Wadsworth Publishing, Belmont, CA.

Revelle, Penelope, and Charles Revelle. 1988. *The Environment: Issues and Choices for Society.* Jones and Bartlett Publishing, Boston.

Sproull, Wayne T. 1970. *Air Pollution and Its Control.* Exposition Press, New York.

Turco, Harold P. 1997. *Earth Under Siege: From Air Pollution to Global Change.* Oxford University Press, NY.

Vesilind, Anne. 1996. *Environmental Engineering.* PWS Publishing, Boston.

Occupational Health

By Rallie Pearson, M.D., MSEH, MPH, and
Shirley L. Morgan, MSEH, EDD, MPH
East Tennessee State University

Key Terms

Aerosol
Biohazards
decibels (dB)
Dust
Gases
Fumes
Industrial health educator

Industrial hygienist
Industrial toxicologist
Mist
Noise
Occupational health nurse
Occupational physician
Primary irritants

Safety engineer
Smoke
Threshold limit values (TLVs)
Toxic effect
Toxicology
Vapor

Objectives

- Discuss the issues surrounding the need for occupational health and safety.

- Identify the rules, regulations, and federal organizations that implement and enforce these regulations.

- Identify and discuss the occupational health team members, their duties, and their roles in today's society.

- Discuss various types of occupational diseases associated with microbial exposure, their occurrence, treatment, and control.

- Identify physical hazards in the environment, their sources, impact on the exposed population, and methods of reduction.

For centuries, employers and employees have recognized the need for health and safety in the workplace. Ever since antiquity, people have described occupational diseases. The Sallier Papyri describe the deleterious effects of certain occupations on ancient Egyptians. Hippocrates (460 B.C. – 360 B.C.) described the toxic properties of lead and the symptoms of "lead colic" exhibited by workers who handled the metal. Other physicians and historians of this era, including Herodotus, discussed the influence of occupation on workers' health.

Pliny the Elder, born in A.D. 23, wrote that workers in certain dusty occupations, especially those involved in mining asbestos, tied makeshift respirators made of animal bladders over their mouth to prevent the inhalation of dust. Galen, a Greek physician practicing medicine around A.D. 162, described diseases unique to miners, tanners, cloth workers, chemists, and workers in other occupations. Agricola and Paracelsus investigated diseases of workers in the 16th century.

Bernardino Ramazzini (1633–1714), an Italian physician, often is considered the patron saint of industrial medicine. He observed, investigated, and described diseases related to occupations. He was appointed professor of medicine at the University Modena, where he wrote his most widely read work, *De Morbis Artificium Diatribe* (The Diseases of Workmen). Ramazzini noted classical descriptions of the signs and symptoms of mercury and lead poisoning. He advised physicians not only to ask patients the routine questions concerning their health but also to inquire of their patients without fail: Of what trade are you? Ramazzini advised physicians to learn the nature of occupational diseases in shops, mills, mines, and wherever workers toiled, declaring that occupational diseases are studied most effectively in the work environment.

The first occupational cancer was described in 1775 by Sir Percivall Pott, an Irish surgeon living in England. He published a paper on cancer of the scrotum in chimney sweeps, which, he noted, occurred with surprising regularity among men of this occupation. Willan, a 15th-century physician, described skin lesions common in bakers; and Charles Turner Thackrah wrote of his observations concerning the diseases of workmen in the manufacturing district of Leeds in 18th-century England.

Dr. Alice Hamilton, daughter of Bernardino Ramazzini, was one of the first American specialists in the field of occupational disease and generally is considered to be the founder of occupational medicine in the United States. In 1910 she began to study the ill effects of dangerous trades. Her famed Illinois Survey investigated the health conditions in the lead industry. The problems she found among felt-hat and lead industry workers were shocking. In completing her study, she remarked that the health effects of new chemicals used in industry were determined by using the workers as guinea pigs. Dr. Hamilton's emphasis on preventing exposure by applying engineering controls to process technology have a powerful impact on the development of the field of industrial hygiene in the United States.

THE NEED FOR OCCUPATIONAL HEALTH AND SAFETY

By the end of the 19th century, large corporations and sweatshops employed and exploited millions of eager immigrants in contemptible jobs. Although the working conditions were appalling, the immigrant workers still were better paid in America than they were in most parts of Europe doing peasant work. Work was extremely hard and dangerous for most workers, and the long working hours were grueling. Because they were non-unionized, the workers typically were unable to resist their employers' demands to increase production. The tremendous gains in productivity per worker after 1890 were accomplished only at an exorbitant cost in human suffering.

During the early part of the 20th century, the industrial revolution ushered in the extensive use of power machinery and equipment. The rapid industrialization of the United States produced a multitude of new dangers for workers. Typically, the machinery and equipment were designed with little or no consideration for operator safety. Workers were untrained and unskilled in the use of the new and often dangerous machines. Workdays of 11 to 13 hours were the norm rather than the exception. The long hours drastically increased the workers' probability of sustaining a life-threatening injury or illness at the workplace.

The situation was worsened by the inadequacies of medical facilities, and medical help seldom was available. As a result, the number of work-related injuries, disabilities, and deaths was at record high levels. A 1904 report in the labor press estimated that 27,000 workers were killed on the job each year. In 1907, the Bureau of Labor reported the annual death toll to be 15,000 to 17,500 (of approximately 26 million male workers).

Work available to women was lower-paying than that for men, and sometimes was more dangerous, particularly in the garment industry sweatshops. On March 25, 1911, in New York City, the upper three stories of a 10-story building, in which the Triangle Shirtwaist Company was located, caught fire. Most of the buildings exits were blocked or locked and had no fire escapes. Of the 500 employees, 145 perished either by burning to death or by jumping from the building.

Increasing rates of on-the-job injuries, disabilities, and deaths attracted considerable government and public attention. At this time safety was primarily treatment-oriented rather than prevention-oriented. Workers compensation laws finally were passed, adding to the emphasis on preventing injuries and illnesses.

LEGISLATION

Modern occupational health in the United States was a result largely of the industrial revolution in 19th-century England. With the rapid development of deplorable work conditions and the exploitation of women and children in its workplaces, various laws were passed to protect workers in that country. England's Factory Act established general standards of heating, lighting, ventilation, and work hours. A period referred to as the American Industrial Renaissance ensued, during which the United States learned from occupational research and legislation in England. A few states even adopted some of the English laws concerning worker protection. During this period of reform, Upton Sinclair's graphic book, *The Jungle* (1906), aroused public sympathy for workers and unions where none had existed before, facilitating passage of laws protecting workers.

The U.S. government became involved in occupational safety and health for the first time in 1890, passing legislation governing safety in coal mines. The government's next significant effort to protect workers resulted in the adoption by the states of workers compensation laws. The first compensation law in the United States was enacted in 1908 for federal employees. In 1910, New York became the first state to institute a workers compensation law. This prompted a period when employees received compensation for medical services, from employers who were made increasingly responsible for the medical care of workers who became injured or ill on the job, as well as for payment of occupational accident and disease compensation. Workers compensation laws also resulted in the most rudimentary health efforts, such as requiring safety helmets in high-risk work areas.

Government attention was directed toward the identification, definition, and diagnosis of occupational diseases, such as silicosis, plumbism (chronic lead poisoning), anthrax, benzol and radium poisoning. Also during the 1910s, occupational health emerged as a medical specialty. In 1914, an Office of Industrial Hygiene and Sanitation was created in the Public Health Service and an Industrial Hygiene Section was established in the American Public Health Association. During the same period, the United States Bureau of Mines was established. In 1937, the American Medical Association created the Council on Industrial Health to coordinate medical efforts in the industrial health field.

Social Security Act

Prior to passage of the Federal Social Security Act of 1935, state health agencies had made little progress in occupational health. Up to that time, only five states had programs designed specifically to aid industrial workers. The Federal Social Security Act made available monies for the expansion of programs to benefit industrial workers. This federal aid resulted in programs for the improvement of the health and safety of all workers in each of the states by 1950. Although the effect of these laws on occupational health promotion in the workplace was indirect, the laws were somewhat useful. Employers were obligated to promote health and safety in the workplace to avoid the prohibitive costs of increased premiums, litigation, and compensation settlements for injured workers. Although a step in the right direction, the state laws regarding industrial inspection and occupational diseases passed in the first two decades of the 20th century proved to be insignificant in preventing accidents and industrial disease.

OSHAct

After 1950 a movement began that would eventually develop into Public Law 91–596, the Occupational Safety and Health Act (OSHAct) of 1970. After years of government neglect, the first comprehensive federal health and safety law was proposed by President Lyndon Johnson in 1968. Industry initially united and defeated the bill, but during the late 1960s and early 1970s, Congress enacted four safety and health laws that had a significant impact on industrial hygiene activities in the United States, including the Federal Metal and Nonmetallic Mine Safety Act of 1966, the Federal Coal Mine Health and Safety Act of 1969, the Occupational Safety and Health Act of 1970, and the Federal Mine Safety and Health Act of 1977. Support for these new laws developed over time from sources such as individual congressmen and senators, professionals in the occupational health and promotion fields, labor unions, foundations, and researchers in the discipline.

Prior to enactment of these laws, governmental regulations of safety and health matters had been largely the concern of state agencies. There was little uniformity of application of codes and standards from one state to another, and almost no enforcement proceedings were lodged against violators of those standards. Some states spent as much as $2.70 per worker, and others spent less than one cent per worker. The federal government had only limited safety and health standards for its contractors. Most federal programs focused only on specific occupations such as railroad workers, longshoremen, federally contracted construction workers and service suppliers, atomic energy workers, and miners. Enforcement of federal safety and health laws was the responsibility of the Bureau of Labor Standards in the U. S. Department of Labor. Although there were thousands of federal contractors, inspection and enforcement activities were extremely limited because of inadequate funding and insufficient staff. Regulations of the OSHAct of 1970 signaled an important shift in governmental involvement in the area of occupational health promotion. The OSHAct moved the focus of employers from treatment-oriented medicine to preventive measures — a strategy deemed necessary to reduce occupational disease.

The OSHAct guaranteed a safe and healthful workplace to all people, recognized the rights of workers, and gave workers the protection of the U. S. government. The act required employers to furnish each employee a place of employment free from recognized hazards that caused or were likely to cause death or serious physical harm to employees and to comply with occupational safety and health standards instituted under the act. The act also granted employees the right to be notified by their employers when they were exposed to toxic materials or harmful physical agents, the right to file confidential complaints with the Occupational Safety and Health Administration regarding unsafe conditions, and the right not to be discriminated against by the employer for exercising any rights granted by the act. It called for inspection of the workplace without prior notice to a company and allowed a representative of the workers to accompany the inspector on the tour. The act carried fines for violations and required employers to maintain records of work-related deaths, injuries and illnesses, as well as exposure to toxic materials and harmful agents. The records were required to be available to the workers and the government. The OSHAct required employees to comply with occupational safety and health standards and all rules issued by the act that were applicable to employees' actions and conduct.

OSHA

The OSHAct also provided for the formation of the Department of Labor's Occupational Safety and Health Administration (OSHA). OSHA was charged with setting standards for safety in the workplace and with maintaining compliance with these standards. OSHA also was given the authority to set and enforce regulations for workplace safety and health through civil penalties. OSHA allowed for any worker to register a complaint and call for an inspection, while protecting the worker from discrimination for using provisions of the OSHAct.

NIOSH

In addition to creating OSHA, the Occupational Safety and Health Act of 1970 resulted in establishment of the Department of Health, Education and Welfare's National Institute for Occupational Safety and Health (NIOSH). The act authorized the NIOSH to conduct research and identify industrial hazards, as well as to promote occupational safety and health through education and the dissemination of information. Since its creation, the NIOSH has researched and published many important criteria documents for industrial exposure, as well as describing risks and protective measures. Industrial situations that NIOSH has studied include occupational exposure to coke oven emissions, asbestos, arsenic, mercury, vinyl chloride, and a number of organic solvents. Passage of the OSHAct and creation of NIOSH represents tremendous progress in the history of occupational safety and health.

Meticulous attention to and support of occupational health programs benefit private enterprises. Labor turnover, absenteeism, and liability compensation for occupational illness and injury are three sources of significant financial loss to business and industry. Industrial health programs are important in decreasing the monetary costs associated with these factors. Healthy workers are more capable, productive, and dependable than an unhealthy workers.

Occupational health programs also benefit the employee and the community. For employees and their dependents, occupational health programs facilitate sustained earnings, lower personal health care costs, increase and extend productivity, and increase job satisfaction and security. In the community, occupational health programs increase prosperity, reduce welfare costs, decrease incidents of labor unrest, and support higher quality community medical and public health services.

THE OCCUPATIONAL HEALTH TEAM

The development of occupational health and industrial hygiene programs in the United States originated in factories, manufacturing plants, and mills and remained exclusive to these industries for many years. Today, occupational health and industrial hygiene programs are found in every type of industry. Members of the occupational health and industrial hygiene team employed by an industry are responsible for operation of the program and delivery of medical care in the workplace.

In general, the occupational health and industrial hygiene program is designed to protect workers from illness and injury on the job, either by law, regulation, or contract. The definition of occupational medicine by the Council on Industrial Health of the American Medical Association is as follows:

> Occupational medicine deals with the restoration and conservation of health in relation to work, the working environment and maximum efficiency. It involves prevention, recognition, and treatment of occupational disabilities and requires the application of special techniques in the fields of rehabilitation, environmental hygiene, toxicology, sanitation and human relations.

A good industrial health program is designed primarily for the benefit of the workers, although employers often gain substantially from the program as well. The Council on Industrial Health of the American Medical Association lists the objectives of an occupational health program as:

1. To protect individuals against health hazards in their work environment;

2. To ensure and facilitate the suitable placement of individuals according to their physical capacities and their emotional make-up in work that they can perform with an acceptable degree of efficiency and without

endangering their own health and safety or that of their fellow employees; and

3. To encourage personal health maintenance.

The Council on Industrial Health further describes the following services that the occupational health team of an industry should provide as:

1. Regular appraisal of plant sanitation;

2. Periodic inspection for occupational disease hazards;

3. Adoption and maintenance of adequate control measures;

4. Provision of first aid and emergency services;

5. Prompt and early treatment for all illnesses resulting from occupational exposure;

6. Referral to the family physician of individuals with conditions requiring attention and cooperation between the patient and the physician to remedy the condition;

7. Uniform recording of absenteeism from all types of disability;

8. Unbiased health appraisals of all workers;

9. Access to rehabilitation services within industry; and

10. Availability of a beneficial health education program.

The number and character of workers engaged in the occupational health and industrial hygiene program in a given industry vary with the number of employees, type of industry, demands of the workers, and philosophy of the management. Like any other major management function, safety and health management requires a defined chain of command ending with an accountable individual at the level of president or vice-president.

Very small plants often make provisions only for first aid, or for a physician to be called in the case of an emergency. Medium-size plants or companies often employ a full-time occupational health nurse who administers routine care. Larger industries may have facilities including an infirmary, eye and dental clinics, X-ray and laboratory services, along with the appropriate number of physicians and technical support staff these facilities require. Large occupational medical staffs usually are supplemented by the work of industrial hygienists, safety professionals, and **industrial health educators** who work together to ensure a workplace that promotes optimum health, safety, and productivity of those who work there.

Occupational Health Nurse

Central to most occupational health programs is the **occupational health nurse**. The role of occupational health nurse varies with the needs of the employers for whom the nurse works. In the past, the occupational health nurse was primarily a first-aid giver. This role has changed during the last decade. Today the occupational health nurse is responsible for the care of illnesses and injuries occurring at the workplace. For workers who require additional or specialized care, the occupational health nurse must provide referrals to appropriate qualified physicians. The nurse must be knowledgeable in the areas of preventive and rehabilitative health. If the industry does not employ an industrial health educator, the occupational health nurse often is responsible for counseling and providing health and safety education. The responsibility for maintaining complex occupational health record systems often rests with the health nurse, in addition to the routine duties of assisting the occupational physician with workers' physical examinations and health screening tests.

Occupational Physician

Most industries do not require the services of an **occupational physician** full-time but, rather, arrange for physicians' services on a contractual basis. The occupational physician may maintain regularly scheduled hours on certain days at the company clinic or may provide care from his or her office. The occupational health physician typically performs pre-employment physicals on prospective employees, treats work-related injuries and illnesses, supervises drug screening, and determines the presence and extent of workers' disability for the company and various government agencies.

Industrial Hygienist

Industrial hygiene activities are defined as the anticipation, recognition, evaluation, and control of environmental factors that have an adverse effect on the health and efficiency of employees or among citizens of the community. The **industrial hygienist** assesses and recommends methodology for controlling environmental hazards and toxic substances such as dusts, gases, vapors, and fumes; physical agents such as excessive noise, heat, and radiation; biological hazards such as enzymes; and other job-related stresses such as monotony. In the past, only the larger corporations typically employed industrial hygienists, but in recent years even small companies employ or contract the services of an industrial hygienist.

Responsibilities of the industrial hygienist include the following:

- Direct the industrial hygiene program;
- Examine the work environment and environs;
- Study work operations and processes, and obtain full details of the nature of the work, materials, and equipment used, products and byproducts, number and sex of employees, and hours of work;
- Make appropriate measurements to determine the magnitude of exposure or nuisance to workers and the public;
- Study and test biological materials, such as blood and urine, by chemical and physical means, when such examination will aid in determining the extent of exposure;
- Interpret results of the examination of the work environment and environs in terms of ability to impair health, nature of health impairment, workers' efficiency, and community nuisance and/or damage, and present specific conclusions to appropriate interested parties such as management and health officials.
- Make specific decisions as to the need for, or effectiveness of, control measures, and, when necessary, advise as to the procedures that will be suitable and effective for both the environment and environs;
- Prepare rules, regulations, standards, and procedures for the healthful conduct of work and the prevention of nuisance in the community;
- Present expert testimony before courts of law, hearing boards, workers compensation commissions, regulatory agencies, and legally appointed investigative bodies covering all matters pertaining to industrial hygiene;
- Prepare appropriate text for labels and precautionary information for materials and products to be used by workers and the public;
- Conduct programs for the education of workers and the public on how to prevent occupational disease and community nuisance;
- Conduct epidemiological studies among workers and industries to discover possibilities of the presence of occupational disease, and establish or improve threshold limit values or standards as guides for maintaining of health and efficiency;
- Conduct research to advance knowledge concerning the effects of occupation upon health and means of preventing occupational health impairment, community air pollution, noise, nuisance, and related problems.

Safety Engineer

The level of education and training of the **safety engineer** traditionally has varied greatly, from technicians who performed simple control procedures to the personnel manager responsible for completing accident reports and other forms required by government agencies and insurance companies. Today, the safety engineer commonly possesses a doctoral degree and has the responsibility of developing complex systems for the analysis and control of occupational hazards. The safety engineer in an industry with diversified processes must be a generalist. He or she must be knowledgeable in a wide range of technical, legal, and administrative areas. The safety engineer is concerned not only with preventing accidents but also with hazard control systems based on environmental and human factor analysis. According to the American Society of Safety Engineers (ASSE), the major functions of the safety engineer are the following:

- Identifying and appraising accident- and loss-producing conditions and practices and evaluating the severity of the accident problem;
- Developing accident prevention and loss control methods, procedures, and programs;
- Communicating accident- and loss-control information to those directly involved; and
- Measuring and evaluating the effectiveness of the accident- and loss-control system and the modifications needed to achieve optimum results.

The safety engineer and associated staff usually are responsible for executing the following safety functions:

- Ensure that federal, state, and local safety laws, regulations, codes, and rules are observed;
- Ensure that OSHA record-keeping and reporting requirements are met;
- Assist management in preparing safety policies and ensure that they are carried out;
- Monitor all activities where accidents could occur that would cause injury to personnel, damage to equipment or facilities, or loss of materials;
- Cease any operation or activity that constitutes an imminent hazard to personnel or could result in loss of equipment or facilities;
- Establish liaison and working arrangements with other activities involved in accident prevention, such as plant security officers, fire prevention workers, and medical personnel;
- Assist in the formation of safety committees and direct their activities;

- Review and approve the safety aspects of plant facility designs and of equipment procured;
- Assure that hazardous areas and dangerous equipment are posted according to standards;
- Control selection and use of hazard monitoring, personal protective and emergency equipment;
- Conduct safety training of personnel at all levels;
- Investigate accidents and hazardous conditions, and prepare necessary reports;
- Disseminate information on safety to all employees;
- Accompany inspectors from governmental agencies and insurance companies at the plant;
- Establish procedures for hazardous operations;
- Make on-site reviews of activities and determine their potential for accidents;
- Inspect emergency supplies; and
- Maintain all records relating to safety activities

Industrial Health Educator

The **industrial health educator** is a recent addition to the occupational health care team. In small industries the occupational health nurse may counsel and educate workers concerning health and safety in the workplace. In other companies, the safety engineer may have the role of health and safety training and education. As government and other agencies increase their scrutiny and documentation requirements of health and safety practices and controls in industry, the occupational health nurse and safety engineer have less and less time to educate employees effectively in the areas of health and safety practices. The industrial health educator may possess a bachelor's, master's, or doctoral degree, and is qualified to execute the following responsibilities:

- Educate workers and the public in the prevention of occupational diseases and injuries such as carpal tunnel syndrome, back injury, dermatitis, and others;

- Counsel workers concerning job-related stress, sexual harassment, drug abuse, and other problems that could affect their job performance and productivity;

- Conduct epidemiologic studies, surveys, and audits to determine the prevalence of certain occupational diseases and illnesses among workers, as well as health and safety attitudes of workers;

- Prepare appropriate text for labels and precautionary information for materials and products to be used by workers and the public; and

- Conduct research to advance knowledge concerning the effects of certain occupations upon health, and determine the means of preventing occupational health impairment.

OCCUPATIONAL DISEASES

Biological Hazards

Biological agents generally represent fewer hazardous exposures than those of a physical or chemical nature. Certain occupations, however, allow a significant number of exposures. These occupations include laboratory, research, and hospital personnel; physicians, veterinarians, and people involved with food and food processing, plants, and animals. Miners and farmers also are at a greater risk than most other workers because of their contact with the soil which may harbor potentially hazardous biological agents.

Biological hazards, also known as **biohazards,** are living organisms that are infectious agents and represent a potential risk to human or animal health. The five types of biological agents that may produce infection in humans are: bacteria, viruses, rickettsiae, fungi, and parasites.

Transmission of biohazardous agents may occur through inhalation, injection, ingestion, or physical contact. Whether a person exposed to the biohazardous agent will contract the

disease depends on a number of factors, including the number of organisms in the environment, the virulence of the organisms, and the person's resistance to the organism. Biohazardous agents may be both synergistic and additive. For this reason, a person exposed to a combination of stresses, such as those of a physical or chemical nature, is more likely to be susceptible to the biohazard and thus contract the disease.

Classification of Biological Hazards

Identification and classification of biohazards are essential to determine the appropriate means of control to prevent infections. The U. S. Public Health Service (USPHS) and the U. S. Department of Agriculture (USDA) contributed to development of standard classifications for evaluating the hazards represented by a variety of biohazardous agents. The standard provides a means of describing minimal safety conditions. The standard defines four classes of biohazardous agents and a fifth class representing animal pathogens that are excluded from the United States by law. Agents comprising Class 1 are less hazardous than those of Class 2, and so on. The standard provides only for the minimum safety conditions considered necessary. The five classes of agents are as follows.

Class 1   Agents of no or minimal hazard under ordinary conditions of handling that can be handled safely without special apparatus or equipment, using techniques generally acceptable for nonpathogenic materials. Class 1 includes all bacterial, fungal, viral, rickettsia, chlamydial, and parasitic agents not included in higher classes.

Class 2   Agents of ordinary potential hazard. Class 2 includes agents that may produce disease of varying degrees of severity through accidental inoculation, injection, or other means of cutaneous penetration but that usually can be contained adequately and safely by ordinary laboratory techniques.

Class 3 Agents involving special hazards or agents derived from outside the United States that require a USDA permit for importation unless they are specified for higher classification. Class 3 includes pathogens that require special conditions for containment.

Class 4 Agents that require the most stringent conditions for containment because they are extremely hazardous to personnel or may cause serious epidemic disease. Class 4 requires special conditions for containment.

Class 5 Foreign animal pathogens that are excluded from the United States by law or whose entry is restricted by USDA administrative policy.

Bacterial Agents

Bacteria are simple, single-cell organisms visible only under the microscope. They multiply by fission or simple division into two parts. Bacteria include *cocci*, which are round and resemble a string of beads; the *rod-shaped* bacilli; and the *corkscrew*-shaped spirilla. Some bacteria are disease-causing, or pathogenic; others are harmless or even useful.

Occupationally induced bacterial infections usually are caused by neglected minor wounds and abrasions in which the integrity of the skin surface is compromised. These infections typically are caused by mixed bacteria, but staphylococci and streptococci most often are the primary offending organisms.

Rickettsia and Chlamydial Agents

The rod-shaped or coccoid rickettsiae are bacterial in nature but smaller in size. As obligate parasites, they rely on their hosts to provide everything they need for growth, reproduction, and even survival. Because rickettsiae can survive only within living cells, these microbes are associated with and transmitted to people via blood-sucking arthropods such as fleas, ticks, and lice. Typhus and Rocky Mountain spotted fever are transmitted by rickettsiae.

Chlamydiae, bacterial in nature, also are obligate parasites. As intracellular microorganisms, they are distinguished from rickettsiae by their smaller size and their more complicated method of reproduction. Chlamydiae usually are transmitted in the air and gain access to the body through the respiratory system. Chlamydiae occur as two species, both of which are pathogenic to humans. The primary source of human infection is birds.

Viral Agents

Viruses are noncellular, parasitic pathogens that are smaller than bacteria, rickettsiae, or chlamydiae. In fact, they are the smallest organism known and can be seen only with the aid of an electron microscope. Viruses are obligate parasites that are neither living nor nonliving, but require association with a living cell to grow, reproduce, and function. Occupationally acquired viral diseases are likely to include animal respiratory viruses, poxviruses, enteroviruses, and arboviruses. Infections may be acquired from the vector or from handling animals or animal products. Laboratory-acquired infections may result from working with the infectious agent, from accidents, animals, clinical or autopsy specimens, from aerosols, or from glassware. In hospitals, viral transmission may occur among patients and staff.

Fungal Agents

Fungi are a phylum of plants derived from algae, of which more than 70,000 species are known. All fungi lack chlorophyll and other pigment. Because they are incapable of synthesizing protein or other organic material from simple compounds, fungi are considered parasitic or saprophytic. Occupationally acquired fungal disease is not significant and is confined mainly to farmers, animal handlers, and other

Environmental Health

outdoor workers. Diagnosis of fungal diseases is made by microscopic identification of the fungus with cultural confirmation. Fungal diseases may be classified according to their effects, which may be systemic, subcutaneous superficial (such as ringworm or athlete's foot), or hypersensitivity effects. Hypersensitivity effects usually are attributable to fungal antigens inhaled with dusts and usually involve pneumonitis with symptoms similar to asthma.

Parasitic Agents

Although microbes such as bacteria and viruses can be parasitic, the classification of parasitic agents generally includes not the microbes but, instead, the parasitic organisms that are either a plant or an animal. Parasites live advantageously in or on another organism to whose welfare they contribute nothing. Protozoa, helminths, and arthropods typically cause infections of occupational significance. Malaria and other blood and gastrointestinal disorders are caused by protozoa. Helminths are responsible for the transmission of schistosomiasis and hookworm. Mites and chiggers are arthropods and may cause simple dermatoses or may act as vectors or hosts for other nonarthropod parasites.

A parasitic disease is any disease resulting from the invasion of the body by parasitic agents. Depending on the virulence of the parasite and resistance of the host, the host may or may not contract the disease.

Control of Biohazards

The effects of biological hazardous agents often are subtle and develop after a lag time. An agent representing a biological hazard may be invisible, odorless, and tasteless. For this reason, workers often are not cognizant that they are being exposed. In addition, when an infection does develop, its origin may be difficult to determine. In light of these characteristics of biohazardous agents, education and training are required to increase awareness of the need for control of biological hazardous agents. Because of the serious potential risks of biohazards, effective biohazard control is essential.

The biological hazard control program usually consists of analyzing biohazards, developing safety regulations, training and educating personnel, inspecting and enforcing safety rules, reporting and investigating accidents properly, and funding programs adequately to carry them out to completion.

The primary emphasis of biohazard control should be at the source of potential contamination. Control practices usually include a health surveillance program, standardized work procedures, education of employees, and environmental control procedures. The primary goal of biohazard control is to prevent illnesses in the worker. Control efforts may be difficult because the results of exposure to a biohazard typically are not clinically evident for a considerable time. Unintended exposure to biohazards often stems from poor working habits of the employees.

Management's role in the control of biohazards is to educate employees about the potential risks of the substances with which they are dealing. Although the degree of hazard to the employee depends primarily upon the biological agent itself and its conditions of use, employees should receive proper instruction concerning the hazards to which they will be exposed each time they work with a biohazardous substance. The employees should assume that every biological agent to which they are exposed presents a hazard and, for this reason, they should exercise every precaution available to them when handling any biohazardous substance.

All new employees should receive a pre-employment physical examination to establish a baseline reference. Workers currently employed by or transferred to the biohazardous area also should receive regular physical examinations. Workers exposed to biohazards include those handling potentially oncogenic, biological, or toxic chemical materials, those responsible for cleaning laboratory glassware, handling experimental animals or their tissues, and those who perform janitorial duties. The current health status of employees should be considered when working with biohazards, as a worker may become more susceptible to infection or harm as a result of change in health status, such as in the case of pregnancy.

Workers likely to be exposed to biohazards should be vaccinated if a satisfactory vaccine exists. The efficiency of vaccines in preventing infection in workers may be less than that of the general population because the worker may receive a higher dose of the infectious microorganisms than the general public would. In addition, the worker may be subject to exposure by a different route than normally would be expected in the general population.

Management should establish and implement an environmental control and personnel safety program that includes biological safety. A safety manual with written safety policies concerning biohazards should be made available to all personnel likely to be exposed. The manual should cover general safe practices and procedures. Also, specific procedures for each department's employees should be made available to workers.

To further control exposure to biological hazards, no person should be admitted to a biohazardous area unless he or she is assigned specifically to work within that area. Eating, drinking, smoking, and gum chewing should be prohibited in areas where work with infectious agents is conducted. Employees who work with biohazardous material should be required to carefully wash and disinfect their hands before and after eating or smoking. All unnecessary materials and equipment should be restricted from the biohazardous area.

Employees and visitors entering biohazardous areas should be required to wear protective clothing commensurate with the level of risk involved. Protective clothing should not be worn outside the work area. The OSHA-required universal biohazard symbol should be used to identify all restricted biohazardous areas. All storage spaces, incubators, refrigerators, and other equipment associated with biohazardous materials also should bear this symbol. All surfaces likely to come in contact with the infectious agent areas should be disinfected with a suitable germicide.

Appropriate precautions should be exercised to reduce the risks associated with processes such as centrifugation, grinding, and other processes likely to generate aerosols. Contaminated wastes should be decontaminated before disposal. Before incineration or autoclaving, dry contaminated wastes should be collected in impermeable bags and sealed. Heat or chemicals should be used to decontaminate wet wastes before discharging them into the sanitary system. For biohazard control to be effective, all personnel involved with biohazards must work together to reduce the amount of potential health hazard by following and enforcing the recommended procedures and guidelines.

Chemical Hazards

Each year more than 5,000 new chemicals are developed, many of which will be used in the workplace. Most chemical substances have the potential to cause injury or illness of the worker who handles them. Chemicals that are not inherently toxic still may pose a potential hazard because of their potential for fire or explosion. Only small amounts of highly toxic substances such as cyanide, arsenic, mercury, and beryllium compounds can produce significant harm. All materials can be relatively safe if the proper precautions are taken while handling them.

The three primary routes by which chemical substances can enter the body are inhalation, absorption through the skin, and ingestion. A less common route of entry is by injection with sharp objects, compressed air, or pressurized liquid.

1. *Inhalation.* The surface area of the lungs ranges from 300 square feet at rest to about 1,000 square feet during inspiration. This allows inhaled chemicals to be absorbed rapidly into the bloodstream and distributed throughout the entire body. Approximately 90% of all industrial poisonings, other than dermatitis, are attributable to inhalation.

   Although many air contaminants are absorbed and distributed throughout the body, several remain in the lungs and cause irritation. This irritation causes pulmonary inflammation and subsequent scarring, also known by the names of anthracosis, byssinosis, siderosis, silicosis and asbestosis.

2. *Absorption.* Absorption of toxic chemicals through the skin usually is slower than inhalation. If the integrity of the skin has been compromised, however, absorption can be rapid. Some chemicals are absorbed readily through the skin and hair follicles. Although the skin has an outer coating of sebum, sweat and keratin that provides a small amount of protection, this coating is washed away easily with soap and water, as well as many organic solvents and bases. Chemicals readily absorbed through the skin include benzene, toluene, nitroglyceride, tetraethyl (organic), lead, mercury, and arsenic. Absorption is facilitated in hot environments and when body oils have been removed by degreasers and solvents. Contact dermatitis accounts for 30% of all worker compensation cases and occupational diseases.

3. *Ingestion.* Chemical substances generally are not ingested intentionally by workers, but accidental ingestion may occur by eating, smoking, or drinking in areas where toxic chemicals exist. Most chemicals are easily absorbed into the bloodstream during digestion. Careful washing before eating and drinking is required to prevent unintentional ingestion of toxic substances. Lead and arsenic are two of the more toxic substances ingested.

Air Contaminants

Excluding dermatitis, inhalation of air contaminants is the leading cause of occupational illnesses. Chemical hazards exist as air contaminants in the following forms.

Mist. A mist is composed of liquid droplets suspended in air and is formed by condensation from a gas to a liquid or by dispersing liquid into tiny particles. Dispersion can be accomplished by various processes, including splashing, foaming and spraying. Chromic, hydrochloric, hydrofluoric, nitric and sulfuric acids often are used in a diluted form in pickling, cleaning, and electroplating operations. These acids frequently are sprayed, causing mists to form. When inhaled, all acid mists are dangerous lung irritants. Adequate ventilation around these operations is necessary to remove any toxic mists that develop, and personal protective equipment, such as appropriate respirators, should be worn wherever acid mists are found.

Vapor. Vapors are the gaseous forms of substances that exist normally as liquids or solids at room temperature and pressure. Vapors generally are present wherever their liquid sources are found. Vapors may be present when using organic solvents, paint thinner, cleaners, and other agents. To determine the relative amount of vapor present and, thus, the severity of a vapor hazard, the vapor pressure of the liquid must be known. The higher the vapor pressure, the greater is the amount of vapors released from a liquid. Vapors generally gain entrance to the body through inhalation, and through skin absorption to a lesser extent. Many vapors present fire and explosion hazards, necessitating that each vapor be evaluated on an individual basis to determine the hazard it presents and to determine its appropriate handling, storage, disposal, and emergency procedures.

Gases. Gases are fluids that take the shape of whatever container is available to them. Gases diffuse and can be converted to a liquid or solid state by increasing the pressure and decreasing the temperature. Gases typically are produced by arc welding, combustion, and other chemical reactions. Each gas has a unique action on lung tissue. Some gases do not harm the lung tissue but, rather, dissolve in the blood and exert toxic effects in some other area of the body. Carbon monoxide, a toxic gas, is an example of this mode of action. It is commonly found in industry and is responsible for more deaths by asphyxiation than any other gas.

Carbon monoxide most often is produced by incomplete combustion of petroleum products in internal combustion engines.

Some gases produce adverse reactions directly on the lung tissue. Phosgene gas, for example, is a highly irritating gas that causes fluid to form in the lungs so the individual literally drowns.

Smoke. Smokes are produced by the incomplete combustion of organic materials such as wood, coal and petroleum products. Smoke consists of particles smaller than 0.1 micron, which are smaller in size than dust particles. Smoke generally contains gases, droplets, and dry particles.

Dust. Dusts are solid particles produced by crushing, grinding, drilling, and otherwise handling materials. Dust particles range in size from 0.1 micron to 25 microns. Those from 0.5 to 5 microns settle deep in the lung and cause most dust-induced illnesses. Larger dust particles usually are filtered by hairs in the nose, pharynx, throat, or bronchi before gaining access to or reaching the alveoli of the lung.

Dust is either organic and inorganic. *Organic dust* is a product of living material, such as grain. *Inorganic dusts* originate from non-living matter, such as minerals and metals. Some dust-induced diseases, such as anthracosis and silicosis, may manifest themselves only after years of exposure. Other dust-induced illnesses, such as those caused by toxic metal exposure from lead and manganese, appear in only days to weeks. Allergic reactions from dust may occur in seconds.

Fumes. Fumes are solid particles created by condensation of a substance from a gaseous state. Fumes generally occur after a molten metal changes from a liquid to a vapor or gas and is condensed in the air. This process usually produces oxides when the vaporized metal reacts with the air. All metal fumes and dusts are irritating, but some cause much more serious harm than simple irritation when inhaled. Fumes and dusts are produced in operations such as smelting, grinding and welding. Metals creating a health hazard include antimony, arsenic, beryllium, cadmium, chromium, copper, iron, cobalt, lead, mercury, selenium, tellurium, thallium, and manganese.

To keep fumes at a minimum, good housekeeping must be practiced, and all employees with significant exposures should be included in a surveillance program that includes monitoring blood and urine for metal levels.

Aerosol. Aerosols are liquid droplets or solid particles that remain dispersed in the air a prolonged time. When deposited in the lungs, aerosols may produce rapid local tissue damage, some slower tissue reactions, eventual disease, or only physical blocking. Some toxic aerosols do not affect the lung tissue locally but are transferred from the lungs into the bloodstream, where they are distributed to other organs. Asbestosis fibers may be considered an aerosol, causing fibrotic growth in the alveolar tissue, clogging the ducts, or limiting the effective area of the alveolar lining.

Absorption

Chemical hazards arise from high concentrations of mists, vapors, gases, or solids in the form of dusts or fumes in the air. In addition to the hazard of inhalation, many of these materials act as skin irritants or may be toxic by absorption through the skin. Organic and inorganic chemicals are the major sources of occupational dermatoses. Most chemical agents are classified as primary irritants.

Primary irritants are likely to evoke adverse reactions in all people. These chemical substances react on contact, dissolving a portion of the skin. The result may range from complete destruction of the skin to burning or inflammation, depending on the concentration of the chemical and the duration of exposure to the skin. Many primary irritants damage skin because they are water-soluble. Even the water-insoluble compounds, of which many are solvents, react with the lipids in the skin. The exact mechanism of primary skin irritation is not completely understood. About 80% of all occupational dermatoses are caused by primary irritants.

Most inorganic and organic acids act as primary irritants. Certain inorganic alkalis, such as ammonium hydroxide and sodium hydroxide, are primary skin irritants. Metallic salts, especially the arsenicals, chromates, mercurials, nickel sulphate, and zinc chloride, produce severe irritant effects on the skin. Organic solvents, representing a large number of substances, irritate the skin because of their solvent properties. Because the skin irritation generally is confined to the area of direct contact, dermatitis caused by a primary irritant is referred to as contact dermatitis. Although a contact dermatitis can be severe, it should not recur as long as the infected person avoids contact with the irritant. This may be accomplished either by a job reassignment or through the use of protective gear that prevents skin contact with the offending substance.

Control of Airborne Chemical Hazards

Because chemical hazards often are airborne, control of air contamination should receive priority. Some common control methods include the following:

1. *Substitution or replacement.* Replacing toxic substances with innocuous substitutes is often possible. Many harmless chemical substitutes perform as well as harmful agents and at a fraction of the original hazard potential.

2. *Isolation of operation.* Isolating the hazard-generating process within an enclosure prevents contamination of the surrounding clean areas. This method includes mechanization or automation of the process so employees are not exposed to the hazards the process generates.

3. *Elimination or reduction of employee exposure.* A work area generating significant amounts of contaminated air is isolated from other working areas. The isolated areas have self-closing doors, no windows, and a slightly negative pressure to prevent contamination of the general work area. When possible, employees are restricted from this hazardous area to minimize exposures.

4. *Local exhaust.* Air contaminants are captured at their sources and removed from the area by using hoods and fans. Local exhaust can be used effectively to rid workers' air of dust, fumes, and vapors.

5. *Ventilation.* A general ventilation system typically is not sufficient to control airborne contaminants that represent significant health hazards. In the case of numerous, widely distributed, and low-toxicity sources of contamination throughout a building, general ventilation is helpful. General ventilation includes opening windows and doors and operating fans.

6. *Wetting methods.* Wetting is especially useful with dust hazards. Wetting reduces or eliminates the amount of dust generated. Cutting, drilling, grinding, and other operations are all rendered less hazardous by wetting control methods.

7. *Housekeeping.* Air contaminants often can be effectively controlled or eliminated by good housekeeping practices, which include sealing stored solvents, wiping up spills, and removing dust as it accumulates.

8. *Personal protective equipment.* Respirators are effective in reducing the hazard associated with airborne contaminants. The type of respirator must be appropriate for the hazard involved. To be effective, respirators must be properly fitted, maintained, and worn. Other protective equipment may include clothing, gloves, boots, and coveralls.

9. *Control of occupational skin disease.* Almost all chemical substances represent a hazard to the skin. Control of occupational skin disease begins with the worker's recognition of those substances related to his or her job that cause skin irritations. Proper precautions should be taken to minimize exposure. Where possible, less irritating or nonirritating chemicals should be substituted. Enclosures, temperature controls, automated handling devices, exhaust hoods, and process changes all are engineering controls that can reduce exposure to irritating substances.

10. *Detailed and accurate labeling* of known irritant chemicals and *strictly enforced standard practices* for their handling and use are effective control methods. Employers

should alert and educate employees about the hazards associated with chemicals the employees use, in addition to the precautions to be taken in their use. Employees can effectively use personal protective equipment, such as gloves and special clothing, to avoid or minimize exposure to skin irritants. For each chemical, employees should use the appropriate protective gear, as some chemicals degrade or dissolve protective gloves and clothing. To provide additional protection to the skin, employees can use barrier creams and ointments with gloves and protective clothing, but they should remove the ointments after the job is completed.

Physical Hazards

Physical hazards include excessive levels of electromagnetic and ionizing radiation, noise and vibration, and extremes of temperature and pressure.

Radiation

More and more industry relies upon radiation for many processes, including nondestructive testing of welds, fastening and other internal structures, medical diagnoses and treatment, examination of packages and baggage, and use in radioactive gauges in quality control. Ionizing radiation consists of alpha, beta, and neutron particles, and X-rays and gamma rays. Each of these may cause injury by producing ionization of the cellular components, leading to functional changes in body tissues. The body's tissues differ in their sensitivity and biological responses to ionizing radiation. The injury resulting from radiation exposure is dependent on (a) time and (b) intensity of exposure. The greater the length of time a worker is exposed to a radiation source, the greater is the injury that can result. The intensity of a dose depends on the strength of the source, distance from the source, and presence and amount of any shielding.

Radiation effects generated during a massive single exposure are acute and can produce both immediate and delayed effects on the body. Low but repeated radiation exposures are chronic and generally have delayed effects. *Acute* exposures typically are caused by accidents. *Chronic* exposures generally are the result of unrecognized hazardous conditions.

The most common way to prevent workers' overexposure to radiation is to closely monitor exposure to radiation. Employers use film badges, film rings, or pocket dosimeters to monitor ionizing radiation exposure. Pocket dosimeters are preferable as they give a continuous reading of ionizing radiation present. Film badges must be removed and processed to determine the dose of ionizing radiation received, thus giving the employee no warning of overexposure. In addition to careful monitoring of radiation exposure, employers should observe the following precautionary measures against ionizing radiation:

1. Permit only qualified personnel to operate and handle any equipment or material that produces ionizing radiation.
2. Prepare and post in the worksite operating and emergency procedures for radiation safety.
3. Restrict access to areas in which equipment or materials produce ionizing radiation.
4. Require personnel entering areas where ionizing radiation is present to wear protective clothing and equipment.
5. Ban the use of edible materials, cosmetics, and cigarettes in areas where ionizing radiation is used.
6. Develop clean-up techniques and procedures for every area using any radioactive material.

Noise Pollution

Noise is defined as unwanted sound. Fourteen million workers in the United States are exposed to hazardous noise. Noise is one pollutant that dissipates when generated, but the effects may linger until death. According to some authorities, the world noise level is increasing by 1 decibel per year. Noise can be an indoor problem or a community concern.

Indoor noise consists of sound generated by the electric home can opener, mixer, knife, air-conditioner fan, radio, television, food blender, garbage grinder, and vacuum cleaner. In offices, the telephone, computer, copier, and whining air conditioner or fan generate noise. Industry has numerous sources of noise, such as engine blades, belts, wheels, and abrasive devices. The first attention was brought to hearing loss in boilermaker factories, where there was much riveting.

Among the various sources of community noise, are trucks, cars, airplanes, tractors, helicopters, and motorcycles. As if those are not enough, we produce off-road bikes, snowmobiles, motor boats, and race cars. At construction and demolition sites vehicles and tools create noise. For example, bulldozers, earth movers, concrete breakers (jackhammers), power saws, pile drivers, pumps and motors and pneumatic riveters all produce high levels of noise. Power lawnmowers, weed eaters, and other home and garden tools generate noise in addition to banging garbage cans, barking dogs and racing three wheelers. In addition, on holidays we shoot firecrackers to make noise. A hundred years ago people thought horses, mooing cows, and crowing chickens were too noisy!

To determine levels of noise, a sound level meter or a noise meter measures sound pressure in **decibels** (**dB**). In noise study, levels are expressed on a logarithmic scale. Thus, 80 dB is 10 times as loud as 70 dB and 90 dB is 100 times as loud as 70 dB, 100 dB is 1000 times as loud as 70 dB, etc.

Exposure to noise levels greater than 85 dB for lengthy periods can result in hearing loss. The hearing loss depends on how loud the noise is and the length of time it is heard. Table 15.1 gives ratings for some common sources of noise.

If noise did not harm the body, it would not be considered an environmental health issue. Vern Knudren from the University of California, Los Angeles, said, "Noise, like smog, is a slow agent of death." It can cause psychological, psychophysical, and physiological damage.

1. Loud noises affect the body *psychologically* in several ways. Hearing a neighbor's television when trying to sleep or a loud radio while studying is not only an invasion of one's privacy but also a source of tension, anxiety, and anger. These reactions could lead to a loss of temper, culminating in quarrels, fights, and even homicide.

2. The *psychophysical* effect pertains to communication interface, such as speech. Particularly loud or unsettling speech can trigger involuntary or voluntary reactions, such as stress or overreaction, which prevent the body from relaxing and disturb rest. Noise also may prevent a person from hearing warning signals, thereby precipitating an accident.

3. Loud noises affect the body *physiologically* in several ways. Generally, hearing loss, the major problem associated with noise, is attributable to the irreversible damage to the inner ear.

Noise causes headaches, gastric ulcers, poor circulation, irregular heartbeat, and stomach spasms. When subjected to loud noises, adrenaline is pumped into the bloodstream, which in turn causes the heart to beat faster and the metabolism rate to increase. As the heart beats faster, the blood vessels constrict (in the brain they dilate, or expand). This causes blood pressure to rise and the heart to work harder, which can precipitate heart problems. Noise causes the ciliary muscles in the eye to tear and the pupil of the eye to dilate, permitting unwanted light (glare) to enter. This glare often causes accidents in noisy environments.

Any one or a combination of these factors can lead to reduced job performance, increased absenteeism and accident rates, poor morale, high labor turnover and increased workers' compensation claims.

Because noise is potentially harmful to the human body, employers should control it. Noise control includes reducing the source, putting distance between the person and the source, and filtering out or attenuating the noise.

1. Employees reduce noise at its *source* by using quieter machines, appliances, auto mufflers, and tires. By using fewer power tools and appliances and by maintaining vehicles and equipment, employees can cut down on noise. Jet aircraft engines can be designed to reduce the noise at the point of its generation. Garbage cans and lids can be quieted by special design. Noise can be reduced by controlling the volume of television sets, radios, and juke boxes.

2. Planning and zoning can increase the *distance* and thus reduce the amount of noise reaching people. Locating nursing homes, hospitals, schools, and homes away from noisy industry, airports, and other noise-generating sources such as interstate highways can help to put some distance between people and noise.

3. If it is impossible to reduce the noise or to put distance between you and the noise, the noise can be attenuated by filtering. Ear muffs and acoustic materials such as glass can prevent sound from entering houses. The purpose of soundproofing buildings where people live, work, and recreate is to attenuate noise. Sound can be absorbed by earth mounds, walls of concrete, and or stonework as barriers, and dense rows of trees along highways. It is better, however, to prevent the noise if possible.

TABLE 15.1 Ratings of Common Noise Sources

Response Criteria	dBA	Sound Source
	150	
	140	Aircraft carrier deck
Painfully loud		
Limited amplified speech	130	
	120	Jet aircraft flyover
Maximum vocal effort		Discotheque (rock band)
	110	Chainsaw
		Riveting machine
Very annoying	100	Motorcycle
Hearing damage (8 hours)		Heavy truck
	90	Power lawn mower
		Snowmobile
Annoying	80	Heavy traffic (50 ft)
Telephone use difficult	70	Freeway traffic (50 ft)
Intrusive		Dishwasher
	60	Conversational speech (3 ft)
Quiet	50	Business office
	40	Average residence
Very quiet	30	Library
	20	Broadcast studio
Just audible	10	
Threshold hearing	0	

Source: Environmental Quality, First Annual Report of the Council on Environment Quality

Environmental Health

Temperature Extremes

Evaluation of the hazards represented by temperature extremes include length of exposure, nature of the work, wind speed, humidity, and the worker's physical condition. Extreme low temperatures may cause tissue damage from hypothermia and frostbite with little warning. Frostbite results from prolonged and severe constriction of the blood vessels at temperatures below 32° F. Severe cold injuries such as those of deep frostbite generally are irreversible, and amputation of the affected body part may be necessary. Continued exposure to extreme cold may cause death.

Heat stress consists of the body's natural responses to stresses brought on by excess heat. Heat stress taxes the cardiovascular system, and can cause cramps, heat exhaustion, heat stroke, and even death. The same degree of exposure to excessive heat may produce different effects depending on the susceptibility of the worker exposed.

Extremes in temperature affect work performance. The extent to which performance is lowered depends on the intensity of heat or coldness, duration of the exposure period, tasks conducted during exposure, physical condition of the worker exposed, and the presence or absence of other stressors.

Control of temperature extremes includes continuous monitoring of the temperatures to which workers are exposed. Employers should provide outdoor workers, such as construction and agricultural workers, with adequate shelter from the heat and cold. Workers in hot environments should have unlimited access to cool water and should be allowed frequent breaks to drink. Employers should provide appropriate clothing and protective gear. For extremely low temperatures they should provide suitable coats, gloves, hats, and boots. For extremely high temperatures, appropriate clothing should be lightweight and permeable clothing and hats.

Employers should limit thier employees' exposure to temperature extremes and carefully monitor employees who are exposed to high and low temperatures. Employees should use the buddy system when they enter extremely cold or hot areas, as loss of consciousness can occur almost immediately. Employers should implement a work-rest schedule to reduce stress peaks and to schedule strenuous work for the appropriate time of day based on temperature. Where possible, mechanical heating or cooling of the environment is effective in controlling extremes in temperature.

INDUSTRIAL TOXICOLOGY

Toxicology is the science that studies poisonous and toxic substances and their mechanisms and effects on living organisms. In and out of the workplace, everyone is exposed to a tremendous array of chemical substances. Most of these chemicals do not present a hazard under ordinary circumstances, but all substances have the potential to cause harm at some sufficiently high level of exposure. Philippus Paracelsus stated, "No substance is a poison by itself. It is the dose that makes a substance a poison." How a material is used is the major determinant of its hazard potential. Any substance contacting or entering the body will have adverse effects at some excessive level of exposure. The potentially fatal condition known as *water toxicity* demonstrates that excessive intake of a substance as innocuous as water can be harmful. By the same token, the body can tolerate any substance without harmful effect at some lower exposure. No substance can be labeled absolutely as toxic or nontoxic.

Toxicity generally is considered the ability of a substance to produce an undesirable physiologic effect when the chemical has reached a sufficient concentration at a specific site in the body. A **toxic effect** is any noxious effect or undesirable disturbance of the body's physiologic function, whether reversible or irreversible. The toxicity of any chemical depends upon the degree of exposure. The **industrial toxicologist** is responsible for defining quantitatively the level of exposure at which harm occurs. The toxicologist also prescribes precautionary measures and exposure limitations so that normal, recommended use of a chemical substance does not result in excessive exposure and subsequent harm.

A material is considered toxic if it demonstrates the potential

— to induce cancer
— to produce long-term disease or bodily injury
— to affect health adversely
— to produce acute discomfort
— to endanger human or animal life through exposure via the respiratory tract, skin, eyes, mouth, or other routes.

The National Institute of Occupational Safety and Health (NIOSH) has listed more than 12,000 toxic materials that meet these criteria, and new chemicals are being introduced into industry at the alarming rate of approximately 500 a year. At this rate, the likelihood of proper experimentation and testing of these materials for toxic properties being conducted is questionable.

The factors that contribute to determining the degree of hazard a toxin may pose are

— route of entry,
— dosage,
— physiological state of the worker at the time of exposure and
— environmental variables.

Toxins vary in their degree of harm within the same person, depending upon the time of day he or she is exposed. Genetic factors and other interacting toxins and stressors also influence an individual's sensitivity to the chemical substance. Many chemical agents are nonselective in their actions on tissues or cells, exerting harmful effects on all living matter. Other chemical agents act only on specific cells.

Harmful effects include local and systemic damage.

1. *Local effects* usually involve injury at the point of contact with the chemical substance: the skin, eyes and mucous membranes of the upper respiratory tract.

2. A toxicant can cause injury *systemically* only after it is absorbed by the organism and distributed to the internal organs of the body.

Common routes of entry into the body are ingestion, injection, skin absorption, and inhalation. The nature and intensity of chemical effects on an organism depend not only on the administered dose but also on other physiologic factors including absorption, distribution, binding, and excretion of the chemical substance in the body.

The extent to which a chemical substance should be controlled depends on the severity of its effect on the body and its established dose-response relationship. The dose-response relationship indicates how a biological organism's response to a toxic substance changes as its exposure to a substance increases. For example, a small amount of carbon monoxide causes drowsiness, whereas a larger dose can be fatal. A dose-response curve relates percent mortality to dose administered. In determining a dose-response relationship, it is assumed that a threshold exposure exists below which no harmful effect occurs. Toxicologists doubt that this threshold concept is valid for radiation damage and carcinogenesis. Radiation damage and the initiation of cancer may exhibit a zero threshold. This means that no dosage can be considered safe; even the most minute exposure has the potential to cause physiologic damage.

Exposure limits called **threshold limit values (TLVs)** have been developed by the American Conference of Governmental Industrial Hygienists and adopted as standards by the U.S. government. Threshold limit values are intended to be used only as guidelines in the control of occupational exposures. TLVs are not meant to protect every worker, even though a safety factor is used subjectively to calculate the TLV so it usually is below the smallest level believed to cause any toxic effect. Strong evidence exists that the mechanisms for radiation damage and carcinogenesis are different from those for ordinary toxic effects. Because exposure to radiation and carcinogens, however small, has the potential to inflict permanent damage, the threshold below which no damage occurs is said to be zero.

ENFORCEMENT OF LAWS

Prior to the enactment of the Occupational Safety and Health Act (OSHAct) on April 28, 1971, governmental regulations regarding safety and health had been the responsibility of state agencies. One of the primary reasons for creation of the OSHAct was that the existing state programs were grossly inadequate and had little uniformity of application of codes and standards from one state to another. In any given state, almost no enforcement proceedings were undertaken against even blatant violators of those standards. In many instances, state safety codes and regulations were inadequate in their provisions and poorly enforced because of insufficient funding of the state programs. Inspectors and enforcement personnel were poorly trained and empowered to enforce the laws.

Although the OSHAct was created as a federal law, it permitted the states to regain sole authority to police occupational safety within its borders if they met specific conditions. A state desiring to regain control over regulation of its industries was required to submit a proposed plan indicating how it intended to execute a program that would be at least as effective as the federal one. The Secretary of Labor then would have to approve the plan and, if approved, the state would pay half of the cost of the approved program and the federal government would pay the other half. The Secretary of Labor is the principal administering officer of the OSHAct. Once the state gained control of the program, the U.S. Department of Labor was required to maintain surveillance over the state program for 3 years to ensure that the state executed its responsibilities properly.

Upon enactment of the OSHAct, a number of states objected to the extreme costs necessary to ensure that OSHAct requirements were carried out. These states declined to assume responsibility for enforcing the OSHAct and relinquished enforcement of the act to the federal government. The states that chose to regain control of enforcement of the OSHAct and standards developed their own enabling legislation and standards. The legislation and standards of the individual states are more stringent than those of the federal government in many cases.

The OSHAct describes responsibilities that employers and employees alike must carry out. Only the employers, however, can be penalized for failing to comply with the law. The employee is obligated to comply with occupational safety and health standards and all rules, regulations, and orders issued pursuant to the act that are applicable to his or her own actions and standards. The employee may file complaints of violations by his or her employer with the Department of Labor. The Department of Labor has the authority to inspect the establishment without notification. If an employee fails to adhere to the prescribed health and safety standards, even willfully, the employer may be cited for violation.

Occupational safety and health compliance officers may conduct inspections of any workplace without prior notification. Compliance officers must be admitted to the worksite, where they have the right to inspect the facilities and safety records. The following priorities may be used in making inspections.

1. An inspection will follow any accidental death or accident in which five or more workers are injured. According to the OSHAct, such an accident must be reported within 48 hours of its occurrence.

2. A worksite will be inspected if a report of an imminent hazard is received. The inspection will be conducted to determine if an imminent hazard indeed exists and to ensure that noted imminent hazards have been eliminated.

3. Industries that are themselves considered inherently hazardous will be inspected at

frequencies and times established by the responsible Occupational Safety and Health Administration (OSHA) office.

4. Other industries will be inspected according to schedules to be established by OSHA offices.

If the compliance officer considers an industry in violation of the OSHA standards, he or she must issue a citation to the employer within 6 months of the violation. The citation will indicate a reasonable time for eliminating or abating the hazard. The four possible types of citations for OSHA standards violations:

1. *Imminent danger.* Any condition or practice that reasonably could be expected to cause death or serious physical harm immediately or before correction can be made through normal procedures.

2. *Serious violation.* Any condition or practice, means, method, operation, or process that has a substantial probability of causing deaths or serious physical harm.

3. *Nonserious violation.* Any condition in which an incident or occupational illness resulting from violation of a standard probably would not cause death or serious physical harm to workers. No permanent injury is likely to result from a nonserious violation.

4. *De minimus* (no penalty). Any condition in which a violation of standard has no immediate or direct relationship to the safety or health of the workers.

OSHA can request the employer to halt immediately any operation that represents an imminent danger. If the employer refuses to halt the operation, the compliance officer will notify employees of the hazard. The Department of Labor then may request a court to shut down the operation.

For any violation, the inspecting compliance officer may propose a penalty of up to $1,000 per day until the condition is corrected. These penalties are mandatory for serious violations. Imposition of the penalties is optional in cases of nonserious violations. Willful or repeated violations each may be assessed a civil penalty of up to $10,000. If the death of an employee results from a willful violation, the employer may be punished by a fine of not more than $10,000, imprisonment of not more than 6 months, or both if he or she is convicted in a court of law. These penalties may be doubled upon subsequent convictions.

The Toxic Substances Control Act (TOSCA) of 1976 was designed to protect workers from chemical hazards. The act requires that sufficient appropriate data be developed on the health and environmental effects of chemicals. Development of these data and information is the responsibility of the chemical manufacturers and processors. The EPA is required to establish the standards to be used for testing chemicals. The chemical tested may be banned or regulated if the EPA considers test information to be insufficient or if the chemical would be widely distributed. The EPA is required to ban or restrict the use of any chemical substance representing an unreasonable risk of injury to health or the environment.

The OSHAct requires the Secretary of Health, Education and Welfare to publish an annual toxic substances list with the purpose of identifying all known toxic substances in accordance with common definitions that may be used to describe toxicity. If a substance does not appear on the list, this does not indicate that it is nontoxic but that its effects may be unknown. A listing on the toxic substances list does indicate that the listed substance has the documented potential of being hazardous if misused.

OSHA is responsible for establishing permissible standards of potentially toxic substances in the workplace. Criteria documents are developed for each significant toxic substance. Criteria documents represent extremely thorough searches of the literature that summarize all significant work related to establishment of the desired standard. To aid OSHA in meeting its responsibility, the National Institute for Occupational Safety and Health (NIOSH) has been charged with developing criteria documents for chemical substances.

In addition to OSHA, other federal government regulatory agencies have enforcement powers.

- *Mining Enforcement and Safety Administration.* Established by the Secretary of the Interior in 1973, it is responsible for administering the enforcement provisions of the Federal Coal Mine Health and Safety Act of 1969 and the Federal Metal and Nonmetallic Mine Safety Act. The Federal Mine Safety and Health Amendments Act of 1977 transferred the authority for enforcement of mining safety and health from the Department of the Interior to the Department of Labor.

- *Nuclear Regulatory Commission (NRC).* Established as an independent regulatory agency under the provisions of the Energy Reorganization Act of 1974, the NRC now is responsible for all licensing and related regulatory functions formerly assigned to the Atomic Energy Commission. The NRC licenses and regulates the uses of nuclear energy to protect public health and safety and the environment. This is accomplished by licensing persons and companies to own and use nuclear materials and to build and operate nuclear reactors. The NRC develops regulations and sets standards for these types of licenses. It also inspects the activities of licensed persons and companies to ensure that they are not in violation of NRC's safety rules.

SUMMARY

The workplace — where people spend 8 hours of a 24-hour day — should be safe and free of the biological, chemical, and physical agents of disease. These agents may be inhaled, injected, ingested, or transferred by physical contact.

Biological hazards, called biohazards, are living organisms classified as bacteria, viruses, rickettsiae, fungi, and parasites. Chemical toxins are found in mist, vapor, gases, smoke, dust, fumes, and aerosol. Physical hazards include radiation, noise pollution, and temperature extremes.

To provide an environment conducive to good health, a variety of occupational specialists are required. These include the occupational health nurse, occupational physician, industrial hygienist, safety engineer, and industrial health educator. Some of these specialists use monitoring devices to quantitatively and qualitatively evaluate the work environment.

Legislation has been enacted to promote workplace health and to establish agencies to oversee compliance. Foremost of these are the Public Health Service and the Occupational Safety and Health Act, which created OSHA, in charge of setting standards for safety in the workplace. The OSHAct also created the National Institute for Occupational Safety and Health (NIOSH).

REFERENCES

Ashford, N. A. 1976. *Crisis in the Workplace: Occupational Disease and Injury.* MIT Press, Cambridge, MA.

Bird, F. E., and G. L. Germain. 1985. *Practical Loss Control Leadership.* Institute Publishing, Loganville.

Brandt, A.D. 1947. *Industrial Health Engineering.* Chapman and Hall Ltd., London.

Daubenspeck, G. W. 1974. *Occupational Health Hazards.* Exposition Press, New York.

Everly, G.S., and R. H. L.

Feldman. 1985. *Occupational Health Promotion.* John Wiley and Sons, New York.

Hammer, W. 1976. *Occupational Safety Management and Engineering.* Prentice Hall, Englewood, New Jersey.

Hanlon, J.J. 1964 *Principles of Public Health*. C.V. Mosby, St. Louis.

Johnstone, R.T., and S.E. Miller. 1961. *Occupational Diseases and Industrial Medicine*. W.B. Saunders, Philadelphia.

Key, M. M., A. F. Henschel, J. Butler, R.N. Ligo, I.R. Tabershaw, and L. Ede. 1977. *Occupational Diseases*. U.S. Department of Health, Education and Welfare, Washington, DC.

Kohn, J.P., M.A. Friend, and C.A. Winterberger. 1996. *Fundamentals of Occupational Safety and Health*. Government Institutes, Rockville, MD.

Kryter, K.D. 1984. *Physiological, Psychological and Social Effects of Noise*. NASA Scientific and Technical Information. Washington, DC.

LaGrega, Michael D., Philip L. Buckingham, Jeffrey C. Evans, and Environmental Resources Management Group. 1994. *Hazardous Waste Management*. McGraw-Hill, Highstown, NJ.

National Safety Council. 1983. *Fundamentals of Industrial Hygiene*. 2d ed. Chicago.

Perkins, Jimmy L. 1997. *Modern Industrial Hygiene*. Van Nostrand Reinhold, New York.

Roberts, J.M. 1976. *OSHA Compliance Manual*. Teston Publishing, Virginia.

Stellman, J.M., and S.M. Daum. 1971. *Work is Dangerous to Your Health*. Pantheon Books, New York.

U.S. Environmental Protection Agency. 1971. *Noise from Construction Equipment and Operations, Building Equipment and Home Appliances*. Government Printing Office, Washington, DC.

Environmental Planning

By Bailus Walker, Ph.D., MPH
Howard University, College of Medicine

Key Terms

Allowances
Objectives

Planning
Planning premises

Priority setting
Risk analysis

Objectives

- Understand the planning process.
- Understand priority setting.
- Understand how to determine alternative courses.
- Understand risk analysis as it relates to planning.

One difficulty inherent in any discourse on planning is that of defining the scope of the discussion. Most simply put, **planning** is advanced thinking as a basis for doing. A more expansive definition of planning is the systematic process by which goals (policies) are established, facts are gathered and analyzed, alternative proposals and programs are considered and compared, resources are measured, priorities are established, and recommendations are made for the deployment of resources designed to achieve the established goals.

Within this broad definition, planning can be either functional or project-oriented. D. C. Ranney points out that planning is *functional* when it develops an appropriate course of action for decision makers in a particular field.[1] *Project-oriented* planning is broader; it involves reconciliation of numerous and diversified functional considerations. Functional and project-oriented planning may be applied to practically every human endeavor.

[1.] Ranney, D. C. 1969. *Planning and the Politics of the Metropolis.* Charles Merrill Publishing, Columbus. OH.

The process of planning for the prevention and control of environmentally provoked diseases and for the protection of ecological systems can be visualized as having three elements:

1. Thinking about what to do (establishing goals and objectives)

2. Thinking about how to get it done (programming)

3. Continuous assessment as the programming unfolds as to whether the objectives and programming are correct.

Most environmental planning situations involve *solutions* to problems, requiring *coordination with others* in relation to a *sequence of future events*. Depending on the setting, coordination may be more or less important than sequence planning, and the planning of content may present a major or a minor challenge. In any given circumstance, all three factors must be given appropriate weight.

It also is important to recognize that the environmental planning process by nature is continuous and cyclical. It follows the pattern of establishment of goals, development of approaches to achieve the goals, reevaluation throughout the implementation process, setting revised or updated goals, revision of approaches, another reevaluation of goals and programs, and so forth. Reevaluation should be allowed for at any point in the program on the basis of newly acquired knowledge or insights, or on the basis of changed events.

ESTABLISHING OBJECTIVES

Objectives are referred to variously as purposes, missions, goals, or targets. **Objectives** or purposes may be used in connection with ultimate things such as reducing serious environmental risks to human health. Goals or targets often carry the connotation of specific qualitative or quantitative ends. These terms, however, are used interchangeably throughout this chapter.

The first step in planning is to identify objectives. This requires careful consideration.

In the United States, setting environmental health objectives has been enhanced significantly by a prevention policy framework for the nation called *Healthy People 2000*. It frames the national goals and objectives for reducing premature mortality and preventable diseases by the year 2000. By defining the mission of public health clearly and ensuring the participation of both the private and public sectors, the *Healthy People 2000* initiative has the potential to strengthen the nation's environmental health system and provide health, social, and economic benefits.

The need for sound information is reflected in efforts to develop measurable objectives. When plans for improved environmental health outcomes and reduced environmental risks include assumable targets for accomplishments, we can be much clearer about what is needed and what is possible. For example, in lead poisoning — a leading cause of neurological disorders in children — if substandard housing is a major source of lead exposure, effective environmental interventions can be crafted to address this issue.

Experience in the development of *Healthy People 2000,* along with studies of the disparities between risk and priorities at national and state levels, makes it clear that measurable objectives significantly strengthen accountability.[2] As implementation of the environmental health plan proceeds, a routine monitoring process can challenge environmental managers and program planners to reshape programs and services to address whatever failure becomes apparent. For instance, the 1990 health objectives for the nation did not identify, with few exceptions, special population groups at highest risk for getting environmentally related diseases. Now there is an obvious need to focus prevention efforts more tightly on the poor, racial minorities, children, and older people. Clearly, the potential for health improvement is the greatest for these population groups, and

---

[2.] Healthy People 2000. 1970. *National Health Promotion and Disease Prevention Objectives.* Department of Health and Human Services, Washington, DC.

communities cannot achieve local health objectives without raising their health status through the prevention and control of environmental hazards to human health.

Periodic review of environmental programs and services consistent with established objectives often reveals new data, new information, and new science that will require changes in goals and objectives. In *Healthy People 2000* an original objective, for example, was to reduce the prevalence of blood lead levels exceeding 15 mg/dL* and 25 μg/dL** among children 6 months through 5 years to no more than 500,000 and zero, respectively. In the 1995–1996 mid-course review of this objective, the targets were revised as a result of the significant progress made in the area of environmental health. Data from lead poisoning prevention screening programs indicate that the prevalence of blood lead levels exceeding 15 and 25 mg/dL have dropped dramatically since the baselines (using 1984 data) were established for the objective. Unfortunately, research also has identified health threats from lead levels at even lower levels than those monitored by the year 2000 objectives (10 micrograms/deciliter) well beyond the goals themselves.

Operationally, *Healthy People 2000* — which includes 17 environmental health objectives covering a broad range of exposure media such as air, water, and soil — offers an invaluable tool for setting priorities, determining program needs, and tracking priorities. Substantively, the objectives build upon the tripartite foundation of health promotion, health protection, and preventive services, including environmental risk reduction programs.

Even though *Healthy People 2000* provides guidance on what is to be achieved at the national level, states and local communities can make their own decisions based on environmental health needs and resources at their level. Using the national objectives as a template, they can select priorities, objectives, and implementation plans to guide their efforts.

MULTIPLE OBJECTIVES

Environmental programs have multiple purposes. To say, for example, that the objective of water resources management is to prevent waterborne diseases is not enough. Much more accurate is to state its objectives as being satisfactory disposal of water-carriage waste products of community activity; to enhance satisfactory stream (river, lake) quantity and quality for intended multiple uses. In sum, the objectives should reflect that inherently water is a multiple-use resource. Each of the individual water uses is important to community health and social and economic well-being. Although not generally recognized as such, a key water resource is the satisfactory ultimate disposal of residual waste products from human activities. The waste assimilation capacity of the stream from which a community takes its water supply becomes a prime water resource asset to be wisely used and developed in efforts to reduce the risk of water-related diseases.[3]

Similarly, the setting of objectives for waste disposal must recognize that conservation of human health and protection of ecological systems require that adverse exposure to constituents of waste be prevented through identification, measurement, biological evaluation, and application of effective control technology.

PLANNING PREMISES

An important step in environmental health planning is to establish critical **planning premises**. These are planning assumptions, the future setting in which planning and implementation take place. If the emphasis is to be on prevention of environmental health problems, consideration must be given not only to the current situation but also to expected future conditions. This entails forecasting, which is important to premising.

The need for adequate forecasting is apparent from the key role it plays in environmental

---

* milligrams per deciliter

** micrograms per deciliter

3. Velz, C. J. *Applied Stream Sanitation.* 1970. Wiley Interscience, New York.

planning. And forecasting has value aside from its use in developing environmental plans. In the first place, environmental managers' making forecasts and reviewing them compel thinking ahead, looking to the future of environmental risk and providing for their management.

Forecasting, especially with wide participation throughout the environmental agency, may help to unify and coordinate plans. Focusing attention on the future assists in bringing singleness of purpose to environmental planning. Even though much emphasis is placed on environmental forecasting, all forecast is subjected to a degree of error, as the best analysis or judgment is not clairvoyance. Guesswork seldom can be omitted from forecast, although it can be reduced to a minimum. Sometimes the margin of error is considerable, although usually it can be brought within tolerable limits.

The political environment in which environmental planning operates is a premise of utmost importance. Government, whether at the federal, state, or local level, controls a number of elements in the environmental management arena. Political stability, however, perhaps is even more important than the extent of government constraints. If the political situation is stable, environmental planners deal with a known condition in making the plan. Conflicting expectations by the different branches of government may create some difficulties in environmental planning. Problems resulting from conflicts between the agendas and goals of the legislative branch and the executive branch can be formidable. Even when the two branches are in some agreement on environmental goals, they may disagree about how to accomplish them. Also, although both branches are powerful in setting the agenda for agencies, they do not necessarily control the alternatives among which choices are made.

Conflicts also arise between federal and local governments, between neighboring states, between regions, and between state and local governments. Any or all of these conflicts may result in insufficient resources for environmental planning and implementation, simple failure to initiate an environmental health program, or a deluge of demands for clarification of new legislation or policy in the face of established, perhaps longstanding policies that move in the opposite direction.

Tension, then, can be constructive, with the opposing parties stimulating each other to perform better environmental planning, or destructive, with the conflict consuming everyone's energy in fights over turf or planning and money rather than efforts to solve environmental problems.

Environmental conditions are related closely to population growth and economic conditions, and hence population trends provide a good basis for establishing planning premises. The main elements that influence population growth are: (a) birth and death rates; (b) migration (immigration and emigration); (c) economic opportunity and; (d) environmental quality.

Reduced population growth rates auger well for lower research consumption and pollution. Higher population growth rates put severe pressure on natural resources and economic growth.

The pattern of economic growth has the potential for reducing environmental pollution, with new plants and new industrial operations having the technological ability to emit fewer pollutants and consume fewer resources than older industries. How any future economic growth affects environmental quality depends on the pattern of growth. Increased investments in businesses should have mostly positive environmental implications. Much of the new capital likely will be invested in relatively "clean industries" with built-in pollution control devices. The possible negative environmental implications of strong economic growth would result primarily from the probable sites of new facilities. These may be built outside established industrial sites, sometimes upsetting the balance of ecological systems.

The U. S. Bureau of the Census projects that the nation's population will grow by another 3.4 million people by the end of the decade of the nineties, with births and deaths expected to remain constant. In making the projections, the Bureau employs the cohort survival approach, which, because it commences with the present population structure and specific birth and death rates and migration, is generally recognized as the most reliable method of population projection for short-range projections. This advantage diminishes when applied to long-range projections. Like any other method, it depends on ensuring changes in birth rates, and migration, which are difficult to anticipate.

Economic base studies can develop quantitative measures of economic opportunities, providing a basis for projecting future growth potential. The economic base consists of those activities that provide basic employment and income on which the rest of the community depends. For several decades, the Bureau of Labor Statistics (BLS) has prepared projections of the U. S. economy.[4] The projections use three alternative scenarios.

1. The moderate-growth labor force scenario is based on the middle population projections and assumes labor force participation growth comparable to past years.
2. The high-growth labor force scenario assumes higher participation rates and uses the Bureau of the Census, high net immigration population projections.
3. The low-growth scenario uses the middle population projections and assumes lower labor force participation rates. BLS disaggregates non-Hispanics, blacks, Hispanics, Asians, and others into 5-year age groups by sex.

The projected participation rate for each age-sex-race group is multiplied by the corresponding population projection to obtain the labor force projection for that group. The group then is summed to obtain the total civilian labor force.

The BLS aggregate economic projections are developed using an econometrics model. The model contains 340 behavioral equations, 668 identities, and 283 exogenous variables, for a total of almost 1,300 variables, which describes all facets of aggregate economic performances. Estimates for exogenous variables are applied to the model and a solution of the behavioral and identity equations is generated. Finally, the results are evaluated with regard to previously formulated targets for various key indicators of economic behavior. The principal exogenous assumptions underlying the model fall into the categories of demographic, fiscal and monetary policy, energy prices, and supply and foreign economic activity.[5]

Unlike the more exact sciences, economic base studies permit disagreement as to the relevant variables. These are employment, population, personal income, and number of new industries.

A PLANNING PROCESS

Historically, environmental planning has been of a piecemeal nature. The environment consists of systems that relate to each other — air, water, land, etc. — and should be planned as a group of systems whenever possible, rather than as categorical areas. For example, climate is a system that affects us all, including those in other environmental areas. The climate determines whether land will grow food, cotton, etc., and thus support human populations. The climate also determines if disease-producing insects, such as flies and mosquitoes, will inhabit an area, as many times in the past, flies and mosquitoes have influenced human habitation. Hence, climate is a factor to be considered in environmental health planning. Some other factors to be considered are: terrain, rainfall, wildlife, industry, transportation and personal considerations—religion, age, sex, ethnic background and socioeconomic level.

A planning process consists of nine steps:

1. Identify the problem.
2. Analyze the problem situation.

[4.] U.S. Bureau of the Census, Current Population Report, No. 1111. March 1995, p. 5.

[5.] U.S. Department of Labor. 1995, Nov. *Monthly Labor Review Notes on Current Labor Statistics.* Government Printing Office.

3. Set a goal.
4. Set objectives.
5. Develop alternative solutions.
6. Test alternatives.
7. Select best alternative solution.
8. Implement the plan.
9. Evaluate the plan.

A planning process is presented in Figure 16.1.

Another approach to planning consists of six steps. In brief, the steps are:

1. Examine the situation.
2. Set goals.
3. Set objectives.
4. Design the program.
5. Implement the program.
6. Evaluate the program.

Examine the Situation

Before developing a new environmental health program or modifying an ongoing one, it is necessary to get a complete picture of the situation. One needs to know the size and nature of the problem. A planner needs information concerning planned activities for public and environmental problem areas, available physical and human resources, and information about the population being served. Successful planners also require information about an area's geography, weather and man-made features (such as industry, highways, public utilities, housing), along with public concerns and opinions. Various agencies provide this information, and they should be involved.

Set Goals

A clear statement of goals is essential to the development of a program. Goals should be broad and attainable.

Set Objectives

Objectives, like goals, must be clearly stated. They should be time-related in order to establish

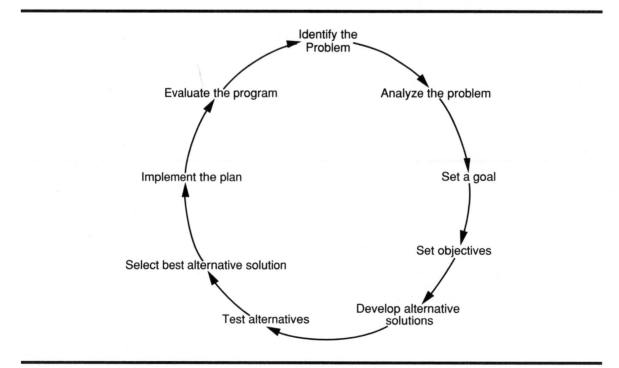

FIGURE 16.1 A planning process.

effort needed. They, too, should be attainable. Objectives may be ranked in order of priority to enhance completion.

Design the Program

In this step, conceive and describe an integrated set of activities, procedures and resources that make attainment of the objectives possible. This may be for a completely new program or a modified version of an existing program. The program should be described in detail, with its requirements in manpower, money, facilities and equipment clearly stated.

Implement the Program

In this phase, the planned program is put into action. This means committing the necessary materials, equipment, personnel and technology. A planner may become frustrated at this step because of shortages of materials, equipment, qualified personnel, and the needed technology, not to mention inflation, which can necessitate additional funds before the program can be completed.

Evaluate the Program

Once the program is under way, it should be continuously monitored and evaluated, so that adjustments can be made to compensate for situation changes, errors in estimates and assumptions, inflation, and spontaneous changes in program operation. Once every year or two planners reconsider the problem for which they planned the program. They may design alternative approaches to assist in meeting the overall goal.

PRIORITY SETTING

The relation of possible goals and objectives to each other is of particular importance in environmental planning because it necessitates the development of some means of determining the relative importance of various environmental health problems. It involves **priority setting** in relation to goals and objectives. Many different environmental problems are present at any given moment or place — usually many more than can be addressed adequately with available resources. Some problems must take precedence over others.

Frequently, environmental decisions are made more on the basis of public perception of risk, expressed through legislative mandates, than on scientific assessments of risk. Evidence of this was found in a study by the Environmental Protection Agency's (EPA) Science Advisory Board. The Board's report showed that EPA's funding priorities were more aligned with public opinion about health and the environment than with scientific assessments. The group concluded that many environmental problems it considered to be of relatively low risk, such as contamination from hazardous waste sites, were receiving extensive public attention and federal resources while problems judged to be of greater risk, such as indoor air pollution and pesticides, were receiving far less attention and resources.[6,7]

Certain fundamental factors should be considered in determining program priorities. The priority-setting technique should be consistent with the purposes intended. It should provide a formal, systematic, and consistent framework to catalog and compare information to help decision makers design strategies, allocate resources, evaluate progress, and inform the public. The factors to be considered include not only potential threats to human health and the environment but also social and economic factors. A properly designed system should be comprehensive enough to accommodate numerous, often competing objectives.

Most important, the method by which information is obtained and used should be objective, explicit, and replicable, so as to preserve the

---

6. Patton, D. The ABC's of Risk Assessment. *EPA Journal.* Jan/Feb/March 1993.
7. Reilly, W. K. Why I Propose a National Debate on Risk. *EPA Journal.* March/April 1991.

SOLID WASTE

The Situation

In a rural county in a mountainous state, one-half of the county is not served by solid waste collection. Houses average one-fourth of a mile apart in the predominantly farming area. Because it is not economically feasible for the poor county to provide solid waste collection, the waste is thrown into streams and into open dumps throughout the area. The improperly disposed waste serves as a breeding place for rats, roaches, flies and other insects. In addition, the county is degrading the environment, by polluting the water, land, and air with open burning of refuse.

The Goal

The goal for the program is to protect the health of the public by collecting and properly disposing of the solid waste to reduce insect- and rodent-borne disease, and improving environmental and ecological conditions.

The Objectives

- To reduce diseases spread by insects and rodents.
- To enhance environmental and ecological conditions by removing the open dumps.
- To reduce the amount of waste thrown into streams.
- To reduce air pollution by stopping burning in backyard incinerators.
- To reduce the county "eyesore" — trash thrown onto the land and into the streams.
- To reduce ground and surface water pollution.

The Program

The distance between houses makes it economically nonfeasible to provide house-to-house refuse pickup. Thus, providing refuse receptacles, the "green box" method of a central receiving area, is the method of choice. At central locations in the rural area, 20 cubic yard bulk refuse receptacles will be provided by the county via tax support. Five locations will be provided as determined by the population and other factors. Citizens will bring their refuse and dump it into the containers. The county will collect and dispose of the refuse from the central sites twice a week. The county will hire two people to monitor the five storage areas and will purchase a front-loader compactor-type collection truck to collect the refuse and transport it to the county sanitary landfill.

Implementation

The county will hire two people to monitor the five receiving sites and will build a shelter at each site to house them. The county will purchase a garbage truck and will hire the driver. The county will purchase the bulk refuse receptacles and place them at the five sites. The community will bring its refuse to the central locations. Trucks will transport the solid waste to the county landfill.

Program Evaluation

The program can be evaluated by:

- Determining the reduction of waste in streams.
- Determining the reduction of waste in open dumps.
- Determining the reduction of waste in backyard incinerators.
- Determining the improvements in the general appearance of the area.
- Determining the reduction of rats and insects and the prevalence of the diseases they spread.

credibility and acceptability of the priority-setting process. Ranking models that provide a framework for analyzing information and presenting results often are used in the process. These models have been used, for example, to rank hazardous waste sites for remediation priority. Developers of the models have attempted to be comprehensive in the set of environmental elements and receptors considered and routes or pathways by which the receptors can be significantly affected. In this sense, the model serves as the organizing structure or checklist for hazardous waste site potential impact. The Hazardous Ranking System (HRS) model is broadly applicable to the types of hazardous waste sites that the EPA and other agencies and organizations must evaluate. It emphasizes long-term risks, and the EPA addresses immediate threats by other methods.[8]

The National Research Council/National Academy of Sciences judged the HRS model to be generally well documented and supported. Despite certain technical limitations, it is generally consistent with accepted scientific knowledge and has been subjected to extensive peer review, public participation, and public comment.

The success of priority setting also hinges on its ability to involve all interested stakeholders in the process. Stakeholders provide information to improve decision-making and help build crucial support for the environmental health planning system. Thus, priority lists must be created with input from the affected, interested, and concerned public, citizen organizations, and many others.

Formal Public Health Assessment

Another approach to setting priorities is through a formal public health assessment — an evaluation of relevant environmental data, health outcome data (e.g., morbidity, mortality) and community concerns associated with an

In the Superfund site remediation, the first step is to nominate a hazardous waste site for remediation and score it using the HRS model. The relative threats associated with contaminant releases from different sites are assessed. The HRS combines various characteristics of the site, wastes, and surrounding environment to compute the overall score. As part of the calculations, separate scores are computed for each of four exposure pathways: groundwater, surface water, soil, and air.

The HRS score, ranging from 0 to 100, is a screening mechanism for determining whether a proposed site is included on the Superfund National Priority List (NPL). The EPA uses other scoring and ranking systems in later phases of the Superfund process, but these systems are considerably less formal than the HRS.

environmental issue. The Agency for Toxic Substances and Disease Registry (ATSDR) has applied this approach to assessing environment and health issues near or in hazardous waste sites. That agency has identified six basic steps in acquiring data and information for public health assessment:[9]

1. Evaluating information on the site's physical, geographic, and operational setting;

2. Identifying health concerns of the affected community(ies);

3. Determining the contaminants of concern associated with the site;

4. Identifying and evaluating exposure pathways (environmental transport mechanisms and human exposure pathways);

5. Determining public health implications based on available community-specific health outcome databases and other medical and toxicological information; and

6. Determining conclusions and recommendations concerning health risk.

Obviously, many factors must go into shaping priorities — the values and perception of

---

[8.] National Research Council. 1994. *Ranking Hazardous-Waste Sites for Remedial Action.* National Academy Press, Washington, DC.

[9.] *ATSDR Public Health Assessment Guidance Manual.* 1992. Lewis Publishers, Ann Arbor, MI.

community members, the constraints of the economy, the culture of governance — but hard science remains a reliable compass in a turbulent sea of environmental concerns. Science can lend a measure of coherence, predictability, authority, order, and integrity to the often costly and controversial decisions that must be made in environmental planning and implementation of programs and services.

Risk Analysis

Using risk as a common denominator in priority setting creates a measurement that helps distinguish the environmental equivalents of heart attacks from indigestion and broken bones from bruises. **Risk analysis,** or risk assessment, is a qualitative and quantitative process used to evaluate hazardous conditions and to characterize the resulting risk. Risk analysis uses tools of science, engineering, and statistics to analyze risk-related information and to estimate and evaluate the probability and magnitude of outcomes adverse to humans and other biota.

As with every methodological risk, analysis as a priority setting tool has limitations. Often, lack of specific data makes it difficult to adequately address critical issues in the risk assessment process. In these cases, resolution of the issues must be based on professional judgment in addition to quantitative scientific knowledge.

Major criticism of the risk-analysis process include the following:

1. The risk assessor might manipulate the risk analysis process to produce a desired conclusion.
2. Many important factors cannot be incorporated adequately into a risk assessment.
3. Risk analysis does not possess a sufficient level of precision to be used in priority setting. The results are based on too much uncertainty.

Despite uncertainties and controversies hovering around the evaluation of environmental risks, comparative risk assessment serves as an excellent guidepost for targeting resources and mobilizing and deploying expertise in an efficient and rational way. It offers a logical framework within which to organize information about complex environmental problems that will assist planners and policy analysts in setting priorities and in making related decisions regarding resource allocation. Comparative risk analysis can provide an explicit estimate of the likelihood of specific human health or ecological impact.

The importance of setting environmental priorities based on risk has been summarized in an especially worthy manner by R. Loehr, in an article in the *EPA Journal:*[10]

> There are heavy costs involved if society fails to set environmental priorities based on risk. If finite resources are expended on lower-priority problems at the expense of higher-priority risks, then society will face needlessly high risks.

Two aspects of potential environmental problems — their temporal and spatial dimensions — must be given considerable weight in setting priorities.

1. The *temporal* dimension is the length of time over which the problem may be caused, recognized, and mitigated. For some environmental problems it can be long. Some pollutants can persist in the environment — and thus pose environmental risks — indefinitely.
2. The *spatial* dimension of an environmental problem is the extent of the geographical area that it affects. Some, such as an elevated level of radon, may be limited to basements of some homes, whereas stratospheric ozone depletion can affect the entire globe. Some long-term and widespread environmental problems should be considered as relatively high-risk. Some environmental risks are potentially so serious, and the recovery time so long, that risk reduction action should be reviewed as a kind of insurance premium.

---

[10] Loehr, R. What Raised the Issue? EPA Journal. March/April 1991.

Environmental Health

While a laudable end, incorporating the concept of relative health and environmental risks into decisions on environmental priorities is nevertheless difficult. The lack of information on risks and benefits, the ethical dimensions of subjecting populations to known risks. and the inevitable value judgment involved — all affect the ability of environmental planners and risk managers to establish priorities that reflect relative risk. In many cases good data to evaluate risk do not exist. This fact complicates efforts to evaluate risk on a consistent basis.

Estimating benefits resulting from environmental interventions is important in priority settings. Four major steps are involved in calculating the economic benefits expected from particular interventions.

1. Determine the effects the interventions will have on specific groups — for example, those being regulated. For example, how many fewer gallons or pounds of pollutants will be discharged as a result of a regulation? The effects of regulations clearly depend on a number of uncertain factors: the attitude of those being regulated, effectiveness of the intervention or control techniques employed, and the vigor with which they are implemented or enforced.

2. Translate the effect of reduction in the offending activity (such as emissions) into improvements in the ambient environmental conditions. The latter depend not only on discharges of pollution, but also on variations in weather and climate, changes of seasons, and synergistic effects between different pollutants. Hence, a given discharge may have little effect on air and water quality at one time of day or year, yet cause serious problems at another.

3. Translate changes in environmental conditions into physical effects. To what extent does cleaner air, for example, mean healthier citizens and fewer materials damaged (corrosion, soiling)? Similarly, cleaner water brings with it increased recreational and commercial fishing, more places for safer swimming, reduced water treatment costs, certain health improvements, and other advantages. Some of the physical effects of reduced pollution may not be difficult to measure. For example, by comparing the outputs of two forms, identical in all respects safe for exposure to air pollution, it is possible to predict how crop yields might increase if air pollution were reduced. Other effects are difficult to isolate. Human health, for example, depends on a whole constellation of environmental, socioeconomic, and other influences. Statistical techniques are beginning to help unravel the effects of specific isolated phenomena such as air and water pollution.

4. Value the physical effects so the benefits of environmental interventions can be expressed in a fashion commensurate with its costs. This step is not only a scientific matter but also a philosophical one. To take an earlier example, suppose that agricultural output will increase by a certain percent following air pollution control. It then is a straightforward process to multiply the added crops by their market price to obtain an adequate estimate of that component of benefits. Similarly, if municipal water treatment costs in a community were to decrease by 1 million annually because of water pollution control upstream, that dollar reduction can serve as a reasonable estimate of that part of the overall benefits.

But what of the much more difficult valuation problems — those involving the prolongation of life or the amelioration of serious illnesses? In these cases can a dollar value be placed on regulatory "outputs?" Well-developed — although hardly conclusive — literature in economics and related disciplines can be found on this subject.

DETERMINING ALTERNATIVE COURSE

An enormous number of strategies exists for the prevention and control of environmentally provoked diseases. These strategies range from education, to publication of research results, to the enforcement of rules and regulations. Because the number of alternative courses in most environmental planning situations is legion and numerous variables and limitations are involved, evaluation can be exceedingly complex.

Risk communication designed to educate the public has been proposed as a form of primary and secondary prevention. The surge of interest in risk communication in government partly reflects a search for alternatives to direct regulatory control of environmental hazards. Government agencies sought ways to control hazardous substances or activities short of banning them. In a democracy, communication is an essential part of all societal decisions. The participants — individuals, groups, and institutions — express their concerns and viewpoints, present facts and arguments to support them, and listen to what other participants have to say. At various points in this ongoing process, elected officials and public servants act in the name of society, sometimes adding their own messages to those already existing.

Contrary to what many analysts think, there is no single overriding problem, and thus no simple way of making risk communication easy. Risk messages necessarily compress technical information, which can lead to misunderstanding confusion, and distrust.

Many scientists, decision makers, and members of the public have unrealistic expectations about what risk communication can accomplish. For example, to expect that improved risk communication always will reduce conflict and result in smooth risk management is mistaken. Risk management decisions that benefit some citizens can harm others. In addition, people do not all share common interests and values, so better understanding of environmental risk may not lead to a consensus about controversial issues or to uniform personal behavior that may limit exposure to environmental hazards. Even though good risk communication cannot always be expected to improve a situation, poor risk communication will nearly always make it

worse. We also would be mistaken to think that if people were to understand and use risk comparisons, they would have an easier time making decisions. Comparing risks can help people comprehend the unfamiliar magnitudes associated with risks, but risk comparison alone cannot establish acceptable levels of risk or ensure systematic minimization of risk.

Factors other than the level of risk — such as voluntariness of exposure to hazards to the degree of dread associated with consequences — must be considered in determining the acceptability of risk associated with a specific activity or phenomenon. Some risk communication problems derive from mistaken beliefs about scientific research on the nature of how risks are assessed and managed and on risk communication itself. Scientific information, for example, cannot be expected to resolve all important risk issues. All too often research that would answer the question about environmental health has not been done or the results are disputed. Although a great deal of research has been done on the dissemination and preparation of risk messages, less attention has been devoted to the risk communication process. In addition, even when valid scientific data are available, experts are unlikely to agree completely about the meaning of these data for risk management decisions. Finally, we cannot expect easy identification and understanding of the values, preferences, and information needs of the intended recipients of risk messages.

Communicating with citizens about risks can increase their desire to participate in or otherwise influence decisions about the control of those risks, thereby making risk management even more cumbersome. The interests of citizens and their motivation to participate in the political process can introduce difficult challenges when the implementation of risk control measures is necessarily decentralized and local preferences preclude solution in the broader interest. Many hazardous waste facilities have operated under these pressures.

Ideally, environmental risk information should use language and concepts that recipients already understand. To present scientific and technical information in everyday language is difficult. Still, the disseminants of information should strive to be sensitive to psychological needs of the recipients and their desire for answers that are as clear and decisive as possible.

Many things compete with risk messages for attention, and getting the impended recipients to attend to the issues the risk communicator thinks are important is often difficult. From the risk communicator's standpoint, the two aspects are (a) stimulating the attention of the ultimate recipients and (b) interacting with news media and other intermediaries. Messages can reach the recipients in several different ways: face-to-face, in groups, through professional or volunteer organizations, through mass media, and through community service agencies.

ECONOMIC INCENTIVES

An essential element of any successful environmental planning strategy must be the design of programs and services that mesh well with economic and other social goals. Experience shows that the environment is best served when government examines existing and potential environmental problems, sets priorities according to the relative risks of these problems, and creates incentives for the private sector to work out the most cost-effective responses to environmental objectives.

In many respects, the Clean Air Act Amendments of 1990 are a product of economic environmental convergence. The amendments authorize the distribution of **allowances** to coal-burning utilities whose facilities emit sulfur dioxide, a precursor of acid precipitation. The federal government will issue these allowances to utilities, which can buy and sell them in the open market. The quantity of allowances is large enough to create an active market, yet limited enough to force continuing reduction of emissions, as emissions in excess of allowances are prohibited.

The marketable allowances system creates incentives to achieve the desired level of emission reduction at least cost. Electric utilities that make larger-than-required emission cuts can save excess emission allowances for future use, or they can sell them to others. Because utilities are free to choose compliance strategies, they can be expected to hold down costs of emission reductions, to the benefit of electric rate payers and utility stockholders. In many cases, a cost-effective emission reduction strategy will mean investments in more efficient technology and conservation, restraining utility emissions.

Economic incentives seek to correct market failures directly by changing the cost faced by private decision-makers to reflect the full social costs of their actions. Incentive-based policies seek to influence but not dictate the actions of the targeted parties. If incentives are designed properly, private actions can approximate more closely the socially optimal use of environmental resources.

Economists long have argued that incentive programs are more likely than command and control regulations to minimize the cost of achieving environmental planning objectives. This is because incentives can be targeted specifically to correct the market failure. Command-and-control regulations can be a clumsy tool for achieving the same objectives. Practical problems of administration, monitoring, and enforcement may make regulation a more effective approach in some applications. Incentive-based approaches, however, offer many potential advantages that should be considered before adopting a regulatory approach.

The most important advantage of incentive approaches is the shift from government decisions to private-sector decisions to achieve policy or program objectives. In theory, regulations can achieve the same results as incentives. In practice, however, optimal regulations are difficult to design because they require detailed understanding of the costs and benefits of numerous activities. The more diverse are the sources and activities a policy addresses, the more difficulty regulators have in achieving optimal outcomes through command-and-control regulation. Incentive approaches can encourage action automatically where the benefits are greatest relative to costs.

In addition, command-and-control require-ments often are not flexible enough to adjust easily to dynamic change in production and pollution control technologies and in market conditions. For example, economic incentives are more likely than are some forms of command-and-control regulations to induce improvements in pollution-control technologies.

Finally, it is important to distinguish between the concept of cost-effectiveness and that of efficiency. A cost-effective environmental program reaches a target at less cost. To maximize net social benefits (efficiency), the right targets as well as the right instruments must be chosen.

ASSESSING PROGRESS

If goals or objectives are definite — accomplish-ments capable of measurement — a system to monitor performance should be in place. Historically, many environmental programs have relied on activity-based measures (i.e., number of enforcement actions taken) because of the inherent difficulty in establishing a linkage between program activity and environmental improvement or the prevention of environmentally related diseases. Evaluating environmental programs and activities and learning from experience are efforts that each participant in environmental efforts — citizens, environmental groups, government, and industry — can share. Three mechanisms can help participants understand environmental activities and accomplishments of goals and objectives: (a) a basic accountability system to monitor environmental indicators; (b) a comprehensive and integrated management information system; and (c) a process for ongoing improvement of the quality of environmental monitoring data.

Environmental monitoring to assess progress in achieving environmental objectives can be divided into three categories, each designed to answer different questions:

Source monitoring: What residuals enter or will enter the environment, and in what amounts?

Ambient monitoring: What concentrations of residuals are present in air, water, soil, or food?

Effects monitoring: What are the consequences of these residuals for humans, animals, plants, and materials?

Source monitoring has a role in enforcing compliance with emission standards; forecasting those activities for production, storage, transportation, use, and disposal that may cause pollution; and taking inventory of emissions from production processes. Ambient monitoring serves in determining changes in levels of current and potential pollutants in the environment, inspecting for compliance with standards of ambient concentrations of pollutants and gathering information for understanding the transport and distribution of residuals. Effects monitoring aids in determining impacts of current and potential pollutants on humans, animals, plants, and materials and evaluating their economic, social, and anesthetic costs.

Environmental trends that result from human-induced ecosystem changes require continuous collection of a consistent set of environmental data over long periods. Although some human activities have obvious effects on the environment, long-term environmental monitoring is necessary to detect long-term trends that result from cumulative impacts. For example, toxic substances can accumulate in stream sediment and salts can build up in soils as a result of continuous evaporation in irrigated agricultural fields. Although short-term data may be useful to describe short-term impacts, environmental trends revealed through monitoring programs over several years provide a very different picture of overall environmental trends.

Because the environment is composed of many biological organisms, non-living substances, and complex interactions among them, any single organization, public or private, would not likely have the expertise or financial resources to conduct monitoring adequately. Thus, assessing progress of environmental plans through monitoring of status and trends of environmental conditions requires the cooperation of local, state, and federal agencies and organizations. Multi-agency cooperation is valuable to minimize the duplication of data collection efforts and ensure effective, efficient data collection, the use of data collection methods, and consistent data quality so data can be compared over time and space in assessing progress consistent with the environmental plan.

Measurement of trends also requires a base from which to measure changes. This base is similar to a control group in a scientific experiment. Some areas do not have enough monitoring programs to establish a base from which to measure changes in environmental quality (i.e., levels or effects of residuals).

Establishing a base for the purpose of detecting changes in environmental quality including changes in levels of residuals in an area, can be accomplished in two ways

1. Monitoring in an area with physical (hydrologic and meteorologic) characteristics similar to the area for which the environmental plan is designed but possessing only minor sources of environmental risks (e.g., manmade pollution).

2. Monitoring in a consistent manner before and after new sources of environmental risk occur or new control programs are established.

These two methods could be combined to compare series. Computers and telecommunications are the instruments of information technology applied to environmental monitoring. The tremendous impact of computers on environmental science and technology as a whole already is reflected in environmental risk assessment and in risk management, and the scope for further impact remains vast. Application of data collection — predictive modeling — can be found in many areas of environmental health and environmental protection. For example, the Ohio River Valley Sanitation Commission has a system of continuous monitoring of streams, which it uses as a tool in managing waste disposal and pollution control. The Ohio River system employs transmitters in field stations for telemetering data to the central headquarters.

The stations provide multiple sensor units, which use electrodes or transducers for measuring water quality characteristics. These data can be used to determine if water quality management objectives are met. Whatever method is used, some monitoring will be required where there are relatively few environmental risks (e.g., relatively few pollution or contamination problems).

The two methods of establishing a base — monitoring in different areas and monitoring at different times — both require measurement procedures capable of being compared. When inconsistent measurements are taken, observed changes in environmental quality could be the result of the different sampling measurement method themselves. Many quality measurement methods for both air and water pollutants differ among agencies, with large variability among results obtained from different analytical laboratories.

If it is to make informed decisions about progress in achieving environmental progress, the environmental program must analyze the data it collects. In particular, the program should attempt to relate its data to data on health and ecological effects gathered by other agencies. This type of study should indicate ways in which monitoring can be improved and may assist in the discovery of relationships between substances released to the environment and their subsequent effects.

In establishing the system it should be recognized that it is often difficult to establish a cause-and-effect relationship between the environmental agency's actions and action of the polluters and changes in environmental conditions. The difficulties arise from factors beyond the environmental agency's control including changes in weather patterns or economic conditions. Also the data needed to understand the relationships are often extensive.

FLEXIBILITY IN PLANNING

Because of future uncertainties and possible errors in even the most expert forecast of environmental conditions, in the area of planning one must be able to change directions when indicated by unexpected events. To many planners, flexibility is the most important principle of environmental planning. The ability to change a plan without undue cost or friction, to detour, to keep moving toward a goal despite changes in conditions related to the environment or even failure of plans, has great value. There are many inflexibilities other than social and economics to consider in planning. Inflexibilities of governmental or organizational policies and procedures and psychological inflexibilities of environmental managers — including those responsible for risk analysis and risk managers — are among those that often plague environmental planners.

SUMMARY

We are living in an increasingly complex, interrelated society in which populations are growing rapidly while resources including food, space, land, energy, and water are becoming more scarce. Each year people become more dependent upon manmade systems for the necessities of life.

The need for a basic philosophy of planning is based on the realization that a piecemeal crisis approach to solving environmental health planning is ineffective. Environmental planning provides a comprehensive approach and a national decision-making process. Planners establish objectives, set priorities, determine alternative courses while considering economic incentives and progress and recognizing the need for flexibility in planning.

Principles of Environmental Health Administration

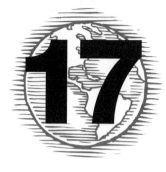

By Larry Gordon, M.S., M.P.H.

University of New Mexico, School of Public Administration

Key Terms

Environmental health and protection
Public health assessment

Risk assessment
Risk communication

Risk management

Objectives

- Describe the health services continuum and the place of environmental health and protection in the continuum.

- Understand the scope of environmental health and protection, and be able to name at least 20 of the programmatic components.

- Discuss why ecological considerations are important to environmental health and protection.

- Describe the mission of environmental health and protection agencies.

- Understand the importance of basing priorities and decisions on sound risk assessment and public health assessment.

- Explain risk communication and how it differs from public information.

- List at least 10 common risk management measures.

- Identify at least 10 federal agencies that have major environmental health and protection responsibilities.

Public and scientific concern regarding quality of the environment and related public health and ecological considerations continue to be intense.[1] This poses a challenge to administer environmental health and protection services that balance public demands with sound, science-based principles.

Environmental health and protection services are integral components of the continuum of health services, essential to the efficacy of the other components of the health services continuum. Other health services include personal public health services (population-based disease prevention and health promotion) and health care (diagnosis, treatment, and rehabilitation of patients

---

Portions of this chapter have been adapted from "Environmental Health and Protection: An Overview," by Larry J. Gordon, in *Principals of Public Health Practice*, edited by F. D. Scutchfield and C. W. Keck, Delmar Publishers, Albany, NY, 1997; and "Risk Analysis," by Larry J. Gordon, in *McGraw-Hill Yearbook of Science and Technology*, McGraw-Hill, New York, 1995.

[1] Gordon, Larry J. 1990. "Who Will Manage the Environment?" *American Journal of Public Health*, August, 80: 904–905.

273

under care on a one-on-one basis).[2] Table 17.1 lists the major components of the health services continuum[3] and gives examples of issues related to each.

Administration of modern environmental health and protection programs is as complex as the nature and causes of the problems, and involves both the public and private sectors. Program administration impacts public health, environmental quality, and the economy. Program

[2] Health Resources and Services Administration, Public Health Service, U.S. Department of Health and Human Services. 1991. *Educating the Environmental Health Science and Protection Work Force: Problems, Challenges, and Recommendations.* Bureau of Health Professions, Rockville, MD.

[3] McFarlane, Deborah, and Larry Gordon. "Teaching Health Policy and Politics in U.S. Schools of Public Health." *Journal of Public Health Policy* 13(4):428–434.

TABLE 17.1 Major Components in Health Services Continuum

Component	Examples of Issues	Component	Examples of Issues
Environmental Health and Protection	Clean air	**Disease Prevention**	Infectious diseases
	Clean water		Clinical prevention
	Toxic chemicals		PKU screening
	Safe food		Glaucoma
	Radiation		Diabetes
	Solid wastes		Osteoporosis
	Occupational health		Cancer
	Hazardous wastes		Suicides
	Risk assessment		Oral health
	Risk communication		Heart disease and stroke
	Risk management		Maternal and child health
	Global degradation		Access
	Land use		
	Noise	**Health Care**	Diagnosis
	Disease vectors		Primary care
	Housing		Case management
	Ecological dysfunction		Outpatient services
	Unintentional injuries		Clinics
	Access		Treatment
			Surgery
Health Promotion	Substance abuse		Long-term care
	Family planning		Acute care
	Nutrition		Rehabilitation
	Health education		Cost containment
	Violence		Health insurance
	Obesity		Mental health and treatment
	Tobacco		Developmental disabilities
	Mental health		Alcohol and drug treatment
	Physical activity and fitness		Managed care
	Access		Access

administration requires properly qualified personnel, an informed and supportive citizenry, environmental health and protection leadership, a sound scientific basis, the data necessary to measure and understand problems and trends, a number of vital support services, rational public and private sector policies and workable legislation, and budgets prioritized to deal with the more significant problems as determined by sound epidemiology, toxicology, risk assessment, and public health assessment, as well as public demands and expectations.[4]

SCOPE

Environmental health, along with personal public health measures, always has been a basic component of the field of public health. The scope of environmental health and protection administration continues to expand and become more complex. The terminology "environmental health and protection," however, has replaced "environmental health" *or* "environmental protection." The latter two terms denoted programs based on organizational settings rather than logical or definable differences in programs, missions, or goals. The distinctions are largely artificial and led to inappropriate organizational confusion, undesirable programmatic gaps and overlaps, and separation of activities that share the common goal of protecting the public's health and enhancing environmental quality. In some cases, the separate terminologies have created divisive administrative barriers rather than building administrative bridges between the organizations involved in the common struggle for environmental quality.[5]

The scope of environmental health and protection administration includes, but is not limited to: ambient air quality, water pollution control, safe drinking water, indoor air quality, noise pollution control, radiation protection, food protection, occupational health and safety, meat inspection, disaster response, cross-connection prevention and elimination, shellfish sanitation and certification, institutional sanitation, housing conditions, recreational area environmental health, poultry inspection, solid waste management, hazardous waste management, vector control, pesticide control, land-use, milk sanitation, toxic chemical control, unintentional injuries, and prevention of ecological dysfunction. Additional global environmental health and protection issues include habitat destruction, species extinction, global warming, stratospheric ozone depletion, planetary toxification, desertification, deforestation, and overpopulation.[6]

DEFINITION

Environmental health and protection is the art and science of protecting against environmental factors that may adversely impact human health or the ecological balances essential to long-term human health and environmental quality. Such factors include, but are not limited to, air, food and water contaminants; radiation; toxic chemicals; wastes; disease vectors; safety hazards; and habitat alterations.[7]

Public health personnel traditionally have justified, designed, and administered environmental programs based narrowly on public health issues. As environmental problems, priorities, public perception and involvement, goals, and public policy have evolved, however, ecological considerations have become increasingly important. Whatever long-term health threats exist, public and public policy leaders also know that pollution kills fish, limits visibility,

[4] Committee on the Future of Environmental Health, National Environmental Health Association. 1993. "The Future of Environmental Health, Part One" *Journal of Environmental Health* 55(4):28–32.

[5] Gordon, Larry J., and McFarlane, Deborah R. 1996. "Public Health Practitioner Incubation Plight: Following the Money Trail." *Journal of Public Health Policy* 17(1):59.

[6] Gordon, Larry J. 1994. "Public Health: A Blurred Vision." *Newsletter, Conference of Emeritus Members of the APHA* 8(2):2–8.

[7] Committee on the Future of Environmental Health, National Environmental Health Association. 1993. "The Future of Environmental Health, Part One." *Journal of Environmental Health* 55 (4):28–32.

creates foul stenches, ruins lakes and rivers, degrades recreational areas, and endangers plant and animal life.[8,9]

The report of the U. S. Environmental Protection Agency's Science Advisory Board states:

> There is no doubt that over time the quality of human life declines as the quality of natural ecosystems declines. [O]ver the past 20 years and especially over the past decade, EPA has paid too little attention to natural ecosystems. The Agency has considered the protection of public health to be its primary mission, and it has been less concerned about risks posed to ecosystems. EPA's response to human health risks as compared to ecological risks is inappropriate because, in the real world, there is little distinction between the two. Over the long term, ecological degradation either directly or indirectly degrades human health and the economy. [H]uman health and welfare ultimately rely upon the life support systems and natural resources provided by healthy ecosystems.[10]

MISSION

Environmental health and protection agencies should have the mission of administering services in such a manner as to protect the health of the public and the quality of the environment. In addition, environmental health and protection administrators should stimulate interest in related areas in which they may not have primary responsibility. For example, it may be desirable to support and promote environmental health and protection-related activities such as long-range community planning, recycling programs, zoning ordinances, plumbing codes, building codes, solid waste systems, economic development, energy conservation, land-use, and transportation systems.

Agencies such as agriculture departments have obvious and appropriate missions of promoting and protecting specific industries or segments of public interest. Conflicts of interest arise when missions are mixed, resulting in the familiar "fox in the henhouse" syndrome. These conflicts of interest result in the public being defrauded rather than receiving the protection it deserves. If environmental health and protection administrators do not articulate and adhere to a mission of protecting the health of the public and the quality of the environment, they may end up actually protecting or promoting the interests of those they are charged with regulating.

GOAL

The goal of environmental health and protection is to ensure an environment that will provide optimal public health and safety, ecological well-being, and quality of life for this and future generations. We do not live in a risk-free society or environment. The goal for environmental health and protection program administrations is not always "zero-risk." The pursuit of zero-risk as a standard or goal is frequently unnecessary, economically impractical, and unattainable and may create unfounded public concern when zero-risk is not attained. Pursuing zero-risk as a goal for one issue also may preclude resource availability to deal with other priorities.

Administrators must understand that the public is barraged with "catastrophe-of-the-week" information regarding environmental risk, coupled with a paucity of critical scientific inquiry. Administrators should recognize that the actual morbidity and mortality statistics would be much larger if all the predicted catastrophes were factual. Finally, administrators should be scientifically critical, routinely questioning existing policies, standards, and regulations as well as proposals to ensure that all measures reflect scientifically valid priorities and needs.

---

[8] Gordon, Larry J. 1995. "Environmental Health and Protection: Century 21 Challenges." *Journal of Environmental Health* 57(6):28–34.

[9] Committee for the Study of the Future of Public Health, Division of Health Care Services, Institute of Medicine. 1998. *The Future of Public Health*. National Academy Press, Washington, DC.

[10] U. S. Environmental Protection Agency, Science Advisory Board. 1990. *Reducing Risk: Setting Priorities And Strategies for Environmental Protection*. U. S. Environmental Protection Agency, Washington, DC.

RISK ASSESSMENT, COMMUNICATION, MANAGEMENT, AND PRIORITIZATION

Risk Assessment

Considering the serious differences in perceived priorities between scientists and those of the public and political leaders, **risk assessment** must be considered an administrative issue to be understood and practiced by all interests involved in protecting the health of the public and the quality of the environment. The U. S. Environmental Protection Agency's Science Advisory Board has defined risk assessment as the process by which the form, dimension, and characteristics of risk are estimated.[11] Utilizing sound scientific principles to assess risk is vital to communicating risk, recommending priorities, designing and administering risk management programs, requesting funds, and evaluating control efforts. Results of risk assessment models may vary considerably depending on the assumptions, data, and models utilized. Serious debate continues over the validity of risk assessment models and methods. These differences may be confusing to public policy makers and may create a credibility gap concerning risk assessment as a useful process.

Many agencies have developed models that utilize the following risk assessment components:

- *Hazard identification* to determine the health, ecological, economic, or quality of life effects of a substance, activity, or problem.

- *Exposure assessment* to evaluate the routes, media, magnitudes, time, and duration of actual or anticipated exposure, and of anticipated exposures, as well as the number of people, species, and/or areas exposed.

- *Amount or dose-response assessment* to estimate the relationship between the amount of the substance and the incidence of adverse effects.

- *Risk characterization* to estimate the probable incidence of an adverse effect under various conditions of exposure, including a description of the uncertainties involved.

Risk assessment always has been utilized informally and even intuitively by public policy makers and environmental health and protection administrators. Utilizing risk assessment mathematical models, however, is a comparatively recent development. Whenever a decision or recommendation has been made to develop a policy or manage an environmental problem based on available information, a risk assessment has been done. Frequently, environmental health and protection administrators must make major emergency decisions based on incomplete but compelling information without having the luxury of waiting until incontrovertible evidence is available.[12] This is done daily by environmental health and protection personnel charged with managing risks such as food, water, air, radiation, toxics, noise, and unintentional injuries.

Most mathematical health risk assessment models have been developed to determine carcinogenic outcomes. Current models reflect single-agent exposure assessment. New models must be developed to assess the effects of multiple incidents of exposures and multiple agents. Increasingly, researchers and practitioners are finding it necessary to develop knowledge and models to determine other types of health and ecological outcomes of various environmental exposures. Besides carcinogenicity, the health outcomes might include mutations, teratogenicity, altered reproductive function, mental health, neurobehavioral toxicity, and other specific organ systems.

Risk assessments generally follow the most conservative estimates that can be defended. Uncertainties in the degree of risk frequently are significant, and many issues in risk assessment can be determined only judgmentally. Taking

---

[11] U. S. Environmental Protection Agency, Science Advisory Board. 1990. *Reducing Risk: Setting Priorities and Strategies for Environmental Protection.* U. S. Environmental Protection Agency, Washington, DC.

[12] Gordon, Larry J. 1995. "Risk Analysis." *McGraw-Hill Yearbook of Science and Technology.* McGraw-Hill, New York.

nearly all relevant information about the test chemicals into consideration, a group of scientists correctly predicted the outcome at a higher success rate than computer-assisted models.[13] Risk assessment remains as much an art as a science, and risk assessment models require significant improvement.

Personnel involved in risk assessment procedures rely on knowledge and skills gleaned from fields such as chemistry, epidemiology, toxicology, biology, engineering, geology, hydrology, statistics, meteorology, and physics. The practice of risk assessment, therefore, is multidisciplinary and interdisciplinary in nature. Risk assessment procedures typically are practiced by a team of individuals representing a spectrum of required competencies.

Many individuals and agencies have recommended developing a uniform model for risk assessment. Others believe this would prevent needed improvements in the available models and would retard progress in risk assessment procedures and public acceptance.

Although all environmental health and protection agencies practice risk assessment modeling to some extent, many believe that formal risk assessment should be separate from environmental risk management programs, to reduce possible politicization of the process. Interesting case studies iterating the politicization of several EPA standards and policies are detailed in the book *The Environmental Protection Agency: Asking the Wrong Questions.*[14]

The U. S. Office of Management and Budget noted that "the need to keep risk assessment and risk management separate has long been the objective of responsible officials."[15] The National Institute of Medicine (IOM), in its report *The Future of Public Health,* recommends that "there should be an institutional home in each state and at the federal level for development and dissemination of knowledge, including research and the provision of technical assistance to lower levels of government and to academic institutions and voluntary organizations." The U. S Public Health Service Bureau of Health Professions publication *Educating Environmental Health Science and Protection Professionals* recommends that the foregoing

> . . . IOM and OMB recommendations could best be accomplished by providing start-up financial incentives for each state to organize and staff an Environmental Health Science and Protection Research and Service Institute within a university. By insuring good environmental epidemiology and risk assessment studies specific to each state, environmental health science and protection issues would be better defined and prioritized. In such a system, program funding could address science based recommendations rather than public hysteria. By basing such institutions in academic settings and separating them from operating agencies, emotionalism would be alleviated.

The Report of The Committee on the Future of Environmental Health[16] recommends that "environmental health and protection research institutes should be established in each state to ensure timely research that addresses local and regional issues."

Risk assessment is only one of the factors to be used to determine priorities. Other vital considerations include public health assessments, social factors, economic factors, political factors, technical feasibility, and community expectations.

Few jurisdictions have adequate multidisciplinary capacity to conduct and implement risk-based decision-making and risk management.[17]

13 Hileman, Bette. 1993. "Expert Intuition Tops in Test of Carcinogenicity Prediction." *Chemical and Engineering News* 71(25):35–37.

14 Landy, Marc K., Marc J. Roberts, and Stephen R. Thomas. 1990. *The Environmental Protection Agency: Asking the Wrong Questions.* Oxford University Press.

15 U.S. Office of Management and Budget. 1990. *Regulatory Program of the United States Government.* Government Printing Office, Washington, DC.

16 Committee on the Future of Environmental Health. 1993, Jan./Feb, Mar. "The Future of Environmental Health." *Journal of Environmental Health,* 55(4, 5): pp. 28–32, 42–45.

17 Burke, Thomas A. 1996, Fall. "Meeting the Educational Needs of Risk Professionals and Professionals in Risk. " *Risk Sciences and Public Policy Institute Newsletter,* Johns Hopkins University School of Hygiene and Public Health, pp. 4–7.

Increasingly, educational programs for environmental health and protection personnel are requiring formal risk assessment and risk communication course content. Programs accredited by the National Environmental Health Science and Protection Accreditation Council now are required to include risk assessment and risk communication as educational competencies. Training in risk assessment and risk communication procedures is available through various short courses and institutes sponsored by various universities, professional groups, EPA, and the U. S. Public Health Service.

The Agency for Toxic Substances and Disease Registry has developed and emphasized the use of **public health assessment** in an effort to better measure public health problems and develop realistic solutions. Public health assessments are being used increasingly to evaluate human health risk. They provide compelling alternatives to risk assessments, as they yield direct measures of human exposures rather than the hypothetical and statistical findings of risk assessments. Public health assessments are based on the data from representative biologic samples and personal monitoring and, therefore, are targeted at actions related directly to the exposure. Public health assessments have enhanced interactions with individuals and communities and have improved public health decisions and actions.[18]

Risk Communication

In the absence of timely and effective **risk communication** to the general public, various interest groups, official agencies, industry, and public policy makers such as elected officials, risk assessment is merely academic. Utilization of risk assessment inherently requires effective risk communication if findings are to be utilized. Administrators must not confuse official pronouncements and the distribution of public information materials with the art of risk communication. As a group, environmental health and protection administrators have been inadequate as risk communicators.

Environmental health and protection administrators must develop and demonstrate effective risk communication skills. Lack of sound communication results in priorities and policies that differ considerably from those based on good environmental health and protection science. Effective risk communication requires complete openness throughout planning and decision making, as well as embracing, including, and involving appropriate interest groups. Failure in risk communication frequently is linked to failure to involve the public early and openly in discussing the needs, assumptions, alternatives, and data on which problems have been assessed and public health assessments conducted.[19] Risk communication, like risk assessment, is multidisciplinary and interdisciplinary, involving disciplinary professionals such as sociologists, political scientists, educators, and marketing professionals.

Effective risk communication requires a continuing relationship between the agency and the public even in the absence of risk communication crises. Risk communication on a single-issue crisis basis is doomed to be less than optimal.

Risk Management

Risk management constitutes those measures designed to deal with risk that has been assessed. Most environmental managers and agencies routinely operate to manage risk, but may not use that terminology. Risk management is the process of integrating the results of risk assessment with economic, social, political and legal concerns to develop a course of action to prevent a problem, or solve an existing problem. Risk management methodologies include developing policies, establishing priorities, enacting statutes,

---

[18] Abraham, John E., and Robert C. Williams, *Enhancing Risk Management and Public Health Decisions Through Exposure Investigations*. Unpublished paper, Agency for Toxic Substances and Disease Registry, Atlanta.

[19] Gordon, Larry J. 1995. "Risk Analysis." *McGraw-Hill Yearbook of Science and Technology*. McGraw-Hill, New York.

promulgating regulations and standards, surveillance, inspection, permitting, epidemiological investigation, public hearings, public information, developing public support, administrative orders, grading, embargoes, citations, regulation, court orders, administrative and court penalties, among others.

The issue of how risk is assessed, communicated and managed is among the most critical environmental problems faced by society. Public perception drives the actions of elected officials. However, public perception of environmental priorities and problems frequently differs from that of environmental scientists. We do not live in a zero-risk society, and it is essential that limited resources be utilized to address the higher priority problems. The environment and the health of the public will be best served by prioritizing problems based on the best of risk assessment measures and experienced professional judgment, coupled with effective risk communication and risk management.

Prioritization

According to the Committee on the Future of Environmental Health, National Environmental Health Association, priority environmental health and protection issues on a global level include species extinction; wastes; desertification; deforestation; global warming and stratospheric ozone depletion; planetary toxification; and, most important, overpopulation.[20] The U. S. Congress, as well as state and local legislative bodies, has authorized and funded the nation's various environmental health and protection programs with little regard for risk, relative risk, or priority. In a December 1991 survey entitled "The Health Scientist Survey: Identifying Consensus on Assessing Human Health Risk," conducted by the Institute for Regulatory Policy of nearly 1,300 professionals in the fields of epidemiology, toxicology, medicine and other

health sciences, more than 81% of the professionals surveyed believed that public health dollars for reduction of environmental health risk were targeted improperly.[21] For many years the U. S. Environmental Protection Agency (EPA) and many other federal, state, and local agencies have been attempting to request and allocate resources on the basis of relative risk, and EPA now is placing increased emphasis on ecological risk.[22]

A Roper poll determined that at least 20% of the U. S. public considered hazardous waste sites to be the most significant environmental issue. At the same time, the report of EPA's Science Advisory Board, *Reducing Risk: Setting Priorities and Strategies for Environmental Protection,* listed, as the major risks to human health, ambient air pollution, worker exposure to chemicals, indoor pollution, and drinking water pollutants as the major risks to human health. Although they are not EPA programs, food protection, unintentional injuries, and childhood lead poisoning (in specified areas) should be added to this list by any reasonable public health priority.

As risks to the natural ecology and human welfare, *Reducing Risk* listed habitat alteration and destruction; species extinction and overall loss of biological diversity; stratospheric ozone depletion; global climate change; herbicides/pesticides; toxics, nutrients, biochemical oxygen demand and turbidity in surface waters; acid deposition; and airborne toxics. Among relatively low risks to the natural ecology and human welfare, the list also included oil spills, groundwater pollution, radionuclides, acid runoff to surface waters, and thermal pollution.

Priorities at local levels may vary considerably. In any case, they should be based on public health assessments, epidemiology, community

[20] Committee on the Future of Environmental Health, National Environmental Health Association. 1993. "The Future of Environmental Health." *Journal of Environmental Health* 55(4):28–32.

[21] Institute for Regulatory Policy. 1991. *The Health Scientist Survey: Identifying Consensus on Assessing Human Health Risk.* Institute for Regulatory Policy, Washington, DC.

[22] U. S. Environmental Protection Agency, Science Advisory Board. 1990. *Reducing Risk: Setting Priorities and Strategies for Environmental Protection.* Government Printing Office, Washington, DC.

risk assessment, cost-benefit analysis, and public demands, as well as legislative delegation of responsibilities.

RELEVANT ORGANIZATIONS

Federal Agencies

In addition to the U.S. Environmental Protection Agency, significant federal environmental health and protection agencies include the Occupational Safety and Health Administration of the U.S. Department of Labor, the U.S. Public Health Service (including the National Institute of Environmental Health Sciences, the Centers for Disease Control and Prevention, the Indian Health Service, the Food and Drug Administration, the Agency for Toxic Substances and Disease Registry, and the National Institute for Environmental Health and Safety), the U.S. Coast Guard, the Geological Survey, the National Oceanographic and Atmospheric Administration, the Nuclear Regulatory Commission, the Corps of Engineers; and the Departments of Transportation, Agriculture, and Housing and Urban Development.

State Agencies

A study conducted by the Johns Hopkins School of Public Health, under contract with the USPHS Bureau of Health Professions, revealed that at least 85% of state-level environmental health and protection activities were being administered by environmental health and protection agencies other than state health departments.[23] Every state indicated that multiple agencies were involved in environmental health and protection activities. Data from the Hopkins study, coupled with data published by the Public Health Foundation,[24] also suggest that states spend approximately as much on environmental health and protection as they do on all other public health activities combined. Another study, conducted by the University of Texas School of Public Health, leads to similar conclusions.[25]

Clearly, environmental health and protection is the largest single component in the field of public health. Regardless of titles, environmental health and protection agencies are components of the broad field of public health as their programs fall within any common definition of environmental health and protection, and are based on achieving public health goals. These agencies have various titles such as environment, environmental protection, ecology, labor, agriculture, environmental quality, natural resources, and pollution control. In general, state environmental health and protection agencies are apt to have responsibility for administering water pollution control, air pollution control, solid waste management, public water supplies, meat inspection, occupational health and safety, pesticide regulation, and radiation protection.[26]

Local Agencies

The majority of local environmental health and protection administration remains the responsibility of local health departments. Local activities tend to differ from those assigned to state agencies; they focus on programs such as food protection, swimming pool inspection, lead in the environment, on-site liquid waste disposal, groundwater contamination, asbestos surveillance, water supplies, animal/vector control, radon testing, illegal dumping, hazardous materials spills, emergency response planning, health impact statements, and nuisance abatement. A

[23] Burke, Thomas A., Nadia M. Shalauta, and Nga L. Tran. 1995, Jan. *The Environmental Web: Services, Structure, Funding.* U.S Department of Health and Human Services, Health Resources and Services Administration, Bureau of Health Professions, Public Health Branch. Rockville, MD.

[24] Public Health Foundation. 1991, Dec. *Public Health Agencies 1991: An Inventory of Programs and Block Grant Expenditures.* Public Health Foundation, Washington, DC.

[25] University of Texas School of Public Health. *The Professional Public Health Workforce in Texas.* Center for Health Policy Studies, Houston.

[26] Gordon, Larry J. 1993. "The Future of Environmental Health, and The Need For Public Health Leadership." *Journal of Environmental Health* 56(5):38–30.

few local jurisdictions administer comprehensive indoor and ambient air pollution control programs. Some local health departments indicate activities in water pollution control, solid waste management, radiation control, and hazardous waste management.[27,28] Most local governments have assigned certain environmental health and protection administration to agencies such as public works, housing, planning, councils of government, solid waste management, special purpose districts, and regional authorities.[29]

Federal, State, or Local?

Environmental health and protection services should be administered as close to the people as possible. Local agencies can do a better job of protecting the local environment than can a distant bureaucracy,[30] according to Energy Secretary Carol Browner. Certain issues, however, have defined the responsible levels of government.

- Problems of an interstate nature, such as interstate protection of food and food products, interstate solid and hazardous wastes transportation, interstate water pollution control, interstate pesticide regulation, and interstate air pollution resolution, are administered by appropriate federal agencies.

- The federal government has retained partial or sole authority to administer many activities that have been federally mandated or funded including, but not limited to, certain aspects of radioactive waste management, water pollution control and facilities

construction, air pollution control, meat inspection, occupational safety and health, and safe drinking water. State and local governments frequently have accepted primacy for administering some of these activities subject to adhering to federal requirements.

- State agencies or special districts may find it easier to administer certain issues on a problem-shed basis rather than on a limited local jurisdiction basis. Examples include water pollution control, air pollution control, solid waste management, and milk sanitation.

- In sparsely populated states as well as rural areas of some states, the state agency may exercise direct administrative authority in all program areas.

- Many state agencies provide technical and consultative support to local environmental health and protection agencies.

- State agencies, as well as federal agencies, may develop criteria, standards, and model legislation for state or local adoption.

- State agencies administer state and federal grant-in-aid funds for local agencies.

- There may be a conflict of interest situation when local environmental health and protection agencies attempt to regulate local government proprietary functions such as public water supplies, solid waste disposal, and sewage treatment.

- Smaller local agencies may not have expertise in certain specialized areas such as epidemiology, toxicology, public health assessment, and risk assessment.

Organizational Diversification

The trend to diversify environmental health and protection programs organizationally will continue in response to the priority of environmental health and protection, demands of environmental advocates, and the trend for many health departments to become involved significantly in health care to the detriment of environmental health and protection and other public health

---

27 National Association of County Health Officials. 1990. *National Profile of Local Health Departments.* National Association of County Health Officials, Washington, DC.

28 National Association of County Health Officials. 1992. *Current Roles and Future Challenges of Local Health Departments in Environmental Health.* NACHO, Washington, DC.

29 National Association of County Health Officials. 1990. *National Profile of Local Health Departments.* National Association of County Health Officials, Washington, DC.

30 Browner, Carol. 1993, Nov. "Public Health — An EPA Imperative." *EPA Insight Policy Paper* (EPA–175-N-93-025). Government Printing Office, Washington, DC.

Environmental Health

priorities. It is unrealistic to develop programmatic relationships between water pollution control, for example, and any one of a number of health care (treatment and rehabilitation) programs. Increased health care responsibilities of federal, state, and local health departments may translate into inadequate understanding, leadership, and priority for environmental health and protection within health departments.[31] In addition, health departments find it difficult to deal with the ecological aspects of environmental health and protection.

Organizational diversification does not mean that environmental health and protection programs are no longer basic components of the field of public health. Even though each community or state has only one health department, every community and state has several other public health agencies including numerous environmental health and protection agencies.

Academic institutions preparing students for environmental health and protection careers should orient students striving for leadership roles in the multitude of agencies involved. Public health leaders should help assure that the programs administered by these agencies are comprehensive in scope; based on sound epidemiology, toxicology, public health assessment, and risk assessment data; and help ensure that they have adequate legal, fiscal, laboratory, epidemiological, and other support resources to be effective.

PROGRAM DESIGN

An environmental health and protection program is a rational grouping of activities designed to solve one or more problems. An environmental health and protection problem is a reasonably discrete environmental issue having an impact on human health, safety, or quality of the environment.

Program activities (risk management activities) include inspection, surveillance, sampling, analyses, public information, environmental health and protection planning, pollution prevention, regulation, epidemiology, public health assessment, risk assessment, education of target groups, demonstrations, consultation, training, research, design and plan review, economic and social incentives, warnings, communication, hearings, permits, grading, compliance schedules, variances, injunctions, administrative and judicial penalties, embargoes, and environmental impact statements.

Prior to designing the program, problems must be defined accurately as to cause, time of day or season, geographic area, nature, intensity, and public health and environmental effects. Program design must stand the scrutiny of critical evaluation to ensure that the design will prevent or solve the problem(s) in an economical and societally acceptable manner.

The net health, environmental, social, and economic impacts of proposed requirements must be evaluated thoroughly prior to implementation. One seemingly desirable measure may result in undesirable problems of a more serious nature than the problem for which the program was intended.

Most environmental health and protection programs have been developed to address a single problem. This has led to unnecessary inefficiencies and ineffectiveness along with poor utilization of personnel and other resources. Properly designed, a program can address components of several environmental problems. This design practice is common in programs such as food protection, institutional environmental control, environmental control of recreational areas, and occupational safety and health.

PROGRAM SUPPORT

All organizations require administrative support elements such as fiscal, audit, purchasing, budget, and personnel. A number of additional support functions are essential to the administration of environmental health and protection services.

---

[31] Committee on the Future of Environmental Health, National Environmental Health Association. 1993. "The Future of Environmental Health, Part One" *Journal of Environmental Health* 55(4):28–32.

Laboratory

Comprehensive laboratory support must be available in quantity and quality for epidemiological investigations, public health assessment, risk assessment, determining environmental trends and needs, developing standards and regulations, enforcement, public information, and program design. These services are available through public health laboratories, environmental laboratories, pollution control laboratories, agriculture laboratories, or, in a few jurisdictions, comprehensive laboratories serving various governmental agencies. At the federal level, more specialized services may be requested from the Centers for Disease Control and Prevention, the Environmental Protection Agency, and the Food and Drug Administration.

Epidemiology

Environmental epidemiology is a specialized epidemiological function dealing with extrapolations and correlations as well as direct cause-and-effect investigations. Early environmental health practice was geared primarily to communicable disease problems. Now it also embraces the impacts of increasing amounts, types, and combinations of non-living contaminants and other stresses. Impacts such as these are more subtle and long range in their effects. There is greater difficulty in measuring effects as well as in precisely isolating and understanding the cause(s).

Some state and local environmental health and protection agencies do not have in-house epidemiological support and must receive these services through another agency, usually a health department. Sound environmental surveillance data and epidemiology are essential to determine needs, trends, and priorities, and to design effective programs.

Legal

Environmental health and protection programs are authorized by legislative bodies at various levels of government and provide for legal remedies when other efforts do not provide for compliance with specified requirements. When regulatory remedies are pursued, the advice, support and involvement of legal counsel is desirable.

Many environmental health and protection agencies have specialized environmental law attorneys. Others may request assistance through the office of a city or county attorney, a state attorney general, or the U.S. Department of Justice, depending on the requirement(s). The involvement of a skilled legal draft person also is essential in drafting legislation.

Public Information and Education

Environmental health and protection is the public's business and will not be understood properly or supported in the absence of continuing public information and educational activities. Even though all environmental health and protection administrators should be involved in these activities, the agency should utilize staff members skilled specifically in assuring a free flow of information and the attainment of new skills by the public, including the news media, target groups, citizen groups, professional groups, elected officials, and other agencies involved in the field of environmental health and protection.

Research

Environmental health and protection programs cannot be properly justified, prioritized, budgeted, designed, implemented, or administered without the benefits of peer-reviewed research. Research is essential to the development of new methodologies for preventing and controlling problems, environmental remediation, analyses, and educating target groups.

Most operating agencies and practitioners are not well equipped to conduct research but should be vital participants in identifying research needs and routinely communicating these needs to appropriate research institutions. The knowledge and skills of practitioners will be enhanced through continuing communication and coalitions with academic programs and individuals involved in environmental health and protection education and research.

Data

Environmental health and protection surveillance and status data currently are inadequate. These data should include environmentally related morbidity and mortality, statistics, specified environmental contaminant and pollution levels, and other environmental/ecological conditions. State-of-the-art environmental health and protection information systems would enhance the level of informed administration at all levels of government and industry.[32]

Fiscal Support

Environmental health and protection administrators are finding it necessary to be creative in funding services. Activities must be evaluated and prioritized to address the more significant priorities within the jurisdiction. Where additional general fund support is not available, administrators must consider reallocating budgets from lower priority activities or developing new sources of revenue such as fees for service or pollution taxes and other market-based incentives.

Prioritizing funding requests requires the best skills in administration, epidemiology, public health assessments, toxicology, and risk assessment. Developing creative funding mechanisms requires that administrators have basic knowledge and skills in public financing and environmental economics. Marketing budget requests requires competencies in marketing, communication, and public policy development.

THE PRIMACY OF PREVENTION

EPA's Science Advisory Board publication *Reducing Risk* states:

> [E]nd-of-pipe controls and waste disposal should be the last line of environmental defense, not the front line. Preventing pollution at its source — through the redesign of production processes, the substitution of less toxic production materials, the screening of new chemicals and technologies before they are introduced into commerce, energy and water conservation, the development of less-polluting transportation systems and farming practices, etc. — is usually a far cheaper, more effective way to reduce environmental risk, especially over the long term . . .

> Pollution prevention also minimizes environmental problems that are caused through a variety of exposures. For example, substituting a non-toxic for a toxic agent reduces exposures to workers producing and using the agent at the same time as it reduces exposures through surface water, groundwater, and the air.

> Pollution prevention also is preferable to end-of-pipe controls that often cause environmental problems of their own. Air pollutants captured in industrial smokestacks and deposited in landfills can contribute to groundwater pollution; stripping toxic chemicals out of groundwater, and combusting solid and hazardous wastes, can contribute to air pollution. Pollution prevention techniques are especially promising because they do not move pollutants from one environmental medium to another, as is often the case with end-of-pipe controls. Rather, the pollutants are not generated in the first place.[33]

Environmental health and protection planning (as different from program planning) is a fundamental prevention function. Although environmental health and protection should be grounded in prevention, the preponderance of efforts and funds currently is devoted to remediation of contamination and pollution created as a result of earlier actions by other interests in the public and private sectors.

Environmental health and protection administrators must have the knowledge, skills,

---

[32] Roper, William L., Edward L. Baker, William W. Dyal, and Ray M. Nicola. "Strengthening the Public Health System." *Public Health Reports* 107 (6):609–615.

[33] U. S. Environmental Protection Agency, Science Advisory Board. 1990. *Reducing Risk: Setting Priorities and Strategies for Environmental Protection.* Environmental Protection Agency, Washington, DC.

and authority to become involved effectively in prevention during the planning, design, and construction stages of energy development and production, land use, transportation methods and systems, facilities, resource development and utilization, and product design and development. Developing the capacity and authority to function effectively in environmental health and protection planning is necessary as environmental health and protection administrators strive to function in a primarily preventive mode rather than secondary prevention or treatment of the environment after the contamination or pollution has been produced and emitted.

BUILDING AND TRAVERSING COMMUNICATION BRIDGES

Effective environmental health and protection administration depends on developing and utilizing constantly traveled communication bridges and network processes connecting a wide variety of groups and agencies involved in the struggle for a quality environment and enhanced public health. A few of these interests are land use, energy production, transportation, resource development, the medical community, public works officials, agriculture, conservation, engineering, architecture, colleges and universities, economic development, chambers of commerce, environmental groups, trade and industry groups, and elected officials. These relationships should be dictated by organizational policy rather than being left to chance or personalities.

PERSONNEL REQUIREMENTS

Like other components of public health, environmental health and protection is not a profession or a discipline. It is a field in which a wide array of personnel practice within a broad and diverse spectrum of individuals, groups, and agencies. The field of environmental health and protection requires the involvement of scores of disciplines as well as interdisciplinarily trained personnel. Personnel function in roles ranging from routine inspection and surveillance levels through administration, policy, education, and research components. Depending on the type of agency and sophistication of programs, effective efforts demand an alliance of physical scientists, life scientists, social scientists, educators, physicians, environmental scientists, engineers, data specialists, planners, administrators, laboratory scientists, veterinarians, attorneys, economists, political scientists, and others in order to fully utilize the variety of environmental health and protection activities.

The Health Resources and Services Administration groups environmental health and protection personnel as (a) environmental health and protection professionals and (b) professionals in environmental health and protection.[34] Environmental health and protection professionals are those who have been educated in the various environmental health and protection technical areas, as well as in epidemiology, biostatistics, toxicology, administration and public policy, risk assessment, communication, public health assessment, risk management, environmental law, and environmental finance. For the most part, these professionals are graduates of environmental health science and protection programs accredited by the National Environmental Health Science and Protection Accreditation Council,[35,36] or of schools or programs accredited by the Council on Education for Public Health.[37]

[34] Health Resources and Services Administration, Public Health Service, U.S. Department of Health and Human Services. 1988. *Evaluating the Environmental Health Work Force.* Bureau of Health Professions, Rockville, MD.

[35] National Environmental Health Science and Protection Accreditation Council. 1993. *Guidelines for Accreditation of Environmental Health Science and Protection Masters Level Graduate Programs.* Denver.

[36] National Environmental Health Science and Protection Accreditation Council. 1992. *Guidelines for Accreditation of Environmental Health Science and Protection Baccalaureate Programs.* Denver.

[37] Council on Education for Public Health. *Council on Education for Public Health: The Accrediting Agency for Graduate Public Health Education.* CEPH, Washington, DC.

Professionals in environmental health and protection include other essential professionals and disciplines such as epidemiologists, biostatiticians, toxicologists, chemists, hydrologists, geologists, biologists, physicians, attorneys, administrators, economists, political scientists, educators, engineers, meteorologists, and social scientists.

The 1990 EPA Science Advisory Board publication, *Reducing Risk*, states:

> The nation is facing a shortage of environmental scientists and engineers needed to cope with environmental problems today and in the future. Moreover, professionals today need continuing education and training to help them understand the complex control technologies and pollution prevention strategies needed to reduce environmental risks more effectively.
>
> Most environmental officials have been trained in a subset of environmental problems, such as air pollution, water pollution or waste disposal. But they have not been trained to assist and respond to environmental problems in an integrated and comprehensive way. Moreover, few have been taught to anticipate and prevent pollution from occurring or to utilize risk reduction tools beyond command-and-control regulations. This narrow focus is not very effective in the face of intermedia problems that have emerged over the past two decades and that are projected for the future.

Competencies for environmental health and protection professionals as practitioners should include:[38,39]

- relevant environmental health and protection sciences such as biology, chemistry, physics, geology, ecology, and toxicology
- technical issues of environmental health and protection

- epidemiology and biostatistics
- etiology of environmentally induced diseases
- risk assessment
- public health assessment
- risk communication
- risk management
- marketing
- interest group interactions
- personnel, financial, and program administration
- organizational behavior
- public policy development and implementation
- environmental health and protection planning
- cultural issues
- strategic planning
- environmental health and protection fiscal impacts
- environmental health and protection law
- federal, state, and local environmental health and protection organizations
- federal, state, and local political processes

Continuing education is an essential component of a career to meet specific needs and to keep current in a rapidly changing environment. Continuing environmental health and protection education should be budgeted, timely, relevant, economical, and convenient, as well as strongly supported by management.

SUMMARY

Within the overall mission to administer services that will protect the health of the public and the quality of the environment, environmental health and protection planning emphasize prevention over remediation. The goal is to ensure an environment that will provide optimal public health and safety, ecological well-being, and quality of life for this and future generations.

---

[38] Committee on the Future of Environmental Health, National Environmental Health Association. 1993. "The Future of Environmental Health." *Journal of Environmental Health* 55(5):42–45.

[39] Sorensen, A., and R. Bialek, eds. 1993. *The Public Health Faculty/Agency Forum: Final Report.* Florida University Press, Gainesville.

Environmental health and protection is the largest single component of the field of public health. At least 85% of state-level environmental health and protection activities are administered by agencies other than state health departments. The total process involves risk assessment, risk communication, risk management, and prioritization.

Environmental health and protection administration will continue to assume a higher priority in our society, and the public will expect and demand greater levels of protection.

Population growth and shifts, resource development and consumption, product and materials manufacture and utilization, wastes, global environmental deterioration, technological development, changing patterns of land use, transportation methodologies, energy development and utilization, and continuing diversification of environmental health and protection agencies will create additional and unanticipated challenges. The competency of properly prepared environmental health and protection administrators will be a critical component.

Summary of Environmental Laws

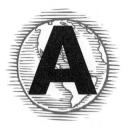

National Environmental Policy Act

The National Environmental Policy Act, signed into law on January 1, 1970, established a framework for the government to assess the environmental effects of its major actions. It required federal agencies to prepare "environmental impact statements" assessing the environmental effects of proposed projects and requests for legislation. The act also created the Council on Environmental Quality (CEQ), a three-member presidential advisory group that is required to prepare an annual environmental quality report for Congress. The council also serves as mediator of disputes among federal agencies over environmental issues. As the administrator of federal pollution control programs, the EPA does not have to comply with the act, but it reviews environmental impact statements prepared by other agencies and makes comments and recommendations on the projects proposed. Environmental Impact Statements (EIS) must include the following:

1. The environmental impact of the proposed action.
2. Any adverse environmental effects that cannot be avoided if the proposal is implemented.
3. Alternatives to the proposed action.
4. The relationship between local short-term uses of the environment and maintenance and enhancement of long-term productivity.
5. Any irreversible and irretrievable commitments of resources that would be involved in the proposed action if it is implemented.

Prior to making any detailed statement, the responsible federal official must consult with and obtain the comments of any federal agency that has jurisdiction by law or special expertise with respect to any environmental impact involved. Copies of the statement and the comments and views of the appropriate federal, state, and local agencies, which are authorized to develop and enforce environmental standards, must be made available to the President, the Council on Environmental Quality, and the public.

Clean Air Act

The original Clean Air Act was passed in 1955, authorizing a research program in the Public Health Service and technical support for local agencies concerned with the abatement of air pollution. Amendments in 1960 directed the Surgeon General to study the problem of motor vehicle pollution. Amendments in 1963 directed research into fuel desulfurization and development of air quality criteria. Amendments in 1965 added the investigation of new sources of pollution.

In 1967 the Clean Air Act was replaced by the Air Quality Act of 1967, although the former name is still used. The 1967 act provided for the designation of air quality control regions, which originally were intended to include only areas with serious air pollution problems. When the Environmental Protection Agency was organized in 1970, it covered all areas of the United States.

The Clean Air Amendment of 1970 required the EPA to set ambient air quality standards to protect public health and welfare and environmental quality, to control emissions from stationary and mobile sources, to control emissions from new stationary sources, and to control hazardous air pollutants.

The 1977 amendments to the act adopted a standardized basis for rule-making regarding criteria for national ambient air quality standards, new source performance standards, hazardous air pollution standards, motor vehicle standards, fuel and fuel-additive provisions, and aircraft emission standards. The amendments established two programs to protect air quality in pristine areas such as national parks, where the air is required to be cleaner than in areas subject to the ambient standards. One program prevents significant degradation of air quality, and the other protects visibility.

Clean Water Act

The basic federal law authorizing regulation to prevent water pollution can be dated from the Federal Water Pollution Control Act of 1956, as amended in 1961, 1965, 1966, 1970, 1972, and 1977. The 1956 act was the beginning of the construction grants program and of the enforcement and research authorizations that form the key parts of the present program. The 1961 amendments increased the funding for construction grants and increased the research program set up under the act.

In 1965 the Water Quality Act created the Federal Water Pollution Control Administration within the Department of Health, Education and Welfare, but this was transferred to the Department of Interior in 1966 under a presidential reorganization plan.

The Water Restoration Act of 1966 authorized research to cover demonstration of industrial waste treatment methods, advanced waste treatment, and joint municipal and industrial treatment. The act required the states to establish standards for all interstate and coastal waters. Federal authority was moved from the Department of the Interior to the Environmental Protection Agency. If the EPA finds the state

standards inadequate, it has the power to set the standards itself.

The Federal Water Pollution Control Act amendments of 1972 replaced the previous language of the Clean Water Act entirely. The act stated the goal of attaining zero discharge of pollutants by 1985, with an interim 1983 goal of attaining water quality to support fish and wildlife and to be suitable for recreation.

The National Pollutant Discharge Elimination System (NPDES) was set up to control pollution from point sources. Facilities are required to have an NPDES permit, negotiated with the EPA or the state water authority, to discharge pollutants into waters. Pretreatment standards for wastes discharged from industrial facilities to publicly owned sewage disposal plants also were provided for. The 1977 amendments strengthened and extended the regulation of toxic substances in water and extended some deadlines written into the 1972 law.

Resource Conservation and Recovery Act

The need to protect groundwater led Congress to enact the Resource Conservation and Recovery Act (RCRA) of 1976. Hazardous raw materials or products are not regulated under RCRA because they are regulated under the Toxic Substances Control Act or there are inherent economic incentives for their careful management. Instead, hazardous wastes have been targeted for regulation, because of their potential impact on groundwater supplies and the absence of an economic motive to ensure responsible management of spent and discarded materials. Shortly after the federal legislation was enacted, states enacted their own laws that greatly resembled RCRA.

Subtitle C of RCRA addresses five major elements for the management of hazardous waste:

1. Classifications of waste and hazardous waste.
2. Cradle-to-grave-manifest system, record-keeping and reporting requirements.

3. Standards to be followed by generators, transporters, and owners or operators of treatment, storage, or disposal facilities.

4. Enforcement of the standards through a permitting program and civil penalty policies.

5. Authorization of state programs to operate in lieu of the federal program.

The EPA took nearly 6 years to develop a near-complete set of regulations to implement the statute. This may explain in part the frequent complaint that the regulations are complicated and difficult to follow.

An entire section of the RCRA law is devoted to defining hazardous waste. This is the most challenging section of the regulations to understand. A waste is defined as "any material resulting from commercial or industrial operations which sometimes is discarded or is accumulated, stored, or treated prior to such abandonment." Recent amendments to RCRA also have included most materials that are recycled or reclaimed in the definition of waste.

Once something has been established to be a waste, the next step is to determine whether it meets the narrower category of hazardous waste. Hazardous waste is defined as any waste that is not excluded from the regulations, and that is either listed or exhibits one or more of the characteristics of hazardous waste.

If the waste is not one of the several hundred ones listed, laboratory analyses must be performed to determine whether it qualifies as hazardous waste by possessing at least one of the four characteristics of hazardous waste: ignitability, corrosivity, reactivity, and EP toxicity. The regulations describe parameters for determining whether a waste qualifies as being characteristically hazardous. *Reactivity* refers to chemical instability or the tendency to release a toxic substance into the air. A flashpoint threshold (less than 140°F) is specified for the *ignitability* characteristic. Specific pH values (greater than 12.5 or less than 2.0) and a steel corrosion rate define the *corrosivity* characteristic. EP *toxicity* involves testing the waste for concentrations of certain soluble heavy metals or pesticides. These wastes are hazardous if extract concentrations are more than 100 times the primary drinking water standards. An array of contaminants may indicate EP toxicity, and wastes exhibiting this characteristic often are denoted for the specific constituent.

Even though they exhibit a characteristic of hazardous waste, several wastes are excluded from full regulation as hazardous wastes. Examples include wastes generated from the processing of ores and minerals, residues remaining in empty containers, certain small quantities of hazardous waste (small quantity generators generate between 100 and 1000 kg/mo), samples, etc.

Generator Standards

A generator is a person, or site, whose act or process produces a hazardous waste, or whose act first causes a hazardous waste to become subject to regulation. Even though generating hazardous waste is not unlawful, a generator must certify that an effort is being made to reduce the quantity of hazardous waste generated. Once a hazardous waste is generated, the generator must notify the EPA (or an authorized state) of that waste. No permit is required to generate hazardous waste, and generators are allowed to store their hazardous waste on site for no more than 90 days without a permit, provided they comply with certain conditions. These conditions include: storing the hazardous waste in either tanks or containers, making or labeling containers or tanks, training personnel, conducting at least weekly inspections, and developing and maintaining a contingency plan for accidents.

When the generator ships the hazardous waste off-site, a hazardous waste manifest must be completed properly. The generator must identify on the manifest the type and quantity of hazardous waste being shipped, the transporters to be used, and the designated treatment, storage, or disposal facility (TSDF). The generator also must ensure that the designated facility received the hazardous wastes shipped. If the manifest is not returned to the generator within 45 days of the date the waste was accepted by the initial transporter, the generator must submit an exception report to EPA or an authorized state. Periodically, generators must submit a summary (annual or biannual report) of the hazardous waste shipped off-site.

Transporter Standards

A transporter's responsibility is summarized best as ensuring that the hazardous waste accepted is received by either the next designated transporter or the designated TSDF. In the event of a hazardous waste discharge during transportation, the transporter must take appropriate and immediate action to protect the public health and the environment. The transporter also has limited responsibility for cleaning up the contaminated area.

TSDF Standards

The owner or operator of every TSDF that receives a regulated hazardous waste for TSD must obtain a permit under RCRA, unless the activity is excluded specifically from the permitting requirements. The permit for TSDF is the key mechanism for reinforcing control of hazardous waste management facilities. The permitting process is structured to allow the EPA or an authorized state to write facility-specific permits. The owner or operator has the opportunity to write facility-specific plans and procedures that are added to the permit as attachments.

Permitting Process

The first major step of the permitting process is the submission by the applicant. After detailed technical review, the EPA or an authorized state determines that the application is complete or makes a tentative decision to either grant or deny the permit. A public notice then is published regarding the tentative decision, allowing the affected community and the owner and operator 45 days to comment. A public hearing may be held if it is requested and warranted. The EPA or an authorized state will respond to comments received and make the final permit decision. This final decision can be appealed.

Authorization of State Programs

From the inception of RCRA, Congress intended to grant states the authority to administer the hazardous waste program, rather than having the EPA implement and manage RCRA on a national scale. A significant amount of federal grant money is appropriated to states each year to facilitate the development and administration of state-run hazardous waste regulatory programs. A state seeking federal authorization is subject to probation under EPA for a period of time, and full delegation is conferred when the state becomes trained and experienced in administering the program. Although a state is never fully autonomous from the EPA, decisions can be made and acted on by an authorized state without lengthy overview by the federal agency.

Comprehensive Environmental Response, Compensation, and Liability Act of 1980

The Comprehensive Environmental Response, Compensation, and Liability Act (CERCLA) of 1980, commonly known as the Superfund Act, was passed by Congress in response to a growing national concern about the release of hazardous substances to the environment primarily at inactive sites but also from actively managed facilities and vessels that are not subject to the Resource Conservation and Recovery Act (RCRA). The key purpose of CERCLA is to establish a mechanism of response for the immediate cleanup of hazardous waste contamination from accidental spills or from abandoned hazardous waste disposal sites that may result in long-term environmental damage.

In general, if a release to the environment is considered a "federally permitted release," it is not subject to CERCLA reporting requirements. A federally permitted release is any discharge that is in compliance with a permit issued under other environmental laws. This exemption applies whether the permit is issued by a federal, state, or local authority. The intent of CERCLA is to provide for response to and cleanup of environmental problems that are not covered adequately by other environmental statutes.

Three basic types of responses may be taken under CERCLA: removals, remedial actions, and enforcement actions. All three actions may be taken at any site. Enforcement actions, either administrative or judicial, always are initiated at the time a site is discovered. The goal of CERCLA is to compel those parties responsible for a non-permitted release to pay for the cleanup of that release. If a potentially responsible party cannot be identified quickly enough to address an imminent and substantial endangerment, the federal government will respond.

The National Priorities List (NPL) is a list of sites that present the greatest danger to public health or welfare or the environment. The list is promulgated by the EPA. The sites on the NPL are prioritized according to the Hazard Ranking System (HRS). Cleanup of the sites must conform to the EPA's National Contingency Plan (NCP).

The NCP specifies the planning, coordination, and communication networks. The NCP requires that each federal region prepare regional contingency plans similar to the NCP. Each EPA region is to have its own regional team and coordinators to oversee responses for removal of oil and hazardous substances, as well as remedial project managers to oversee remedial activities involving hazardous substances. Releases of oils, PCBs, or hazardous substances in excess of reportable quantities must be reported to the National Response Center.

CERCLA has been amended four times. The most recent amendment, the Superfund Amendments and Reauthorization Act of 1986 (SARA), was signed on October 17, 1986. SARA is the first major revision of CERCLA since it was enacted. Some of the major issues addressed by SARA include:

- Cleanup standards — Adopted to discourage moving waste from one location to another without reducing the long-term threat.

- Fund replenishment — Provides for an $8.6 billion, 5-year replenishment of the Superfund.

- Settlement provisions — Deal with provisions that facilitate voluntary settlements by offering a variety of techniques for carrying out such actions.

- Liability — Defines four categories of people as liable for response costs incurred as a result of the release or threat of release of hazardous substances:

  1. The current owner or operator of a vessel or a facility.

  2. The owner or operator at the time of disposal.

  3. Any person who by contract, agreement, or other arrangement is responsible for the disposal or treatment of hazardous substances at, or transported to, a facility from which a release has occurred.

  4. Transporters who selected the disposal facility. SARA also provide a new defense for innocent landowners who acquire property without knowledge that it was used previously for waste disposal.

- State participation — Requires states to provide assurances to the EPA that they have sufficient treatment and disposal facilities complying with RCRA that are adequate to meet the state's needs for 20 years.

- Public participation — Gives the public an opportunity to comment both on a proposed remedial action and on the consent order settling a case. The EPA must respond to these comments. Furthermore, a citizen suit provision is established. Private persons may petition the EPA to have risk assessments performed on any site, and technical assistance grants to Superfund site community groups may be made.

- Health-related authorities — Greatly expands the expertise in health risk assessment to be utilized at Superfund sites. Responsibility for implementing many of these requirements rests with the Agency for Toxic Substances and Disease Registry (ATSDR) in consultation with the EPA. The

ATSDR is required to perform health assessments at all NPL sites. Upon request of a state or the EPA, these assessments must be conducted at other sites. Citizens also are allowed to petition directly to ATSDR for health assessments.

- Federal facilities cleanup program — Makes each department, agency, and instrumentality of the United States subject to CERCLA in the same manner as any nongovernmental entity.
- Radon Gas and Indoor Air Quality Research Act — Emphasizes coordination of efforts and gathering of data.
- Underground storage tank (LUST) trust fund — Establishes a comprehensive corrective action program for releases of petroleum from underground storage tanks. The fund is financed at $600 million from a new tax on fuel.

Toxic Substances Control Act

Passage of the Toxic Substances Control Act (TSCA) in 1976 culminated 5 years of intensive effort by Congress to provide a regulatory framework for dealing comprehensively with risks posed by the manufacture and use of chemical substances. Prior to passage of TSCA, these substances were largely unregulated. TSCA was enacted in large part because of the discovery of widespread contamination by polychlorinated biphenyls (PCBs) and the EPA's lack of regulatory tools to control PCB material. TSCA authorizes the EPA to:

- Obtain data from industry regarding the production, use, and health effects of chemical substances and mixtures.
- Regulate the manufacture, processing, and distribution in commerce, as well as use and disposal, of a chemical substance or mixture.

Premanufacture Notification (PMN)

In May 1977, the EPA published its initial inventory of chemical substances. Any chemicals not listed were considered new chemicals subject to premanufacture review as of July 1, 1979. As new chemicals complete premanufacture review and begin to be manufactured, they are added to the inventory.

If a chemical is not listed already on the inventory, a premature notification (PMN) must be submitted. This notification, among other things, must identify the chemical, provide information on use, method of dispersal, production levels, worker exposure, and potential byproducts or impurities. In addition, the manufacturer must provide data on health and environmental effects of the product and a description of known or reasonably ascertainable data. After submittal of the PMN, the EPA has 90 days to complete the review and either approve production of the chemical or act to ban or otherwise restrict manufacture or use. The EPA may extend the review period for an additional 90 days. If additional time is needed, the EPA and the manufacturer may interrupt the 180-day review to develop additional data.

Testing Requirements

If the EPA determines that data are insufficient to evaluate whether a chemical poses unreasonable risk to health or the environment, it can require testing of the material. Some studies that may be required include: carcinogenicity, mutagenicity, teratogenicity, behavioral modification, synergisms, and various types of toxicity. An Interagency Testing Committee composed of representatives from eight federal agencies select chemicals for testing. Once selected, these chemicals or groups of chemicals are placed on a priority list for testing that may never contain more than 50 chemicals or chemical groups.

Data Gathering

For the EPA to perform an adequate risk assessment of a chemical substance, the agency must have access to all available data regarding the substance. TSCA authorizes the EPA to require industries to provide these data. The agency requires four types of reporting under this section.

1. General data collection: Data must be submitted on chemical substances as they are added to the list.
2. Health and safety studies: Manufacturers test their chemicals routinely for efficiency and safety. Health and safety studies allow the EPA to require a manufacturer to provide copies of these studies. In addition, if the company has copies of, knows of, or reasonably could determine that other reports or studies exist, regardless of their origin, it also must provide copies or lists of these reports.
3. Notification of substantial risk: Industry is required to notify EPA if any evidence of substantial risk is identified.
4. Significant adverse reactions: Industry is required to maintain records of significant adverse reactions alleged to have been caused by a chemical because they "may indicate a tendency of a chemical substance or mixture to cause longlasting or irreversible damage to health or the environment." Records relating to possible health reactions of employees must be kept for 30 years. All other allegations must be kept for 5 years.

The EPA may move to ban the manufacturing and distribution in commerce, limit the use, require labeling, or place similar restrictions on specific chemicals. It also may issue public warnings, require situational notification, record-keeping, reporting, or other measures as the agency deems appropriate.

PCB Regulation

Regulation of PCBs (polychlorinated biphenyls) represents the full extent of powers granted to the EPA under TSCA. Nowhere else in environmental statutes is a substance banned by name. Further, what started out to be a rather simple ban on manufacturing and use has developed into a complex set of regulations restricting PCB use, requiring inspections, reporting, and record-keeping; establishing labeling and marking requirements, and outlining disposal criteria.

Hazard Communication Standard (Right-to-Know Law)

Numerous state and municipal governments' worker right-to-know law resulted in the promulgation of a federal right-to-know law entitled the Hazard Communication Standard. The objective of this law is to communicate to the worker the presence and effects of hazardous chemicals in the workplace that are known to be present in such a manner that employees may be exposed under normal conditions of use or in a potential emergency. With a few exceptions (labeling on pesticides, foods, distilled spirits and consumer products, and total exemptions on regulated hazardous wastes, tobacco, wood and foods, drugs and cosmetics intended for personal use), all workers must be informed. Training for worker identification evaluation and protection was required to be in place by May 25, 1986.

To accomplish this training, each employer must establish a hazardous chemical list. This list is defined in a written hazard determination program developed by each employer. The chemical list required of each employer is composed of two parts:

1. A list of hazardous chemicals as determined from the Material Safety Data Sheet (MSDS) from chemical manufacturers, distributors, and importers, in the "hazardous ingredients" section.
2. A list of in-house reaction products such as welding fumes, carbon monoxide from lift trucks, wood dust, and chemical intermediates.

A MSDS should be requested from suppliers for all incoming materials used and developed and evaluated for reaction products by a qualified person such as a chemist or industrial hygienist. Physical hazards of chemicals, as well as health hazards, must be addressed.

Employee recall is perhaps the most effective measurement of communication. The required information must be in simple and understandable language, as used by the worker. The MSDS probably cannot be used directly as the medium of communication because the language often is too technical. The information must be simplified, summarized, and communicated. In some parts of the country, 20% of the workforce cannot read or write effectively. Written information transfer is not the preferred method. Supervisor-to-worker communication is essential, using visual aids and dialogue.

The basic areas of the employee knowledge are: purpose, what, where, effect on body, detection, protection, and written program and MSDS.

Employers are not only responsible for preparing a written plan for determining whether chemicals they use or store are hazardous (which must be shown and explained to the worker), but they also must develop a written program of the plan they will use to effect the hazard communication program. This plan should designate a person in charge of the various responsibilities and generally explain how they will be carried out. These responsibilities are: provision and maintenance of MSDS, preparation and maintenance of labels, execution and sources for a good training program, production of a hazardous chemical list, description of the methods the employer will use to inform employees of the hazards of non-routine tasks, and description of the methods the employer will use to inform any contractor employees working in the employer's workplace of the hazardous chemicals they may be exposed to while performing their work, and any suggestions for appropriate protective measures.

Safe Drinking Water Act

The Safe Drinking Water Act was passed in 1975 (and amended in 1986) to protect groundwater and drinking water sources. The law requires the EPA to establish recommended maximum contaminant goals (RMCG) for each contaminant that may have an adverse effect on the health of an individual. Two types of drinking water standards were established to limit the amount of contamination that may be in drinking water:

1. Primary standards with a maximum contaminant level (MCL) to protect human health;
2. Secondary standards that involve the color, taste, smell, and other physical characteristics of drinking water sources.

The Safe Drinking Water Act stipulated 83 contaminants for which regulations were required to be developed by 1989. These include:

14 volatile organic compounds
29 synthetic organic compounds
13 inorganic chemicals
4 microbiological contaminants
2 radiological contaminants

A second major provision of the Safe Water Drinking Act for the purpose of protecting groundwater is the regulation of underground injection of toxic chemicals. Injection of liquid wastes into underground wells is used as a means of disposal. Controls were needed to assure that this means of disposal did not damage the quality of aquifers. The act established five classes of underground injection wells. Class IV wells, where hazardous wastes are injected into or above a formation within one-quarter mile of an underground source of drinking water, were to be phased out. Under the 1986 amendments, states must adopt a program for protecting wellheads. The program must include the surface and subsurface surrounding a well or well field through which contaminants are reasonably likely to move toward a well.

Coastal Zone Management Act of 1972

In 1972, Congress declared that it is national policy to preserve, protect, develop and, where possible, restore or enhance the resources of the nation's coastal zone. The Coastal Zone Management Act declared that it is public policy to:

— encourage and assist the states to exercise effectively their responsibilities in the coastal zone through the development and implementation of management programs that will achieve wise use of the land and water resources of the coastal zone, giving full consideration to ecological, cultural, historic, and aesthetic values, as well as needs for economic development.

— encourage the preparation of special area management plans that provide for increased specificity in protecting significant natural resources, reasonable coastal-dependent economic growth, improved protection of life and property in hazardous areas, and improved predictability in governmental decision-making.

— encourage participation and cooperation of the public, state and local governments, and interstate and other regional agencies, as well as the federal agencies having programs affecting the coastal zone.

The management program for each coastal state must include each of the following requirements:

- Identification of the boundaries of the coastal zone subject to the management program.
- A definition of what constitutes permissible land uses and water uses within the coastal zone that have a direct and significant impact on the coastal waters.
- An inventory and designation of areas of particular concern within the coastal zone.
- Identification of the means by which the state proposes to exert control over land uses and water uses, including a listing of relevant constitutional provisions, laws, regulations, and judicial decisions.
- Broad guidelines on priorities of uses in specific areas, including specifically those of lowest priority.

- A description of the organizational structure proposed to implement a management program, including the responsibilities and interrelationships of local, areawide, state, regional, and interstate agencies in the management process.
- A definition of the term "beach" and a planning process for the protection of, and access to, public beaches and other public coastal areas of environmental, recreational, historical, aesthetic, ecological, or cultural value.
- A planning process for energy facilities likely to be located in, or that may significantly affect, the coastal zone, including, but not limited to, a process for anticipating and managing the impacts from such facilities.
- A planning process for assessing the effects of shoreline erosion and studying and evaluating ways to control, or lessen the impact of, such erosion, and to restore areas affected adversely by such erosion.

Occupational Safety and Health Act of 1970

The Occupational Safety and Health Act (OSHAct) was enacted in 1970 "to provide for the general welfare to assure so far as possible every working man and woman in the nation safe and healthful working conditions and to preserve our human resources." The act grants the Secretary of Labor the authority to promulgate, modify, and revoke safety and health standards; to conduct inspections and investigations and to issue citations, including proposed penalties; to require employees to keep records of safety and health data; to petition the courts to restrain imminent danger situations; and to approve or reject state plans for programs under the act. The Secretary's authority includes right of access to the records of other federal agencies, and a shared responsibility with other federal agency heads for the adequacy of programs in the organizations reporting to them.

The act authorizes the Secretary to have the Department of Labor conduct short-term training of personnel involved in performance of duties related to their responsibilities under the act, and in consultation with the Department of Health, Education and Welfare, and to provide training and education to employers and employees. The Secretary and his or her designees are authorized to consult with employers, employees, and organizations regarding prevention of injuries and illnesses. The Secretary, after consultation with the Secretary of Health, Education and Welfare, may grant funds to the states for identification of program needs and plan development, experiments, demonstrations, administration, and operation of programs. In conjunction with the Secretary of Health and Human Services, the Secretary of Labor is charged with developing and maintaining a statistics program for occupational safety and health.

The OSHAct sets out two duties for employers and one for employees. The general duty provisions are:

1. Furnish to each employee a place for employment that is free from recognized hazards that are causing, or are likely to cause, death or serious physical harm to employees.

2. Comply with occupational safety and health standards under the act.

3. Each employee shall comply with occupational safety and health standards and all rules, regulations, and orders issued pursuant to the act that are applicable to the employee's own actions and conduct.

Health standards are promulgated under the OSHAct by the Labor Department with technical advice from the National Institute for Occupational Safety and Health (NIOSH) in the Department of Health, Education and Welfare. NIOSH provides information and data in the area of health hazards, but the final authority for promulgation of the standards remains with the Secretary of Labor.

Consumer Product Safety Act

The Consumer Product Safety Act of 1972 created the Consumer Product Safety Commission (CPSC), whose mission was to reduce product-related injuries to consumers by regulation of product design, labeling, and use instructions. The CPSC is a five-member independent commission with authority to set safety standards for consumer products and to ban those providing an unreasonable risk of injury. The commission also has authority to recall products. The only consumer products not covered were those governed by other regulatory agencies, such as aircraft, automobiles, food, drugs, and pesticides. The CPSC has been provided with a substantial budget to undertake its legal and administrative processes, test products, gather medical statistics pertaining to product-related injuries, and disseminate information to consumers.

Congress included a provision that requires manufacturers and sellers of covered consumer products to report to the CPSC the existence of any substantial product hazards. Rulemaking, rather than administrative adjudication, was to be the principal means by which the CPSC would ensure rapid decision making. Stiff penalties imposed upon violators of the standards set forth in the rules were intended to ensure effective compliance.

Establishment of safety standards was to involve an "offeror process" under which the commission was required to solicit draft standards from outside parties.

In 1981, the act was amended to abolish the offeror process. The CPSC was directed to rely on voluntary rather than mandatory safety standards wherever voluntary standards would "adequately" reduce risk — a potentially major curtailment of its authority.

Selected Environmental Organizations

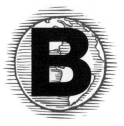

American Public Health Association

An association for the enhancement of public health.

1015 15th Street, NW
Washington, DC 20005–2605
(202) 789-5600

Congress Watch Lobbying

Consumer health and safety, pesticides.

215 Pennsylvania Ave., S.E.,
Washington, DC 20003.
(202) 546-4996

Environmental Action, Inc.

Lobbying, education, grassroots organizing: energy efficiency and conservation, toxics reduction, right-to-know laws, transportation, solid waste, solar energy, deposit legislation. Offers internships.

6930 Carroll Ave., Suite 600
Takoma Park, MD 20912
(301) 891-1100

Environmental Defense Fund

Research, litigation, and lobbying: cosmetics safety, drinking water, energy, transportation, pesticides, wildlife, air pollution, cancer prevention, radiation.

257 Park Avenue South
New York, NY 10010
(212) 505-2100

League of Conservation Voters

Political arm of the environmental community. Works to elect candidates to U.S. House and Senate who will vote to protect the nation's environment, and holds them accountable by publishing the National Environmental Scorecard each year, which can be ordered for $6 and is free to students.

1707 L Street, N.W., Suite 550
Washington, DC 20036
(202) 785-8683

National Environmental Health Association

Professional organization for environmental health professionals, and offers registration services for environmental health specialists.

720 S. Colorado Blvd. Suite 970, South Tower
Denver, CO 80222
(303) 756-9090

Planned Parenthood Federation of America

Education services, and research: fertility control, family planning.

810 7th Ave.
New York, NY 10019
(212) 541-7800

Population Reference Bureau, Inc.

Engaged in collection and dissemination of objective population information. Excellent publications.

1875 Connecticut Ave., N.W., Suite 520
Washington, DC 20009
(202) 483-1100

U.S. Environmental Protection Agency, Public Information Center
Provides general information about environmental topics.

401 M Street, S.W.
Washington, DC 20460
(202) 260-7751

World Watch Institute
Research and education: energy, food, population, health, women's issues, technology, the environment.

1776 Massachusetts Ave., N.W.
Washington, DC 20036
(202) 452-1999

Glossary

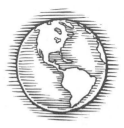

Activated sludge Sewage sediment that contains a heavy growth of microorganisms, resulting from vigorous aeration.

Acute Having a sudden onset and rapid recovery.

Acute toxicity A response to a chemical that occurs within minutes, hours, or days of exposure.

Aeration Introducing oxygen (in air) to water to encourage bacterial growth and decomposition of organic material.

Aeration tank digestion The tank in which aeration takes place.

Aerobic Requiring free oxygen.

Aerosol Liquid droplets or solid particles that remain dispersed in the air a prolonged time.

Anaerobic Living in environments void of free oxygen.

Anthropogenic Refers to air pollutants that may adversely impact human health.

Aquifer A porous stratum that stores water underground.

Arachnids A class of Arthropods in which the head, thorax, and abdomen are unified in one body region.

Arthropods Animals belonging to the phylum Arthropoda, meaning "jointed foot."

Asbestos The mineral chrysotile, used for making incombustible or fireproof articles.

Ashes Combusted materials that have been burned to total breakdown.

Avalanche A sliding mass of ice and snow.

Backsiphonage The backflow of used, contaminated, or polluted water from a plumbing fixture or vessel or other source into a potable (or clean swimming) water supply as a result of negative pressure in the pipe/system.

Bar screen Device that strains out large materials that may damage a wastewater treatment plant.

Biochemical oxygen demand (BOD) Amount of oxygen microorganisms require while stabilizing decomposable organic matter under aerobic conditions.

Biohazards Living organisms that are infectious agents and represent a potential risk to human or animal health.

Biosphere Air, water, and land.

Bored well a well in which a mechanical device bores into the ground to reach water; limited by underlying consolidated bedrock or impervious strata.

Box and can A self-contained, above-ground chamber to collect urine and feces that can later be disposed of properly; sometimes termed "port-a-john" or "portable toilet."

Canning Process of sealing a metal container of food with the microorganism potentially in it and heating the can to kill the organism.

Carbon monoxide Colorless, odorless, poisonous gas, CO, which burns with a pale blue flame, produced when carbon burns with insufficient air.

Carrier A person who harbors and spreads disease without necessarily showing symptoms of the disease.

Catalytic converter Device installed in automobiles to control volatile hydrocarbons and carbon monoxide exhaust.

Causative agent

CERCLA Comprehensive Environmental Response, Compensation and Liability Act, known as Superfund, passed in 1980 by the U. S. Congress to clean up and monitor hazardous waste.

Channel of infection Portal of entry of a causative agent of disease.

Chemical oxygen demand (COD) Test that allows measurement of waste in terms of total quantity of oxygen required for oxidation to carbon dioxide and water.

Chronic Refers to diseases that linger and often become worse over time.

Chronic toxicity A response to a chemical that occurs after years or nearly a lifetime of exposure.

Cistern a tank for storing rainwater from a catchmant area or for storing water hauled in from some outside source.

Coliform group Microorganisms whose presence indicates that contamination is entering a water supply.

Communicable Infectious, contagious.

Comminuter A unit that grind up the large solids to prepare them for digestion by microorganisms in a wastewater treatment plant.

Composting Taking biodegradable materials and, through natural processes, producing humus.

Conduction The transfer of heat between the human body and surrounding substances or objects by direct contact.

Convection Transfer of heat from one place to another by moving fluid (gas or liquid). Natural convection results from differences in temperature. As related to hypothermia and frostbite, the difference in heat in the fluid is caused by fluid in contact with the (human) body gaining heat from the body.

Corrosive Having a pH below 2 or above 12.5; capable of eating away living tissues or nonliving materials through chemical reaction.

Cyclo-propagative Refers to a condition in which the disease agent undergoes a change in form and increase in number within the vector.

DNA The genetic instructions for cell survival and reproduction.

decibels (dB)

Deep wells Wells dug deep into the earth where hazardous waste is injected as a means of disposal.

Deforestation Permanent decline in trees in an area to less than 10% of its original extent; usually denotes human activity.

Dermatitis A skin condition caused by the mite called chiggers, or redbugs.

Desiccation *See* drying.

Digester A large sealed unit in a wastewater treatment plant where anaerobic decomposition takes place.

Disease deviation from the normal physiological state of the host.

Dissolved oxygen (DO) Factor in liquid wastes that determines whether biological changes are brought about by aerobic or by anaerobic organisms.

Dose-response relationship The percentage of subjects exhibiting a response to a chemical as the dose increases.

Doubling time Time required for a population to double its size.

Drilled well Well that is drilled mechanically through rock and compacted areas; not limited to depth of rock. Water is less subject to reduced flows in times of drought and less subject to biological contamination.

Driven well Well created by driving a pipe with a special screened point into the ground until reaching water; limited to areas where soil particles are large and coastal regions with shallow water tables.

Drying Process that removes the moisture from a product to kill the bacteria; also termed *desiccation*.

Dug well Well constructed by digging straight down into the earth manually until reaching water; limited by the depth of the dense bedrock.

Dust Solid particles produced by crushing, grinding, drilling, and otherwise handling materials.

Ecological system A natural association of populations of plants and animals that persists over time.

Electrostatic precipitator Air pollution control device in which particles are electrically charged, then collected on metal plates that are oppositely charged.

Endemic Refers to diseases with the expected number of cases for a specific human population at a specific time.

Environmental health and protection The art and science of protecting against environmental factors that may adversely impact human health or the ecological balances essential to long-term human health and environmental quality. Includes, but not limited to, air, food and water contaminants; radiation; toxic chemicals; wastes; disease vectors; safety hazards; and habitat alterations.

Environmental health practice Study of the relationship between environment and health.

Epidemic Refers to diseases with a greater than normal rate of disease in a population.

Epidemiology Study of the distribution and determinants of diseases and death in specified populations.

Epidermis Outer layer of skin.

Evapotranspiration Plants' drawing water from soil by capillary action, where it evaporates into the air.

Evaporation Physical transformation of a liquid to a gaseous state at any temperature below its boiling point.

Facultative having the ability to exist either aerobically or anaerobically, depending on the surrounding environment.

Fermentation Action of specialized bacteria or yeast to produce alcohol or acid byproducts that prevent the growth of flora.

Fomites Any inanimate objects that provide a "resting place" for causative agents of disease.

Frostbite Damage to or destruction of bodily tissue as a result of exposure to extremely cold air or objects.

Fumes Solid particles created by condensation of a substance from a gaseous state.

Garbage Organic putrescible matter resulting wherever people live, work, travel, and recreate.

Gases Fluids that take the shape of whatever container is available to them.

Greenhouse effect The effect produced by certain gases, such as carbon dioxide, on a planet's atmosphere by raising the temperature of the surface of the planet, thus preventing the outward transmission of long-wave radiation from the surface but permitting the inward transmission of short-wave radiation from the sun to the surface.

Grinder *See* Comminuter.

Grit chamber A basin that slows the water entering a wastewater treatment plant just enough to allow time for heavy particles to settle out.

Growth rate Difference between live birth rate and death rate in a given population.

Half-life The time required for half of the atoms of a particular radionuclide to decay.

Humidity Humid condition; dampness.

Hypertonic environment a condition in which the environment surrounding the cell contains a greater saline concentration than that within the cell.

Hypochlorous acid (H_OC_1) An unstable acid with excellent bactericidal and algicidal properties.

Hypothermia Abnormal, potentially dangerous, low body temperature (= or > 95°F). Most commonly caused by loss of body heat as a result of contact with cold air or objects.

Hypotonic environment a condition in which the saline content within the cell is greater than that of the surrounding environment; allows moisture to enter cell by osmosis.

Industrial hygienist Person assesses and recommends methodology for controlling environmental hazards and toxic substances for a company.

Industrial health educator Person who educates workers in the prevention of occupational diseases/injuries; counsels workers; and conducts health and safety surveys.

Industrial toxicologist A toxicologist who practices toxicology in an industrial setting.

Ignitable Refers to liquids having a flashpoint below 60°C or nonliquids liable to cause fires via friction, moisture absorption, or spontaneous chemical change.

Immunity The quality or state of being immune to a disease.

Incineration Burning waste at high temperatures.

Incubation period The time that elapses between the organism entering the body and appearance of the first symptoms.

Injury Physical damage to the body that results when energy is transferred to the body in amounts greater than it can withstand

Ionizing radiation Radiation that interacts with matter to produce charged particles.

Isotonic environment A condition in which the saline solution surrounding a cell has the same salt concentration as that within the cell and provides optimum growth potential.

Joules Gram in any specified material.

Lead (Pb) A heavy, comparatively soft, malleable, bluish-gray metal, sometimes found in its natural state but usually combined as a sulfide.

Loose-snow avalanche An avalanche that starts at the point or side of a slope when unattached snow crystals slide downward, growing in size, and the quantity of snow involved, as it descends. Loose snow moves as a formless mass with little internal cohesion.

Maggot The larva form of the housefly.

Mass gathering Precise legal definition varies by state and may be determined on basis of a minimum number of persons in attendance, time duration of the activity, its sponsorship, or its location. In general, an assembly of people requiring planning in aspects such as sanitation, emergency preparation, and environmental health precautions to ensure a safe and recreational experience for those in attendance.

Maximum contaminants levels (MCLs) The concentration of water pollutants that may have adverse effects on human health, according to EPA standards.

Mesophilic refers to organisms that grow in a medium range of temperatures, from about 69°F to 113°F.

Metamorphosis Life cycle of arthropod from egg to adult with various stages.

Minimum separation distance the distance that the health department allows between drinking water wells and pollution sources.

Mist Composed of liquid droplets suspended in air and formed by condensation from a gas to a liquid or by dispersing liquid into tiny particles.

Mode of action The interaction between the chemical and a specific cell structure that results in a response.

Myiasis Invasion of the flesh of the host animal by the larva of the fly.

NPDES National Pollutant Discharge Eliminations System, established to control wastewater discharges.

National Electronic Injury Surveillance System (NEISS) An electronic system that monitors admissions to selected hospital emergency rooms daily for injuries involving consumer products.

Nitrogen oxides Compounds formed by the fixation of nitrogen at high temperatures, as in furnaces and internal combustion engines. Primary product is nitric oxide (NO), which slowly oxidizes in air to nitrogen dioxide (NO_2)

Noise Unwanted sound.

Objective Something toward which effort is directed.

Occupational health nurse A nurse responsible for the care of illnesses and injuries occurring at the workplace.

Occupational physician A medical doctor who typically performs pre-employment physicals, treats work-related injuries and illnesses, supervises drug screening, and determines the presence and extent of workers' disability.

Ootheca The egg-containing pouch carried from the abdomen by the German cockroach.

Ozone A form of oxygen (O_3) produced by a reaction of photochemical smog and in electrical discharges; a powerful oxidizing agent, toxic to plants and animals at relatively low concentrations.

Ozone layer That portion of the stratosphere surrounding the earth that shields the earth's surface from the sun's harmful ultraviolet rays.

Pandemic Refers to diseases with a greater than normal rate of disease in the human population covering several countries, maybe worldwide.

Particulate air pollution Small particles suspended in the atmosphere, such as smoke from industrial processes.

Pasteurization Time-temperature process that destroys the pathogenic organism.

Pediculosis Infestation with lice.

Phagocytosis The ingestion and destruction of particlelike matter by cells, especially of infectious microorganisms in man.

Pharmacology The study of drugs and their actions.

Photochemical smog Air pollution derived mainly from emissions from automobiles and other sources interacting in the atmosphere in the presence of sunlight to create ozone and other oxidants.

Physiological needs Physical needs of humans such as light, space, favorable temperature and ventilation.

Pit privy Underground area where urine and feces can be deposited and retained in a sanitary manner.

Planning Advanced thinking as a basis for doing.

Planning premises Assumptions forming the basis for planning and implementation that will take place in the future.

Plasmolysis Shrinking of *bacterium cytoplasm* as a result of loss of water.

Plasmoptysis The bursting of protoplasm from a cell, resulting from the rupture of the cell wall because of high osmotic pressure within the cell.

Playground A recreational area encompassing program activities, play apparatus, and an open-space area designed to focus on the physical and social development of children.

Potable describes water of good taste, odor, and microbiological quality.

Primary clarifier A device, also called a settling basin, through which water moves slowly, allowing a large amount of suspended solids to accumulate on the bottom, producing sludge.

Primary irritants Material that exerts little systemic toxic action.

Priority setting Determining the relative importance of various problems under consideration.

Proboscis Collective mouthparts of the insect.

Proventriculus Gizzard in some insects, where food is ground into smaller particles.

Psychrophilic "Cold-loving"; organisms that grow in a range from 19°F to 68°F.

Public health assessment A process by which human exposure to environmental agents determined through environmental sampling at the point of exposure, and through human biologic testing, personal monitoring, and reviewing existing medical information.

RAD The dose of any form of ionizing radiation that produces energy absorption of 1×10^{-5}.

REM Major unit of exposure to radiation based on dose equivalency in the U. S. customary set of units.

Radiation The emission through space, or through a medium such as air, of energy, as related to human body temperature, specifically heat energy.

Radioactivity Characteristic of an isotope such that it emits radiation.

Radon A dense gas that is radioactive and may enter buildings from the earth.

Reactive Capable of exploding and generating toxic gases when combined with air or water.

Refuse Waste material composed of garbage, rubbish, and ashes.

Resistance to disease Ability to ward off disease such as by immunity.

Risk analysis A qualitative and quantitative process used to evaluate hazardous conditions and to characterize the resulting risk.

Risk assessment The process by which the form, dimension, and characteristics of risk are estimated.

Risk communication A process whereby individuals, groups, or the public are informed and involved concerning the existence, nature, form, severity, and/or acceptability of risks.

Risk management The process of integrating the results of risk assessment with economic, social, political, and legal concerns to develop a course of action to prevent or solve a problem.

Rubbish Combustible and noncombustible solid waste generated from people's activities; includes paper, beverage cans, yardwork trimmings, and many other materials.

Safety engineer Person who has the responsibility of developing complex systems for the analysis and control of occupational hazards.

Sanitary landfill Site where solid waste is buried systematically in sections and covered with soil.

Scabies A mite infestation by *Sarcoptes scabiei*.

Secure landfill Site for hazardous waste disposal consisting of ground excavation and some sort of insulation to prevent waste from escaping into air, water, and land.

Settling basin *See* Primary clarifier.

Sick building syndrome Term used for buildings that spread the causative agent of disease.

Slab avalanche An avalanche that starts when a solid area of snow breaks away at once, leaving a well-defined fracture line where the moving snow has broken away from the stable snow. Slab avalanches are characterized by the tendency of snow crystals to stick together and may contain angular blocks and/or chunks of snow.

Sludge Suspended solids that accumulate in a wastewater treatment plant.

Smog Combination of the words *smoke* and *fog* to describe polluted air.

Smoke Incomplete combustion of organic materials such as wood, coal, and petroleum products.

Snowmobile A self-propelled vehicle steered by skis, runners, or caterpillar treads, and designed to be used principally on snow or ice.

Sporadic diseases Those diseases that occur in scattered cases, such as rabies.

Spring a surface water supply arising from a groundwater source.

Storm sewer Wastewater system that collects surface runoff only from rainwater.

Sulfur oxides Products of the oxidation of fuels containing sulfur; include both sulfur dioxide (SO_2) and sulfur trioxide (SO_3) and the acids formed by their combination with water. Sulfuric acid (H_2SO_4) is of principal interest.

Superfund *See* CERCLA.

Synanthropic referring to the close association of the fly with humans.

Threshold limit values (TLVs) Guidelines in the control of occupational exposures.

Thermal inversion A layer of the atmosphere in which the temperature increases with height; may prevent air pollutants from dispersing, leading to high concentrations of pollutants, which may impact human health.

Thermophilic "heat-loving"; microbes that grow in the range of around 113°F to 167°F.

Toxic Potentially poisonous to humans.

Toxic effect Any noxious effect or undesirable disturbance of the body's physiologic function whether reversible or irreversible.

Toxicology The study of poisons.

Transovarian transmission Transmission of pathogenic organisms from one stage to the next stage in the life cycle of the arthropod.

Transstadial transmission Transmission of pathogenic organisms from one stage to the next stage in the life cycle of the arthropod.

Tumbler Pupa form of the mosquito.

Turbidity Cloudy looking water resulting from particles suspended in the water.

Undertow A current resulting from waves breaking upon a beach, then receding toward the lake or ocean. If the waves are large enough and the beach has a slope, the undertow will have a force great enough to pull a person into the water.

Vapor Gaseous forms of substances that exist normally as liquids or solids at room temperature and pressure.

Vector An organism that transmits a pathogen.

Vehicle of infection Mode of transport from one individual or group to another; water, food, insects, and inanimate objects.

Venturi meter A device for measuring the rate of flow through a wastewater treatment plant.

Volatile organic compounds (VOCs) Organic matter capable of being vaporized or evaporated quickly.

Waste to energy (WTE) Burning solid waste and generating energy or steam or electricity.

Wastewater stabilization pond Water body engineered to utilize biological decomposition as a means of wastewater disposal.

Wetland An area that is partially or completely saturated or occasionally inundated with water. Examples are swamps, marshes, bogs, fens, estuaries, intertidal mud flats, and river deltas.

Winter white-out Condition existing when an overcast sky or snow precludes shadows, causing the horizon to be indistinguishable from the terrain.

Wriggler Larvae form of mosquito.

Years of potential life lost (YPLL) a measure of the impact of premature death on a population, calculated as the sum of the differences between some predetermined minimum or desired life span and the age of death for individuals who died earlier than that predetermined age.

Zoonoses Diseases of animals that are transmitted to people.

ZPG Zero population growth; no overall growth or decline in the total population.

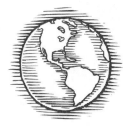

About the Author

Dr. Monroe T. Morgan, Sr., grew up on a farm near Mars Hill, NC. After graduating from Mars Hill Junior College, he earned the B.A. degree from East Tennessee State University, and later the M.S.P.H. from the University of North Carolina and the Doctor of Public Health from Tulane University. He worked as an environmentalist in Fairfax County, VA., and later as Training Officer for the State of Virginia. He developed and chaired for 22 years, the *first* academic department of environmental health in the United States to offer B.S.E.H. and M.S.E.H. degrees, which became the first two such programs to become professionally accredited.

Dr. Morgan has served as a consultant to the National Institutes of Health, the World Health Organization, and the National Academy of Science to study the U. S. Environmental Protection Agency. He served as president of the National Environmental Health Association (NEHA) in the mid-1970s. He received the National Environmental Health Association's highest honor — the Walter S. Mangold Award in 1979 and is the recipient of the NEHA Outstanding Award for Leadership to the Environmental Health Profession.

Dr. Morgan has 34 years of teaching experience, teaching students from the 50 states, including those from most American Indian tribes, and students from 56 countries. He chaired the first Earth Day Forum at ETSU on April 14, 1970.

About the Contributing Authors

Darryl B. Barnett, Dr.P.H.

Dr Barnett has been an Associate Professor in the Environmental Health Science Department at Eastern Kentucky University, Richmond, since 1991. He completed the B.S. in Environmental Health (1970) at East Tennessee State University and the M.P.H. (1977) and doctorate in Public Health (1993) at Oklahoma University Health Sciences Center in Oklahoma City. He retired from the Commissioned Corps of the U. S. Public Health Service in 1991, specializing in Institutional Environmental Heath in the Indian Health Service. He now is Chair of the Faculty Forum of the National Environmental Health Association.

Franklin B. Carver, Ph.D., R.S.

Dr. Carver is currently the Director and a Tenured Associate Professor of the Environmental Health Science Program, Ohio University, Athens, Ohio. He also holds the rank of Commander in the U. S. Navy Reserves as an Environmental Health Officer. With more than 20 years of experience in the environmental health field, Dr. Carver holds the B. S. degree in Health Education from Fayetteville State University (N.C.), the Master of Science in Environmental Health from East Tennessee State University, and the doctorate degree from Ohio University. Dr. Carver worked in industry for three years as an Occupational Health and Safety Officer, and in Liberia, West Africa for four years in environmental health.

He has taught at the University of Liberia, Mississippi Valley State University, and Western Carolina University. He has served as a councilman on the National Environmental Health Science and Protection Accreditation Council for colleges and universities. Currently he is Technical Editor of the *Journal of Environmental Health*. Dr. Carver has received many honors including an invitation to the White House, where he was honored by President Bill Clinton for recruiting qualified candidates in the health profession for induction into the U.S. Navy.

Lawrence R. Curtis, Ph.D.

Dr. Curtis earned the B.S. and M.S. degrees from the University of South Alabama, majoring in biology. He completed the Ph.D. in pharmacology at the University of Mississippi Medical Center in 1980 and joined the faculty of Oregon State University that same year. In May 1995, Dr. Curtis moved to East Tennessee State University, where he is now Professor and Chair, Department of Environmental Health. He has published 47 research papers in peer-reviewed literature. Past-President of the Pacific Northwest Chapter of the Society of Toxicology, Dr. Curtis served on the Continuing Education Committee of the Society of Toxicology during 1992–1996, and is a former Chair, Oregon State University Interdisciplinary Toxicology Program.

Trenton G. Davis, Dr.P.H.

Dr. Davis is a Professor in the Department of Environmental Health, East Carolina University. He received the B.S. degree from East Tennessee State University, the M.P.H. degree from Tulane University, and the doctorate in Public Health from the University of Oklahoma. During his 33 years in public health and academics, he has held a number of positions including Sanitarian; Professor of Environmental Health, East Tennessee State University; Associate Vice Chancellor for Academic Support, East Carolina

University; Interim Dean, School of Industry and Technology, East Carolina University; and Associate Dean, School of Allied Health Sciences, East Carolina University.

Dr. Davis is the recipient of numerous awards including the Walter Mangold Award (National Environmental Health Association), the Walter Snyder Award (National Sanitation Foundation/National Environmental Health Association), the William Broadway Award (North Carolina Public Health Association) and the Trenton G. Davis Award (Eastern District, North Carolina Public Health Association). On the national level he has served as President of the National Environmental Health Association and as technical editor of the *Journal of Environmental Health*. He has written papers for publication in the *Journal of Environmental Health*, the *North Carolina Medical Journal*, the *Oklahoma Medical Journal*, the *North Carolina Public Health Forum*, and other journals.

Larry Gordon, M.S., M.P.H.

Mr. Gordon has been Visiting Professor at the University of New Mexico School of Public Administration since 1988. Previously he was the New Mexico Cabinet Secretary for Health and Environment; Deputy Secretary for Health and Environment; State Health Officer; New Mexico Scientific Laboratory System Director; New Mexico Environmental Improvement Agency Director; Albuquerque-Bernalillo County Environmental Health Department Director; and a Commissioned Officer in the U.S. Public Health Service.

He has served as President of the American Public Health Association; Chair of the National Conference of Local Environmental Health Administrators; President of the New Mexico Public Health Association; and President of the New Mexico Environmental Health Association. He founded the Council on Education for Public Health and has been a member of the National Environmental Health Science and Protection Accreditation Council.

A few of the numerous honors and awards he has received are:

- Distinguished Public Administration Award, from National Society for Public Administration, 1996
- Distinguished Alumnus Award, from University of Michigan School of Public Health Alumni Society, 1995
- Distinguished Leadership in Environmental Management Award, from American Society for Public Administration, 1994
- Lester Breslow Award for Distinguished Service in Public Health, from County of Los Angeles, 1994
- Sedgwick Award, from American Public Health Association, 1987
- Wagner Award, from American Academy of Sanitarians, 1984
- Snyder Award, from National Environmental Health Association, 1978
- Mangold Award, from National Environmental Health Association, 1961

Gordon planned and gained legislative authorization to create the Albuquerque Bernalillo County Environmental Health Department (the nation's *first* local environmental health department), the New Mexico Scientific Laboratory System, the New Mexico Environmental Improvement Agency, and the New Mexico State Health Agency. He also has contributed to enactment of numerous state and local environmental health and protection laws. He earned the M.S. at the University of New Mexico, and the M.P.H. at the University of Michigan School of Public Health. He has written for more than 200 publications.

Albert F. Iglar, Ph.D.

Dr. Iglar holds the B.S. degree in Chemical Engineering and is a licensed Professional Engineer. After undergraduate study, he was employed in water-related programs by the Pennsylvania Department of Health for four years. He obtained the M.P.H. and the Ph.D. degrees from the University of Minnesota, where he also was

a junior faculty member. Since 1970, he has held professorial rank in the Department of Environmental Health at East Tennessee State University. He probably holds the U. S. record for directing more M.S.E.H. theses than any other academician. Among diverse professional contributions, he has focused on radiological health and hazardous waste management.

Shirley L. Morgan, M.S.E.H., E.D.D., M.P.H.

Dr. Morgan, Professor of Public Health at ETSU, received the M.S.E.H. and Ed.D. from ETSU and the M.P.H. degree from the University of North Carolina. Her primary teaching responsibilities have been in Industrial Health Education, Health Administration, and Human Resource Management.

Rallie McAllister, M.D., M.S.E.H., M.P.H.

Dr. McAllister received the M.S.E.H., M.P.H. and M.D. degrees from ETSU. She is a practicing physician in Kingsport, TN.

Bailus Walker, Jr.

Dr. Walker, a native of Springfield, TN., received the B.S. from Kentucky State University, the M.P.H. from the University of Michigan, and the Ph.D. from the University of Minnesota. He has held various academic positions, from adjunct faculty to Dean, at many universities. Including the universities of New York, Minnesota, George Washington, Harvard, Massachusetts, Boston, Michigan State, Kansas, Howard, and Meharry Medical College. He was Dean of the College of Public Health at the University of Oklahoma. His professional experience includes the roles of Director of Public Health and Welfare, New Jersey; Environmental Health Administrator for the government of the District of Columbia; Director, Directorate of Occupational Health Standards, OSHA, U. S. Department of Labor; Commissioner of Public Health for the state of Massachusetts; Director of Public Health for the state of Michigan (the *first* non-physician to be appointed commissioner).

Dr. Walker's service to organizations and agencies includes: President of the American Public Health Association (1987–88), membership on several task forces, consultant to the National Academy of Science, where he served or serves on 10 different committees; consultant to the U.S. Department of Health and Human Services, where he served on five committees, including Chair of the Agency for Toxic Substances and Director of the Registry's Board of Scientific Counselors. Also, he has served as a consultant to the U.S. Department of Energy. Further, he has served on 37 state and national commissions and councils including the U.S. President's Council on Environmental Quality.

Dr. Walker has received more than 24 awards and honors, a few of which are: Environmental Health Scientist of the Year Award; Mangold Award; U.S. Attorney General's Special Commendation for Outstanding Service; Editor's Award by the *Journal of Environmental Health*; and the Joseph E. Cannon Award for Excellence in Public Health Services. He has written three books and has contributed to at least 61 publications including *Public Health Responsibilities, Rules, and Realities*; *Public Health Policy Forum: Environmental Health and African Americans*; and *The Future of Public Health*.

Index

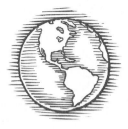

Centers for Disease Control and Prevention, 118, 200, 203, 281, 284
CERCLA, 125
CFCs, 227, 228
Chadwick, Edwin, 21
Chemical(s)
  agricultural, 164-165
  body, 24
  food, 160-162, 169
  hazards, 19, 51, 122, 244, 246, 251, 254
  poisoning, 177
  toxic, 141, 142-143, 145, 177, 192
  waste, 91
  methods of waste disposal, 119, 124
  in the workplace, 144, 245
Chemical oxygen demand (COD), 103
Chiggers, 45, 138, 243
Child Protection and Toy Safety Act, 202
Chlorine and chlorination, 17, 31, 33, 60, 63, 64, 84-85, 170, 228
  in medical waste treatment, 119
  in swimming pools, 77-78, 81
  in therapeutic pools, 83, 84
  in wading pools, 84
  in wastewater treatment, 101, 102, 104
Cholera, 31, 45, 51, 53, 107, 169, 171
Chrysotile, 188
Cigarettes. See Tobacco
Cistern, 55, 56
Clean Air Acts, 222, 269
Climate, 261, 267
Coal
  burning, 226, 227
  gasification, 220
Cockroaches, 30, 31, 32, 49-50, 110, 132, 135-136, 167, 177, 179, 186
Coliform testing, 60, 76, 102
Communicable diseases, 2, 15, 18, 27, 28-29, 165, 184, 185, 186, 284
Composting, 117

Consumer Product Safety Act/Commission, 202-203, 206, 208
Contamination. See also Pollution
  air, 191, 245-248
  of bathing places, 75-76
  fecal, 171-172
  of food, 30, 31, 158, 164-165, 167, 169, 177
  milk, 180
  radiation, 153, 164
  at waste sites, 265
  of water supply, 59, 60, 92, 155, 171, 186
Coors Brewery, 112
Corps of Engineers, 281
Council on Education for Public Health, 286
Council on Environmental Quality, 222
Council on Industrial Health, 235-236, 238

DDT, 48, 145
Deforestation, 229-230, 275, 280
Desertification, 229-230
Developing countries, 2, 9, 33
Digestive system, diseases of, 23, 24
Diphtheria, 34-35
Disease
  causative agents, of, 18-20
  chronic, 27, 29, 144
  defenses against, 21-23
  foodborne, 30, 169, 178, 179
  fungal, 243
  heart, 19, 20,, 200, 219, 249
  infectious/communicable, 14, 15, 18, 27, 28, 29, 165, 184, 185, 186, 284
  from medical waste, 118
  occupational, 118, 218, 234, 235, 241
  prevention, 22, 23, 24, 29, 258, 268
  respiratory, 186, 192, 193, 219
  skin, 245, 246, 347-248
  vector-borne, 127
  waterborne, 83, 186
Disinfection, 17, 36, 39, 60
  in food sanitation, 168

in swimming pools, 77, 78, 84
in wastewater, 94
Dissolved oxygen (DO), 102-103
Dosimeter, 152, 248
Dose-response, 194, 252, 277
Doubling time, 2
Drowning, 208, 209
Drying of food, 160
Dumps(ing), open, 110-111, 130
  chemical, 122, 123
Dust pollution, 39, 91, 92, 167, 218, 227
  in workplace, 233, 243, 246, 247
Dysentery, 31-32, 51, 134, 172

E. coli, 173
Economic
  development, 9
  incentives, 269-270
Ecosystem, 107, 144-145, 258, 259, 270, 275, 280, 283
  aquatic, 226
Effluent, 12, 101, 102, 104, 111, 218
Electrostatic precipitator, 221, 222, 226
Emissions. See Carbon monoxide
Emphysema, 219
Encephalitis, 41-42
Energy
  body, 200, 201
  conservation, 185
  efficiency, 191, 195, 220, 226
  -related pollution, 219
Energy Reorganization Act, 255
Environment(al)
  degradation, 1, 7
  health, 14-15, 18, 21, 23, 24, 70, 71, 144, 145, 179, 199
  influences, 29
  management, 12, 29, 260
  monitoring, 270-271
  occupational, 28, 29
  planning, 258, 259, 261-262, 271-272
  pollutants/hazards, 20, 268
  programs, 259, 270, 271, 275
  quality, 260, 271, 275, 276
  safety, 15
  trends, 270-271, 284

institutional, 36
personal, 32, 36, 137, 138, 171, 172, 179, 185
Hypothermia, 72-73, 251

Immunity, 21, 22, 34
Immunization, 2, 21, 32, 34, 35, 36, 38, 39, 200
Incineration, 45, 107, 108, 111, 113
of medical/hazardous waste, 120, 121, 124
Indian Health Service, 281
Industrial health educator, 238,240-241
Industrial hygienist, 239
Industrial revolution, 234
Industrial toxicologist, 251-252
Infectious. *See also* Communicable diseases
diseases, 14, 27-28, 29
waste, 118, 121
Influenza, 36, 192
Injuries, 185, 199. *See also* Accidents
accidental, 200, 207, 277
bicycle, 203
childhood, 204, 205, 206, 207, 208, 210, 211
to elderly, 204, 205, 206, 208, 211, 212
from falls, 204-205
fatal, 208
fire and burn, 205-206
from firearms, 207
head, 204, 205, 209, 210, 211, 212
intentional, 200
lawnmower, 208
motor vehicle, 200, 211
from poisoning, 206-207
prevention, 200, 201, 277
Insect, 23, 127, 132, 165, 170
breeding places, 109, 110
contamination, 40
control, 15, 115, 169, 184
Insecticides, 40, 43, 44, 47, 48, 49, 134, 137, 138, 167, 177, 218-219
Ionization, gas, 151-152

Jenner, Edward, 2

Johnson, President Lyndon B., 9, 236
Jungle, The, 235

Koch, Robert, 157
Kwashiorkor, 6, 19

Landfills, 45, 101, 108, 111, 112, 119
sanitary, 113, 115, 117
secure, 124
Land use, 15
Lead poisoning, 177, 195, 196, 206, 233, 234, 237, 245, 258, 259
Lead Poisoning Prevention Act, 196
Legionnaire's disease, 193
Leprospirosis, 39
Lice, 40, 47-49, 132, 137, 242
Lifestyle, 14, 28-29
Lister, Joseph, 157
Local health departments, 281-282
Lyme disease, 43-44

Malaria, 41-42, 107, 132, 243
Malthus, Thomas, 6
Mass gatherings, 71
Maximum contaminants levels, 64
Medical self-help, 14
Medical waste, 118, 119-121, 123-124
Mercury poisoning, 234, 237, 245
Mesophilic organisms, 16
Metazoa, 19
Mice, 129, 138, 143, 170, 179
Microorganisms, 157-158, 159, 191
controlling, 18
requirements of, 15-16
Midgley, Thomas, 228
Milk. *See* Pasteurization; Sanitation
Minerals, in water, 55, 60
Mining Enforcement and Safety Administration, 255
Mist, 245
Mites, 40, 44, 132, 137, 138, 243

Molds, 158, 159
Mosquitoes, 41-42, 70, 110, 132, 133
controlling, 134, 179
Mothers Against Drunk Driving (MADD), 213
Mucous membranes, 22, 24, 34, 35, 39, 184, 194
Mushrooms, poisonous, 175
Mutations, 143, 277

Nader, Ralph, 213
NASA, 229
National Academy of Sciences, 227, 265
National Ambient Air Quality Standards, 222
National Electronic Injury Surveillance System, 203
National Environmental Health Association, 280
National Environmental Health Science and Protection Accreditation Council, 279, 286
National Highway Traffic Safety Administration, 211, 212
National Institute for Environmental Health and Safety, 281
National Institutes of Health, 219
National Institute of Medicine, 278
National Institute of Occupational Safety and Health, 192
National Oceanic and Atmospheric Administration, 229, 281
National Research Council, 265
National Safety Council, 203
National Sanitation Foundation, 168
Needs, human, 184-185
NIOSH, 237, 252, 254
Nitrates/nitrites, 61, 162, 176
Nitrogen oxides, 219, 223, 224
Noise, 184, 248-249
control, 15, 71, 185, 250
Nuclear
fission, 150
power/energy, 70, 148, 154-155, 226, 255